Applying the socio-
framework to the B
Admissions Test (BMAT)

Insights from language assessment

Also in this series:

The Impact of High-stakes Examinations on Classroom Teaching: A case study using insights from testing and innovation theory
Dianne Wall

Impact Theory and Practice: Studies of the IELTS test and *Progetto Lingue 2000*
Roger Hawkey

IELTS Washback in Context: Preparation for academic writing in higher education
Anthony Green

Examining Writing: Research and practice in assessing second language writing
Stuart D. Shaw and Cyril J. Weir

Multilingualism and Assessment: Achieving transparency, assuring quality, sustaining diversity – Proceedings of the ALTE Berlin Conference, May 2005
Edited by Lynda Taylor and Cyril J. Weir

Examining FCE and CAE: Key issues and recurring themes in developing the First Certificate in English and Certificate in Advanced English exams
Roger Hawkey

Language Testing Matters: Investigating the wider social and educational impact of assessment – Proceedings of the ALTE Cambridge Conference, April 2008
Edited by Lynda Taylor and Cyril J. Weir

Components of L2 Reading: Linguistic and processing factors in the reading test performances of Japanese EFL learners
Toshihiko Shiotsu

Aligning Tests with the CEFR: Reflections on using the Council of Europe's draft Manual
Edited by Waldemar Martyniuk

Examining Reading: Research and practice in assessing second language reading
Hanan Khalifa and Cyril J. Weir

Examining Speaking: Research and practice in assessing second language speaking
Edited by Lynda Taylor

IELTS Collected Papers 2: Research in reading and listening assessment
Edited by Lynda Taylor and Cyril J. Weir

Examining Listening: Research and practice in assessing second language listening
Edited by Ardeshir Geranpayeh and Lynda Taylor

Exploring Language Frameworks: Proceedings of the ALTE Kraków Conference, July 2011
Edited by Evelina D. Galaczi and Cyril J. Weir

Measured Constructs: A history of Cambridge English language examinations 1913–2012
Cyril J. Weir, Ivana Vidaković, Evelina D. Galaczi

Cambridge English Exams – The First Hundred Years: A history of English language assessment from the University of Cambridge 1913–2013
Roger Hawkey and Michael Milanovic

Testing Reading Through Summary: Investigating summary completion tasks for assessing reading comprehension ability
Lynda Taylor

Multilingual Frameworks: The construction and use of multilingual proficiency frameworks
Neil Jones

Validating Second Language Reading Examinations: Establishing the validity of the GEPT through alignment with the Common European Framework of Reference
Rachel Yi-fen Wu

Assessing Language Teachers' Professional Skills and Knowledge
Edited by Rosemary Wilson and Monica Poulter

Second Language Assessment and Mixed Methods Research
Edited by Aleidine J Moeller, John W Creswell and Nick Saville

Language Assessment for Multilingualism: Proceedings of the ALTE Paris Conference, April 2014
Edited by Coreen Docherty and Fiona Barker

Advancing the Field of Language Assessment: Papers from TIRF doctoral dissertation grantees
Edited by MaryAnn Christison and Nick Saville

Applying the socio-cognitive framework to the BioMedical Admissions Test (BMAT)

Insights from language assessment

Edited by

Kevin Y F Cheung
Research and Thought Leadership Group
Cambridge Assessment Admissions Testing

Sarah McElwee
Research and Thought Leadership Group
Cambridge Assessment Admissions Testing

and

Joanne Emery
Consultant
Cambridge Assessment Admissions Testing

CAMBRIDGE
UNIVERSITY PRESS

CAMBRIDGE
UNIVERSITY PRESS

University Printing House, Cambridge CB2 8BS, United Kingdom

One Liberty Plaza, 20th Floor, New York, NY 10006, USA

477 Williamstown Road, Port Melbourne, VIC 3207, Australia

4843/24, 2nd Floor, Ansari Road, Daryaganj, Delhi – 110002, India

79 Anson Road, #06–04/06, Singapore 079906

Cambridge University Press is part of the University of Cambridge.

It furthers the University's mission by disseminating knowledge in the pursuit of education, learning and research at the highest international levels of excellence.

www.cambridge.org
Information on this title: www.cambridge.org/9781108439312

First published 2017

20 19 18 17 16 15 14 13 12 11 10 9 8 7 6 5 4 3 2 1

A catalogue record for this publication is available from the British Library

ISBN 978-1-108-43931-2

Contents

Acknowledgements

This book is a result of collective efforts from many individuals. It represents a great deal of thought and work from academic and practitioner communities in educational assessment, and in medical education. Numerous people have been involved in preparing the manuscript and we would like to take this opportunity to acknowledge their contributions.

First and foremost, we must thank the authors who have contributed to chapters in this volume: Brenda Cross, Paul Crump, Amy Devine, Mark Elliott, Molly Fyfe, Tom Gallacher, Karen Grant, Nick Saville, Mark Shannon, Lynda Taylor and Juliet Wilson. Their expertise, collaboration and hard work were instrumental in completing this project and producing the final text.

The need for a volume on the validity of the BioMedical Admissions Test (BMAT) was originally identified by Hanan Khalifa (Deputy Director of Partnerships, Projects & Policy) and Simon Beeston (former Director of Cambridge Assessment Admissions Testing) over four years ago, so the genesis for this book came from them jointly. In the final stages of completing the work that concludes this lengthy project, we are grateful that they were unrelenting in their desire to see this volume finished. Similarly, we appreciate Andy Chamberlain's (Head of Cambridge Assessment Admissions Testing) continuing support for the production of this volume, which has been instrumental for getting the text to print.

Special thanks must go to Professor Martyn Partridge (Professor of Respiratory Medicine and Patient Centred Care at Imperial College London) and Dr Paul Dennis (Director of Graduate Entry Medicine at University of Oxford and Supernumerary Fellow at Brasenose College), who kindly agreed to serve as external reviewers once the manuscript was assembled. They are both seasoned academics with extensive experience at the coal-face of medical education, and this showed through in their insightful comments. Their constructive criticism has been invaluable for improving the text and ensuring that it is useful for medical educators. Therefore, their sound advice has contributed significantly to the quality of this volume.

We are also grateful for Professor Cyril Weir's (University of Bedfordshire) review as the joint Series Editor of Studies in Language Testing (SiLT). His comments prompted interesting discussions between us as editors, the contributing authors and experts across Cambridge Assessment. The resultant revisions have enhanced the final volume's potential contribution to the educational assessment community. Furthermore, Cyril's support for including the volume in the SiLT series has been a source of encouragement whilst compiling the final drafts of the manuscript. We must also thank Dr Evelina Galaczi (Head of Research Strategy, Cambridge English Research & Thought Leadership Group) for the insightful suggestion that this volume would be suitable for SiLT.

There were also a large number of people within Cambridge Assessment Admissions Testing and Cambridge English who helped the authors by providing input to chapters. Demographic data for tables in Chapter 2 was supplied by Alice Gresham (Senior Validation Analyst, Validation & Data Services). Colleagues in the Assessment division provided items that are included in Chapter 3 as examples of BMAT tasks: Graeme Bridges, Dr Jane Buckle, Lesley Hay, Dr Mike Housden, Dr Uma Phillips and Dr David Robson (Senior Assessment Managers). Colleagues from these teams also gave feedback on the question paper production processes outlined in Chapter 4 to ensure they were accurately described: Dr Jane Buckle and Lesley Hay (Senior Assessment Managers). Also for Chapter 4, details of the procedures for managing test centres were provided by colleagues from the Network Services division of Cambridge English: Claire McCauley (Network Services Group Manager) and Jonathan Scholey (Inspections Support Officer). The Cambridge Assessment Admissions Testing teams that liaise with BMAT users described the processes discussed in various chapters to authors: Tori Helmer (Customer Experience Group Manager) and Annie Page (Customer Experience Manager). Dr Gad Lim (Principal Research Manager, Research & Thought Leadership Group) commented on the overall structure and layout of chapters at various stages of drafting. Completing this volume relied on the co-operation of all those mentioned above. We are thankful for their willingness to share knowledge and for their generosity with time taken from busy schedules.

In preparing chapters, the authors also consulted with technical expertise from across the Cambridge Assessment exam boards. In particular, conversations with Tom Bramley (Director of Research, Assessment Research and Development) and Dr Stephen Cromie (Senior Assessment Advisor, Cambridge International Examinations) informed the approaches to scoring validity outlined in Chapter 5, and we are indebted to them for their thoughtful reflections.

Publication of this volume was only possible with the support of many colleagues from the Research & Thought Leadership Group: Dr Ivana Vidakovic's (Senior Research Manager) efforts as Managing Editor of SiLT and John Savage's (Publications Assistant) eye for detail were crucial to preparing the final drafts. Ewa Child (Research Support Administrator) and Mariangela Marulli (Administrative Assistant) carried out painstaking work to construct indexes; without their careful and diligent efforts, the volume would be incomplete. Jenny Hunt and Ella Pope's (Research Support Administrators) help co-ordinating external reviewers and co-authors was also vital to the project's smooth progress. Finally, we would like to acknowledge the support of Dr Nick Saville (Director of the Research & Thought Leadership Group and joint Series Editor for SiLT); his encouragement and guidance has played an essential role in completing this book.

To all of the above, we extend our sincerest thanks and appreciation.

Kevin Y F Cheung
Sarah McElwee
Joanne Emery
June 2017

Series Editors' note

The socio-cognitive framework for test development and validation research is a systematic attempt to formulate a coherent approach to these activities, which combines social, cognitive and evaluative (scoring) dimensions of language use and links these in turn to the context and consequences of test use. The socio-cognitive framework identifies the evidence required to develop a transparent and coherent validity argument, while at the same time addressing the interaction between different types of validity evidence.

This volume about the BioMedical Admissions Test (BMAT) is the sixth volume in the Studies in Language Testing (SiLT) series to explicate the socio-cognitive approach used by Cambridge Assessment to validate its tests. The uniqueness of the latest volume is that, unlike the other volumes, it is not concerned with language testing per se but with a different construct viz the theory that the test is based on. For BMAT, this is the theory of the cognitive skills, the core scientific reasoning and the written communication abilities that will enable a student to cope with the demands of a rigorous biomedical degree. BMAT assesses an applicant's readiness for the demanding, science-based study required in medicine and other biomedical courses. BMAT has three elements: a domain-general Aptitude and Skills section, a section based on Scientific Knowledge and Applications, and a short communicative Writing Task. The volume thus represents a pioneering attempt to apply the socio-cognitive framework to an assessment field premised on constructs other than language.

An important outcome of the study has been that it demonstrates clearly how the socio-cognitive approach can be used successfully in the wider education field both to develop and validate examinations, thereby demonstrating its flexibility as a model for test evaluation. It demonstrates how a multidisciplinary approach spanning language testing and admissions testing can be beneficial.

The earlier 'construct' volumes in the SiLT series were concerned with testing English language abilities. The first was SiLT 26, *Examining Writing* by Shaw and Weir (2007), the second was SiLT 29, *Examining Reading* by Khalifa and Weir (2009), the third was SiLT 30, *Examining Speaking* by Taylor (Ed) (2011), the fourth was SiLT 35, *Examining Listening* by Geranpayeh and Taylor (Eds) (2013), and this year will see the arrival of SiLT 47, *Assessing Young Language Learners* by Papp and Rixon (forthcoming 2017). The first four of these volumes covered the examinations that formed the Cambridge English Main Suite of general English examinations, and the fifth was focused on young learners. *Assessing Young Language Learners* completes the set of 'construct' volumes on Cambridge English language examinations; together these five volumes constitute a significant endeavour in academic and publishing terms, representing more than 15 years of dedicated work among academics and practitioners working in the field of language test validation with and within Cambridge English.

The volumes are testimony to the academic rigour, experience and scholarship, as well as to the enormous expertise that resides within Cambridge English and among its external consultants, as well as to the organisation's continuing commitment in the 21st century to generating validity evidence on how language constructs are measured by their language examinations.

Together with the current volume, they represent a significant contribution in the assessment field to our theoretical understanding of the nature of the abilities we are seeking to measure and to the practical approaches that test providers can adopt to achieve that goal with integrity, building a systematic, transparent and defensible body of validity argumentation in the process.

Foreword

Professor Martyn R Partridge

National Heart and Lung Institute, Imperial College London

The health professions globally face a number of challenges at the present time: an increasing health burden associated with a shift from a burden of acute illness to a burden of long-term disease, increasing longevity which is often not disease free, increased public expectations, and increased costs in excess of those of normal inflation. Despite this, entry to the professions which deliver healthcare remains a popular choice amongst young people.

In many respects this is an enviable position but those charged with selecting those to be trained to deliver healthcare have a responsibility and desire to be both transparent and fair, and to select those who can best complete an often rigorous course of study, and be those most capable of tackling these health challenges over a 40-year career.

Thus fair and transparent selection involves identifying those who can complete the course and those who have the most appropriate perceived attributes to fit their eventual profession. In that process we wish to avoid waste and disappointment associated with drop-out from courses, and recognise that we are not necessarily identifying *one* uniform ideal health professional, but recognising the diversity of attributes that may be desirable, in the process perhaps identifying those characteristics not suitable in any branch of the profession.

An admission process concerned with ability to cope with the course of study and defining desirable attributes will involve review of an individual's past track record. This can be difficult if achievements are in a form that is not comparable, and the process also needs to take into account whether the individual had an equal opportunity to succeed. Admissions tests, such as the BioMedical Admissions Test (BMAT), can play an important role in supporting tutors dealing with these issues. Attributes of empathy, compassion, optimal communication skills, ability to reflect, teamwork and leadership skills may all be sought. In addition, and sometimes overlooked, we need to acknowledge the diversity of opportunity open to health professionals and need to look for scientific inquisitiveness if we are to maintain a stream of top-rate clinical scientists. As delivering optimal care becomes harder we also need to consider whether we can identify those with staying power.

To do all of this well can appear to be an impossible task. In the wider field of medical science we are often blessed with a plethora of large-scale studies which permit us to determine the best way forward, but other disciplines are not always so well served. However we are now getting and sharing much more about how best to teach, how best to learn, how best to motivate and how best to assess those for entry into a healthcare profession and their ability to succeed. This book collects together, in large part for the first time, a body of evidence regarding admissions testing. The framework within which this has been done is robust and few can be anything but impressed by the development processes, validation, contextual study and continual review and evaluation that Cambridge Assessment uses in BMAT.

London
May 2017

Preface

The BioMedical Admissions Test (BMAT) was first administered in 2004, but Cambridge Assessment, or the University of Cambridge Local Examinations Syndicate (UCLES) as it was known, has been involved in admissions testing since the first Law Studies Test was administered 30 years ago (Chapman 2005). This initial foray into admissions testing was followed by formation of the MENO Thinking Skills Service – a collaboration between a number of higher education institutions that was research driven and governed by steering groups made up of various stakeholders (Hamilton 1993).

MENO projects were conducted by Cambridge Assessment researchers and the initiative explored aptitude testing for university admissions in the UK, informed by work on standardised testing in the US. However, the research conducted by MENO informed a shift in focus by the mid-1990s. The aim was not merely to produce a psychometric aptitude test; instead, the attention turned towards identification and definition of thinking skills crucial to success in higher education and to professional work, and the creation of instruments which would assess those skills directly. Additionally, it became clear that the work of test developers should include a wider understanding of the assessment instrument's purpose. These principles underpinned development of the Medical and Veterinary Admissions Test (MVAT), which along with the Oxford Medical Admissions Test (OMAT), is a predecessor of BMAT (James and Hawkins 2004, Massey 2004).

Although not all of the editors of the present volume were working on BMAT research during the early years of development described above, an understanding of BMAT's origins is useful for contextualising our work in the division responsible for BMAT today – Cambridge Assessment Admissions Testing. While working at Cambridge Assessment, Joanne Emery began collating together historical work on BMAT. This formed the basis for the present volume. Research continues to underpin the evaluation of assessments, and a collaborative approach ensures that the test developers understand the context of a test's use, and the issues that impact on various stakeholders. For BMAT, engagement with stakeholders is achieved through the BMAT stakeholder liaison group – a twice-yearly meeting of representatives from departments that use the test. Some of the research in the present volume was conducted at the request of these stakeholders and is included here with their permission.

Although it will be clear to readers of the following chapters, it is useful to point out here that BMAT is not an IQ test. In line with the original work of MENO, tests developed by Cambridge Assessment Admissions Testing assess skills useful for higher education study, and in the case of BMAT, for biomedical study in particular. This was made explicit by Dr Alec Fisher when reporting early work on another Cambridge Assessment test – the Thinking Skills Assessment (TSA), which is used across a range of academic disciplines. He compared TSA with the widely used SAT produced by the Educational Testing Service (ETS) in the US:

> One of the most important differences between the SAT and the TSA is that the skills assessed in the TSA are teachable skills which are valuable in higher education. The SAT on the other hand has long claimed to measure "innate" or "native" ability (Fisher 2005:12).

At the time that Alec Fisher made this distinction between Cambridge Assessment's and ETS' approaches, ETS was already moving away from the aim of testing innate cognitive ability (Zwick (Ed) 2004). Since then, the SAT has been revised substantially to recognise the importance of linking assessment to instruction and preparation (College Board 2015). Contemporary perspectives on assessment recognise that standardised tests and examinations are not pure measures of innate ability; instead, they measure a combination of natural talent, learned skills and environmental factors (Kuncel and Hezlett 2010).

This conceptualisation of testing forms an important part of the Cambridge Assessment approach to developing assessments for selection purposes, and we recognise that the constructs assessed by BMAT reflect this complexity. Detailed consideration of a test's theoretical construct is essential to evaluating its validity, but this also needs to be supplemented with an understanding of the test's purpose, and how scores are used to make decisions in practice.

The selection of medical, dental and veterinary students is an important and complicated task. UK medical schools have high applicant-to-place ratios, and applicants often have similar prior academic attainments (the highest A Level grades or equivalent). Medical schools have found it increasingly difficult to differentiate between applicants with strong academic achievement, giving rise to the need for additional measures of their potential for the future course of study. There is also the question of whether students from higher and lower performing schools (or from different school types) are as likely to succeed on a course of study given the same A Level grades, and whether grades from mature students are equivalent to those of school leavers.

For institutions selecting non-UK applicants the comparison of different national examinations is complex and an assessment that provides a common metric for all applicants is of value. Currently, in the UK at least, the A Level (or equivalent) results required for course entry are not available at the time of university application. Selectors therefore have to rely on teachers' predictions of applicants' grades, which can be unreliable. This provides another reason to value results from an additional assessment of applicants' ability.

To be useful to selecting institutions, such an assessment should provide additional information on applicants' ability and must be fair to *all* applicants regardless of their background, culture, schooling, etc. It should also relate to applicants' future performance in some demonstrable way: it would be beneficial if its performance could be shown to permit the selection of those who would achieve most, or to identify which applicants would struggle most with the course. The aims of medical student selection are far from universally agreed but, in general, universities wish to recruit students who are most likely to succeed on the course of study and least likely to struggle with it or to drop out. Other procedures, such as multiple mini-interviews, may be additionally undertaken to select those with attributes thought to be desirable in future doctors, dentists or veterinarians.

Given the high-stakes nature of the medical student selection process, and the government and media scrutiny of student admissions, it is essential that the selection process is both transparent and fair, and *perceived* to be fair by applicants themselves. The under-representation of students from lower socio-economic groups in medical study continues to be an issue, and the UK 'Widening Participation' agenda has seen a government drive to increase medical school entries from state school students and those from particular social groups (Medical Schools Council 2014). The high A Level requirement is a major obstacle to access, with students from areas of social deprivation less likely to demonstrate the high educational attainment seen as a prerequisite for the application process and subsequent admission to study. Nonetheless, it is essential that additional selection assessments do not exacerbate this by acting as a further barrier to entry for certain applicant groups, or as a deterrent to them applying in the first place.

These issues form the background to our standard work conducting research on admissions tests. At times we are required to consider specific parts of the admissions context when interpreting results or planning analysis. Research studies are often designed to investigate a particular aspect or impact of selection for medical study. However, it is only in compiling these chapters together that we have been reminded of the complexity present in this context, particularly when the various challenges are viewed together. By sharing research and practice conducted with BMAT, we hope to inform the work of admissions tutors and other researchers working in similarly complicated contexts.

Kevin Y F Cheung
Sarah McElwee
Joanne Emery

Notes on contributors

Kevin Y F Cheung is a Chartered Psychologist and Senior Research Manager at Cambridge Assessment. He holds a PhD from University of Derby where he researched the role of identity in academic writing and plagiarism. Prior to joining Cambridge Assessment, he lectured in Individual Differences and Quantitative Research Methods at Loughborough University, and Social Psychology at Birmingham City University. His previous research focused on higher education pedagogy, scale development and cognitive processes in hypothesis testing. He currently co-ordinates research activities essential to the quality of Cambridge Assessment's admissions tests. His research interests include construct validity in admissions testing, non-cognitive assessment for healthcare contexts and the role of standardised testing in multi-method selection processes.

Brenda Cross was the Faculty Tutor for the University College London Medical School (UCLMS) and Sub-Dean (Student Support and Welfare) for 22 years until 2016. During her time in these roles, she managed undergraduate admissions and represented UCLMS at the BMAT stakeholder liaison group. Brenda has been involved with medical education for over 38 years and in student selection for medical and biological science courses for over 30 years.

Paul Crump is an Assessment Group Manager in Cambridge Assessment Admissions Testing, where he is responsible for the production of thinking skills and written components of tests, including Section 1 and Section 3 of BMAT. Prior to joining the team, he worked in Cambridge English Language Assessment, where he was responsible for development and production of tests of General and Business English. He holds an MSc in Philosophy from the University of Edinburgh, a first class BA in Philosophy from the University of Hull, and an MA in Applied Linguistics and TESOL from Anglia Ruskin University.

Amy Devine is a Senior Research Manager at Cambridge Assessment, where she is a member of the team working on admissions testing research. She holds a PhD in Psychology from the University of Cambridge and an MA from University of Otago. Her previous research examined the interaction of maths and test anxiety in children, the impact of developmental dyscalculia, and socio-biological explanations for gender differences in maths performance. She currently conducts research on a number of admissions tests provided by Cambridge Assessment Admissions Testing, including BMAT, focusing on their predictive validity and group differences in test performance.

Mark Elliott is a Senior Validation Manager at Cambridge Assessment, where he currently leads operational data analysis for tests administered by Cambridge Assessment Admissions Testing. He holds an MA in Mathematics from the University of Cambridge and an MA in English Language Teaching and Applied Linguistics from King's College London. Mark has nine years of experience in managing quality assurance of high-stakes tests, and expertise in item response theory, malpractice and statistics.

Joanne Emery holds a PhD in Psychology from the University of Newcastle upon Tyne. She is currently a Research Associate at the University of Cambridge School of Clinical Medicine, in the Department of Public Health and Primary Care. She was previously a Senior Research Manager at Cambridge Assessment, with experience of investigating the selection of students into undergraduate medicine; the social, demographic, emotional and cognitive predictors of school achievement; and reforms to A Levels.

Molly Fyfe is a Senior Research Manager at Cambridge Assessment, where she conducts research on issues related to admissions testing. She holds a Master's in Public Health from the University of California, Berkeley, and an MA in Education from the College of Notre Dame. She has research interests in medical education and is studying for a PhD at King's College London. Her current work at Cambridge Assessment focuses on widening participation in medical study and the societal impact of selective admissions methods, including admissions tests.

Tom Gallacher is a Research Analyst at Cambridge Assessment, where he works on admissions tests. He is responsible for statistical analysis that supports research and validation activities for BMAT. He holds an MSc in Organisational Psychology from the Manchester Business School and an MA in Psychology from Edinburgh University. Prior to joining Cambridge Assessment, he worked on Situational Judgement Tests used in the selection of UK clinicians.

Karen Grant is Director of Admissions and a Deputy Director of Medical Studies at Lancaster University. She delivers pharmacology teaching for Lancaster's undergraduate medicine course and is engaged in medical education research. In particular, she is interested in evidence-based admissions procedures in medical selection and the role of outreach programmes in widening access.

Sarah McElwee holds a PhD in Cognitive Development from Queen's University Belfast. Currently, she is a Principal Research Manager responsible for managing the research team working on Cambridge Assessment's admissions tests. Prior to joining the group, she was a post-doctoral researcher in psychology at the University of Oxford, where her research focused on development of tests of verbal and spatial reasoning for children.

Her current research interests include the cognitive processes elicited by test tasks, the consequences of high-stakes testing and the role of test developers in supporting medical education.

Nick Saville is the Director of the Research and Thought Leadership Group at Cambridge English Language Assessment and Secretary-General of the Association of Language Testers in Europe (ALTE). He holds a PhD in language test impact from University of Bedfordshire, as well as degrees in Linguistics and Teaching English as a Foreign Language from the University of Reading. Before joining Cambridge Assessment in 1989, he taught at the University of Cagliari, Italy, and managed test development projects in Tokyo. Nick has specialised in educational assessment since 1987 and has published extensively on a range of topics, such as the impact of assessment on policy; the application of frameworks in test validation; and the role of assessment in learning.

Mark Shannon is currently responsible for admissions test content in components that have science and maths elements, such as Section 2 of BMAT. Before becoming an Assessment Group Manager with responsibilities for test production, he was a member of the original research team that worked on the development of BMAT. He previously studied Education and Biological Sciences at the University of Cambridge and holds an MSc in Social Research Methods.

Lynda Taylor is Visiting Professor of Language Assessment at the Centre for Research in English Language Learning and Assessment (CRELLA), University of Bedfordshire. Her research interests include using qualitative research methods in assessment research, the impact of linguistic variety on assessment and ethical issues, including the provision of testing accommodations. Lynda holds an MPhil and a PhD in applied linguistics and language testing, both from the University of Cambridge, UK. She was formerly Assistant Director of the Research and Validation Group at Cambridge English Language Assessment, and has over 30 years' experience writing on theoretical and practical issues in high-stakes international assessment.

Juliet Wilson is Director of Assessment at Cambridge English Language Assessment, which is the division that manages production of examination materials. She has extensive experience in managing high-stakes testing and was formerly Director of Network Services, which managed the test centre network used to administer tests. Before joining Cambridge Assessment in 1998, she taught English to adults and children in the UK, Colombia, Hong Kong and Portugal. She holds a BA in French and German, a Master's degree in TESOL from the Institute of Education, University of London, and a Certificate in Management from the Judge Institute, University of Cambridge.

List of abbreviations

AAMC	American Association of Medical Colleges
ACER	Australian Council for Education Research
ACT	American College Test
AQA	Assessment and Qualifications Alliance
BM	Bachelor of Medicine
BMA	British Medical Association
BMAT	BioMedical Admissions Test
CB	Computer-based
CCTDI	California Critical Thinking Disposition Inventory
CEFR	Common European Framework of Reference for Languages
CFA	Confirmatory Factor Analysis
CGP	Coordination Group Publications
CriTT	Critical Thinking Toolkit
CTT	Classical Test Theory
DfE	Department for Education
DIF	Differential Item Functioning
EFA	Exploratory Factor Analysis
ESOL	English for Speakers of Other Languages
ETS	Educational Testing Service
FA	Factor Analysis
FHS	Final Honour School
FYGPA	First Year Grade Point Average
GAMSAT	Graduate Medical School Admissions Test
GCSE	General Certificate of Secondary Education
GMC	General Medical Council
GPA	Grade Point Average
HEFCE	Higher Education Funding Council for England
HESA	Higher Education Statistics Agency
IB	International Baccalaureate
ICC	Item Characteristic Curve
IQ	Intelligence Quotient
IRT	Item Response Theory
ISC	Independent Schools Council
JCQ	Joint Council for Qualifications
LKC	Lee Kong Chian School of Medicine
MCAT	Medical Colleges Admission Test

MCQ	Multiple-choice Question
MH	Mantel-Haenszel
MMI	Multiple Mini-interviews
MSC	Medical Schools Council
MVAT	Medical and Veterinary Admissions Test
NS-SEC	National Statistics Socio-economic Classification
OCR	Oxford, Cambridge and RSA examinations
OFFA	Office For Fair Access
OMAT	Oxford Medical Admissions Test
ONS	Office for National Statistics
PB	Paper-based
POLAR	Participation of Local Areas
QAA	Quality Assurance Agency for Higher Education
RVC	Royal Veterinary College
SAT	Formerly the Scholastic Aptitude Test or the Scholastic Assessment Test (currently not recognised as an acronym)
SEM	Standard Error of Measurement
SME	Subject Matter Expert
TESOL	Teaching English to Speakers of Other Languages
TOEFL	Test of English as a Foreign Language
TSA	Thinking Skills Assessment
UCAS	Universities and Colleges Admissions Service
UCL	University College London
UCLES	University of Cambridge Local Examinations Syndicate
UCLMS	University College London Medical School
UKCAT	United Kingdom Clinical Aptitude Test
UKMED	UK Medical Education Database
WJEC	Welsh Joint Education Committee
WP	Widening Participation

1 The Cambridge Approach to admissions testing

Nick Saville

Cambridge English Language Assessment

1.1 Purpose of the volume

Admission to study medicine is highly competitive and medical degree courses are among the most oversubscribed in the world. Many applicants that submit themselves to the multi-stage selection processes used for admissions have the highest school-leaving qualifications achievable. In the UK, these pressures led to development of the BioMedical Admissions Test (BMAT), which at the time of writing has been used for over a decade in the selection of students to medicine, veterinary medicine, dentistry and biomedical sciences courses. Originally commissioned for use by a small number of universities, BMAT has been increasingly employed by institutions around the world, partly due to growing trends for medical courses to use English as the medium of instruction.

In the UK, a report commissioned by the regulatory body for doctors, the General Medical Council (GMC), recommended that medical schools include standardised testing alongside other selection methods (Cleland, Dowell, McLachlan, Nicholson and Patterson 2012). Since the publication of this report, use of BMAT and other admissions tests has become more widespread in the UK, and there has also been more research focused on selection processes. This volume contributes to the body of research on selection for medical study, by presenting work on BMAT that has been conducted in over a decade of research and validation. Historically, this research and validation work has informed test construction and been used to respond to specific stakeholder queries. More recently, the results of research have been made available for medical schools and departments considering use of BMAT in their admissions process, many of whom have since adopted BMAT. Therefore, much of the research in the present volume will be familiar to members of the BMAT stakeholder group; however, this is the first time that this work has appeared together in one collection, and been made available for the wider medical education community.

The process of validating a test to show that it is fit for purpose involves a process of building an argument. As Kane (2013:1) has noted, 'public claims require public justification'. The intention of the collection of studies and procedures in the chapters that follow are offered in the spirit in which

Kane suggests – to make public the validation arguments that support use of BMAT. The studies presented are a mixture of published research, conference papers and internal Cambridge Assessment reports. They are not an exhaustive list but represent key examples and summaries of research work (spanning the earliest years of BMAT to the present day) that covers a broad range of validity evidence. The volume has been compiled for readers involved in selecting students for medicine or biomedical courses, from policy-makers to anyone wishing to better understand the evidence base for the test.

In addition to collecting together research on BMAT, this volume articulates a multi-faceted conceptualisation of test validity – the socio-cognitive approach – and applies it to the admissions testing context of BMAT. This theoretical framework of assessment is used for in-depth analysis of validity in high-stakes language testing, and has been adopted by Cambridge Assessment Admissions Testing because of the comprehensive and structured treatment it provides of multiple aspects in the testing process. Some of the work presented in the following chapters predates Cambridge Assessment Admissions Testing's use of the socio-cognitive model in validation; however, all of the studies included map onto areas identified in the socio-cognitive approach, demonstrating the framework's suitability for the admissions testing context, and potentially for other contexts across educational assessment.

1.2 The Cambridge Approach

Cambridge Assessment Admissions Testing is part of the Cambridge Assessment Group, Europe's largest educational research and assessment agency, and a department of the University of Cambridge. We recognise that this brings with it a high level of responsibility and a requirement to ensure that our assessment systems not only deliver fair and dependable results for test takers, but also have positive effects and consequences for society at large. We work with national governments and other organisations to develop learning and testing solutions that meet their precise needs and, where these needs cannot be met using our existing services, we develop tailored solutions.

In order to ensure that all forms of assessment are of the highest quality and are appropriate to their context and intended uses, Cambridge Assessment has developed a set of common standards known as the *Cambridge Approach* (Cambridge Assessment 2009). This approach sets out an overarching framework for assessment, reflecting the University's broad goal 'to contribute to society through the pursuit of education, learning and research at the highest levels of excellence'.

While Cambridge Assessment Admissions Testing adheres to the Cambridge Approach in general, it also looks at best practice in assessment taking place within the three examination boards that make up the Cambridge Assessment Group, to ensure the quality of the assessments it delivers. In particular,

Cambridge Assessment Admissions Testing uses principles developed by Cambridge English Language Assessment (which provides over 5 million tests a year for speakers of English as a second language) to guide test development, production and research. The Cambridge English *Principles of Good Practice* document provides an accessible and concise overview of the key concepts, together with examples of how the principles are put into practice (Cambridge English 2016). The four guiding principles are: fitness for purpose, communication and collaboration, quality and accountability, validity and validation.

Below we focus mainly on the principles of fitness for purpose and validity and validation to explain why these are relevant to this volume. A brief overview of communication and collaboration is presented and we also summarise how quality and accountability impacts on the work of Cambridge Assessment Admissions Testing.

Fitness for purpose

Central to the validity of BMAT as an admissions test for biomedical study is establishing that it is fit for purpose. Fitness for purpose is a multi-faceted idea that incorporates not only the more traditional aspects of validity and reliability, but also the practicality of the test, its impact on stakeholders, and the quality management system that underpins it to ensure that the standard of the assessment is consistent over time. We discuss these issues below with

Figure 1.1 Elements of fitness for purpose in test validation

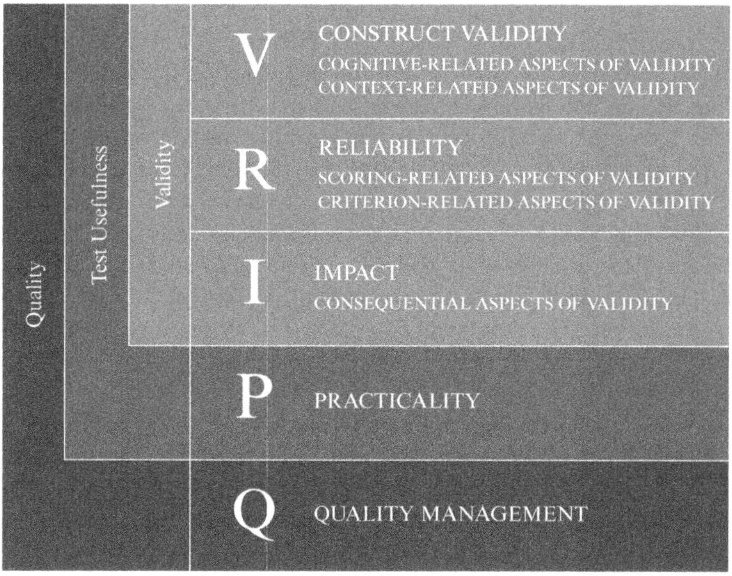

reference to practicality and impact. Figure 1.1 illustrates our approach to achieving fitness for purpose, and shows how developments in testing theory and quality management have been incorporated into a coherent framework that guides our assessment practices.

Impact by design

High-stakes assessment has important effects and consequences within an educational system and on society more widely. These effects are referred to as *impact.* Test takers in particular are affected because the results of tests are used to make important decisions about them which can affect their lives. In developing and administering our tests we adopt the principle of *impact by design*: we strive to achieve positive impact in the contexts in which our assessments are used and we undertake to investigate this through our validation processes. We seek to design and develop test features that promote positive effects on learning (Saville 2012). The principle of impact by design is useful for considering the constructs assessed by BMAT, and how preparing for the test might benefit the test taker.

The individual qualities of validity, reliability, impact and practicality cannot be evaluated independently; rather their relative importance must be determined in order to maximise the overall 'fitness for purpose' of the exam (see Saville 2003).

Practicality considerations

Practicality can be defined as the extent to which an examination is practicable in terms of the resources necessary to produce and administer it to the highest standard in its intended context and use. It affects many different aspects of an examination and we regularly consult relevant stakeholders during test development and revision processes on the practical aspects of using an admissions test. Test length is one such example; while longer tests can increase reliability because they capture more measurement data, they may be impractical to administer. In addition, an overly long exam could induce fatigue in candidates, which in turn could introduce error into the measurements. If some candidates are more susceptible to fatigue than others, this can result in score differences unrelated to the attribute being assessed. This example illustrates how practicality can impact the validity of the inferences based on a person's score responses; therefore, some practical aspects overlap with contemporary conceptualisations of validity (e.g. Messick 1995).

Other practicality considerations are concerned with the locations where an examination is administered and the processes for getting materials to and from these places securely (either digitally or physically). BMAT uses an international network of test centres maintained by the three exam boards across Cambridge Assessment. We work with centres to make sure that the systems we use are up to date and flexible enough to allow effective and efficient administration. Finally, in line with our educational mission, we wish to maintain access for the widest proportion of candidates possible, which means we strive to hold costs at a reasonable level, whilst ensuring that the test is available internationally.

Communication and collaboration

Our approach recognises the importance of communicating and collaborating with the organisations and individuals that use assessments to make decisions. This enables a test developer to have an understanding of the contextual issues that impact on a programme of assessment. Cambridge Assessment Admissions Testing works to ensure that it is receptive to the needs, opinions and knowledge of key stakeholders. In the context of BMAT, these are primarily the biomedical and dental departments that use the test to select students from their applicant pools.

Information and liaison

We constantly liaise with organisations that use our admissions tests, in order to provide support and information. For BMAT, a liaison group meets twice annually to discuss test sessions and general issues related to healthcare admissions. Although hosted by Cambridge Assessment Admissions Testing, meetings are chaired by one of the stakeholders; this changes on a rotating basis. The meeting chair occasionally uses the meeting to identify a specific agenda point, which can prompt a day of discussions and talks that focus on an area of interest. All organisations that use BMAT are invited to the meetings, and attendees typically include the admissions tutors for individual departments or courses. The forum provides an opportunity for BMAT users to discuss operational issues and topics of academic interest. Members of Cambridge Assessment Admissions Testing's research team attend these meetings to present updates and discuss possible areas for future research.

Cambridge Assessment Admissions Testing researchers also attend academic conferences that focus on a wide range of areas, such as educational assessment, higher education policy and medical education. Cambridge Assessment engages in policy discussions regarding the use of admissions tests in various international contexts, and also hosts events to lead discussions around healthcare selection and bring together institutions from the UK and overseas. Most recently, the Optimising Admissions conference held at the Royal College of Physicians in April 2017 featured presentations from the General Medical Council (GMC), medical schools from the Netherlands and healthcare educators from around the UK.

Research collaborations

Cambridge Assessment Admissions Testing works with many organisations throughout the world, including universities, government departments, major commercial organisations and many others. As part of Europe's largest assessment agency, which is also a department of the University of Cambridge, we have a research capacity that enables delivery of joint international projects. These researchers also develop and manage relationships with key stakeholders, often by collaborating with them.

Recently, Cambridge Assessment's collaboration with the GMC has been influential in advancing the UK Medical Education Database (UKMED) project, which will include BMAT data for research purposes. This initiative supports medical education research by linking data together from multiple sources and making it available securely and anonymously. Research into admissions testing is also supported using funded research programmes. A recent round awarded funding for three BMAT-related projects, to researchers from Lee Kong Chian School of Medicine (LKC), University of Leiden Medical School and Imperial College School of Medicine.

Quality and accountability

Quality control and assurance supports an assessment organisation to achieve fitness for purpose consistently. Cambridge Assessment Admissions Testing, like Cambridge English Language Assessment, adopts a process approach to ensuring quality. Processes are defined and agreed so that quality control and quality assurance procedures can be carried out. Many of the processes related to BMAT question paper production are described in Chapter 4 of this volume. These procedures are constantly reviewed as part of the test development and validation cycle.

The test development and validation cycle

To ensure fitness for purpose we employ an explicit model for the *test development and validation process* which incorporates continual improvement cycles. This is applied to all our admissions tests, including BMAT.

As shown in Figure 1.2, the process begins with a perceived need for a new or revised test, and is then broken down into three phases: planning, design and development. The first task in the planning phase is to define the intended *context and use* of the prospective test by identifying stakeholders and their needs, and considering both theoretical and practical issues in meeting these needs. The original BMAT stakeholders were the medical and veterinary schools at University of Cambridge and University of Oxford. As BMAT was designed to meet the needs of these stakeholders at their request, they were consulted throughout the planning, design and development of the test.

Figure 1.2 A model of the ongoing test development validation cycle

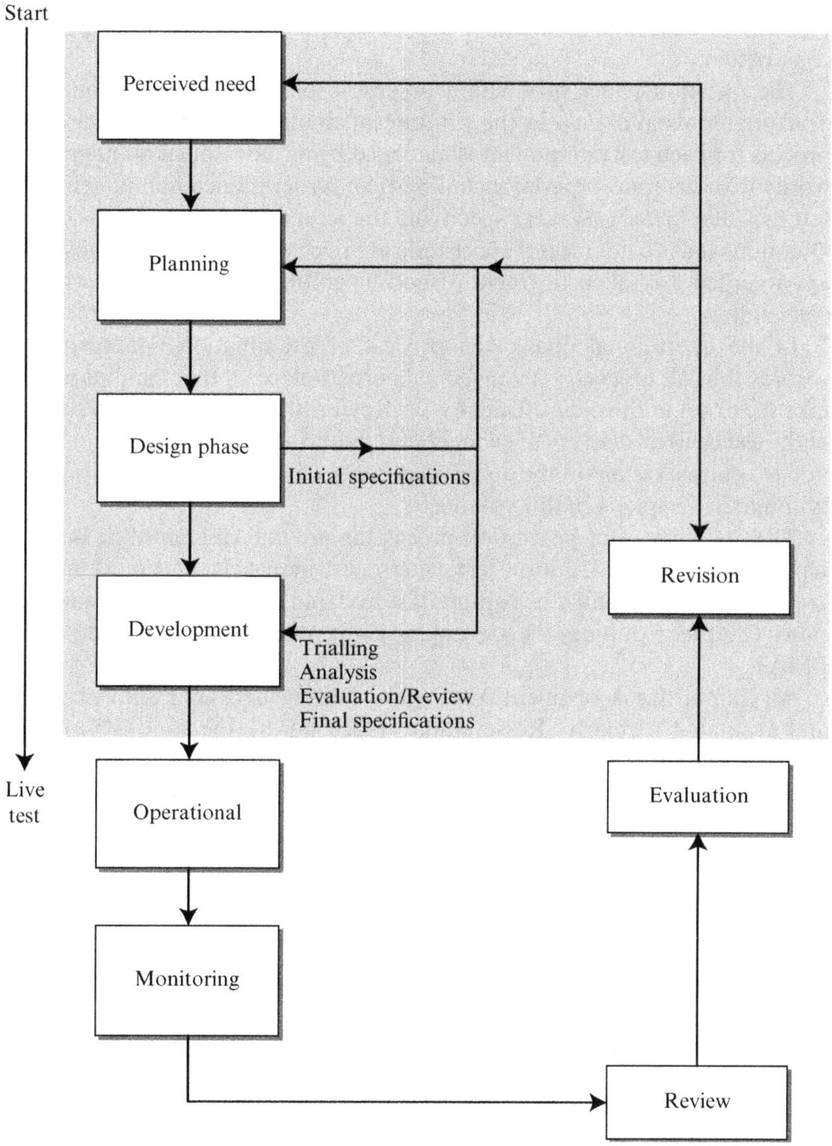

The output of the development stage is a set of test specifications – a document or documents defining the test, its validity argument and its operational requirements. The specifications act as a 'blueprint' for the operational production of tests. The most up-to-date test specification for BMAT is available on the Cambridge Assessment Admissions Testing website. Chapter 3 of this volume describes the original planning phase of BMAT and Chapter 4 outlines how the test specification informs the way that BMAT papers are constructed.

The question paper production process begins with commissioning of draft materials and ends in the printing of the final question papers. The process for each test component is managed by an assessment manager who works with external experts, including item writers. Each component of a test has *item writer guidelines* specifying the requirements of each task type. Questions that do not meet these criteria are rejected or rewritten. Those that are accepted are taken through a rigorous editing process by experienced consultants.

In the operational phase, the process of examination administration ensures that all necessary arrangements are in place so that candidates can take the exam in the most efficient way. Key tasks include quality assurance of the test centres, delivery of exam materials and administrative documentation to centres. Details of the quality assurance of BMAT administration can be found in Chapter 4 of this volume.

The main stages of post-exam processing are marking, grading and the reporting of results. Data on test takers, test materials, and marking and grading procedures must be captured, stored and analysed for all exam sessions. Chapter 5 outlines the scoring, marking and reporting procedures for BMAT.

All Cambridge Assessment Admissions Testing assessments are reviewed and evaluated regularly. Review takes place during the routine monitoring of operational processes, and typically, improvements are implemented in an ongoing manner. All facets of the test's fitness for purpose are evaluated, including its practicality. Although the primary purpose of BMAT has changed little, some contextual factors have changed substantially. For example, the first time BMAT was administered, demand for a biomedical admissions test was limited to a small number of institutions in the UK, whereas now, BMAT is used by 17 institutions in seven countries to support their selection procedures. These developments impact on operational and theoretical considerations that are monitored and adjusted for. An example of this is presented in Chapter 4 as a case study: a revision of BMAT Section 2, which ensured BMAT's fitness for purpose in the face of science curriculum changes and an increasingly international candidature.

If necessary, a major revision project is initiated which, in essence, loops back to the planning phase of the cycle. Cambridge Assessment Admissions Testing involves BMAT stakeholders in the routine monitoring described above, to include their evaluations regarding the need for major revision. The current format and structure of BMAT is outlined below, along with some context regarding the test's purpose and use.

The BioMedical Admissions Test

BMAT is a pen-and-paper test – available at schools and colleges worldwide – that assesses an applicant's readiness for the demanding, science-based study required in medicine and other biomedical courses. It is intended to supplement, rather than replace, the information provided by prior examination results, standardised application forms (such as UCAS), and interviews. Institutions differ in their use of BMAT scores, with some using scores as a hurdle to the interview stage and others not. It is often used in a compensatory manner with other selection criteria, meaning that low-scoring applicants are not always rejected and high-scoring applicants are not always offered a place.

BMAT has three elements: a domain-general aptitude and skills section, a section based on scientific knowledge and applications, and a short communicative writing task. A summary of the sections is provided in Table 1.1.

Table 1.1 Summary of BMAT sections

Section 1 **Aptitude and Skills**	This element tests generic skills often utilised in undergraduate study: problem solving, understanding argument, and data analysis and inference skills. There are 35 items in 60 minutes.
Section 2 **Scientific Knowledge and Applications**	This element tests whether candidates have the core knowledge and the capacity to apply it, which is a pre-requisite for high-level study in biomedical sciences. Questions are restricted to material typically included in non-specialist school Science and Mathematics courses but require a level of understanding appropriate for such an able target group. There are 27 items in 30 minutes.
Section 3 **Writing Task**	This element tests the ability to select, develop and organise ideas and to communicate them in writing, concisely and effectively. A selection of questions on topics of general, medical, veterinary or scientific interest are available, one of which must be chosen. The response is limited to one A4 page in 30 minutes.

BMAT Sections 1 and 2 are in multiple-choice format (objectively marked) and all items are worth one mark. Scores are reported on a calibrated, 9-point scale to one decimal place. The Writing Task is marked by a team of expert markers at Cambridge Assessment. An image of the response is also supplied to each institution to which the candidate has applied. This provides the institution with an example of each applicant's writing skill that has been completed under exam conditions, unlike other samples of writing that are commonly made available as part of the application process. Admissions tutors are therefore confident that applicants authored the Section 3 essay, which can be further reviewed qualitatively if needed. Past

BMAT papers and sample materials are available on the BMAT website: www.admissionstestingservice.org/for-test-takers/bmat

Institutions want to be confident that they have selected the right applicants and deselected those who are least likely to succeed. The utility of BMAT is demonstrated by studies to date, which have shown that BMAT scores relate to applicants' future performance on their course of study. Despite the difficulties involved in making predictions about future behaviour, high BMAT scores are associated with high course outcomes, and low scores (especially for the Scientific Knowledge and Applications section) are associated with poor course outcomes for those admitted, despite their high A Level grades.

A further benefit to institutions is that they are able to use BMAT to deselect applicants for interview if there is sufficient evidence, from usage of the test, that applicants with low scores have very little chance of being offered a place of study (when their scores were unseen by those doing the selecting). Where the selection process begins before A Level results are available (as it does for most) we have also shown that BMAT results can predict those likely to achieve weaker A Level outcomes (importantly, these are applicants failing to meet their conditional offer grades despite high predictions).

Of course, no *single* assessment will be ideal in the selection of those for a career in medicine, dentistry or veterinary medicine and the non-academic attributes thought to be desirable in applicants, such as personal qualities, will need to be assessed in other ways. For this reason a multifaceted approach to medical selection is widely accepted and recommended (Cleland et al 2012). When used alongside other selection criteria, BMAT can usefully aid admissions tutors in choosing applicants who can cope with the academic demands of their future course of study and thrive in the intellectually rigorous environment required. This volume presents work conducted to ensure that BMAT remains fit for purpose in a complex and important environment, where an understanding of the test's validity is crucial.

Validity and validation

Validity has generally been defined as the extent to which an assessment can be shown to produce scores and/or outcomes which are an accurate reflection of the test taker's true level of ability. It is concerned with the appropriateness and meaningfulness of inferences made when using the test results within a particular social or educational context. Validation is the process of accumulating evidence to support these interpretations. We endorse this view and in doing so draw on internationally recognised standards such as the *Standards for Educational and Psychological Testing* (American Educational Research Association, American Psychological Association and National Council on Measurement in Education 2014), which is hereafter referred to as the *Standards* (2014).

Cambridge Assessment Admissions Testing's view of validation draws on a *socio-cognitive approach* to defining the abilities which are to be tested by an assessment system. This theoretical framework of learning and assessment is used for in-depth analysis of the validity of our tests, including BMAT. The model was developed by Cambridge English Language Assessment researchers in collaboration with Weir (2005), and draws on the work of Messick (1989), who stressed the interacting nature of different *types of validity* evidence (and also Bachman 1990, Bachman and Palmer 1996).

The approach is described as socio-cognitive in that carrying out tasks in real life is a social phenomenon and the underlying abilities which enable these actions are mental constructs (the cognitive dimension). A valid test seeks to engage the mental capacities in an authentic way so that appropriate inferences can be drawn from the test score.

In the case of potential for biomedical study, it is important to make explicit what is meant by this notion and to account for the ways in which test results can be used to make dependable decisions about the test takers' ability. In other words, we need to have confidence that high scores reliably reflect more potential than lower scores. This point highlights a fundamental issue of validity – the nature of the *constructs* which are at the heart of our tests and how we account for them. The construct of a test is the theory that the test is based on. For BMAT, this is the theory of the cognitive skills, the core scientific reasoning and the written communication abilities that will enable a student to cope with the demands of a rigorous biomedical degree. Within the socio-cognitive approach, we account for the test construct by considering six 'aspects' of validity for which supporting evidence must be provided.

Figure 1.3 illustrates the principal direction of hypothesised relationships between elements of the socio-cognitive framework. It shows that, while all aspects of validity need to be considered at test development stages, some types of validity evidence cannot be collected until after the test event – particularly those aspects which relate to the effects and consequences of using the results.

This view treats the aspects of validity outlined above as component parts of overall validity. This unitary conceptualisation of validity requires a comprehensive *validity argument* to be presented. A validity argument is a well-reasoned rationale in which the examination provider presents an overall evaluation of the intended interpretations and uses of the test which is being validated. This is consistent with the definition of validation as: 'the ongoing process of demonstrating that a particular interpretation of test scores is justified' (Bachman and Palmer 1996:22).

This approach to validation underpins contemporary work in language testing contexts, but validation of admissions tests have tended to focus on reliability, which is a narrow aspect of scoring validity, and predictive

Figure 1.3 The socio-cognitive validation framework (adapted from Weir 2005)

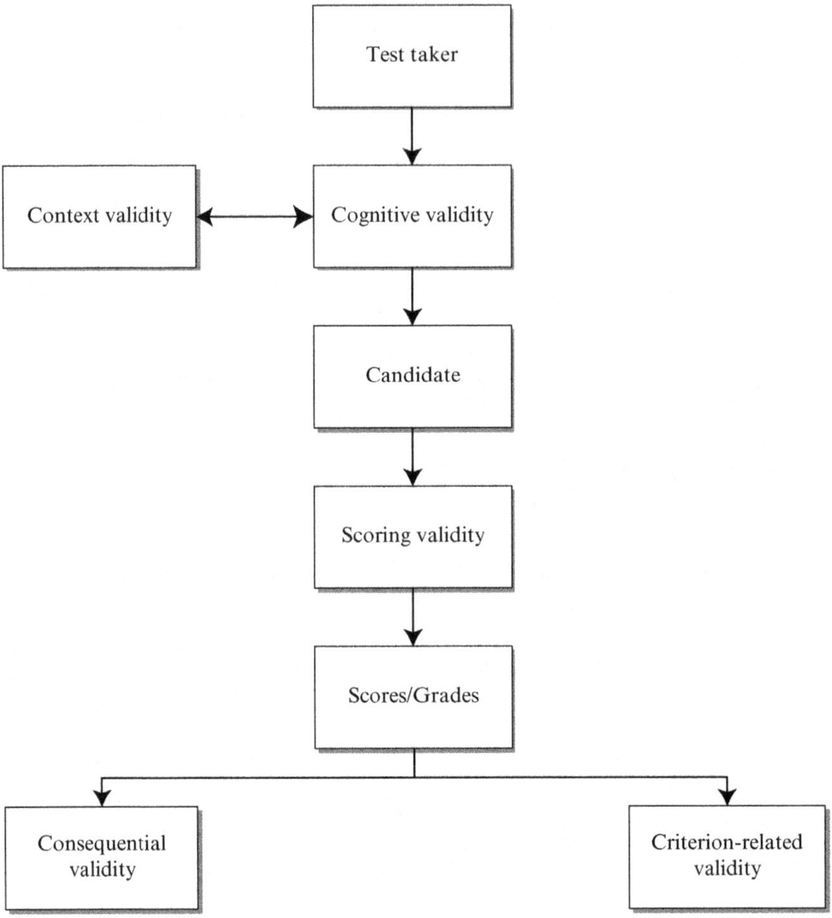

validity, a form of criterion-related validity (Soares 2012). There is growing consensus that the predictive and scoring validity of admissions tests should be supplemented with other forms of validity (Atkinson and Geiser 2009, Linn 2009). By applying the socio-cognitive model to BMAT, this volume provides an example of how various aspects of validity can be considered in relation to an admissions test. In building and presenting a validity argument we seek to:

- set out our claims relating to the usefulness of the test for its intended purpose
- explain why each claim is appropriate by giving reasons and justifications

- provide adequate evidence to support the claims and the reasoning behind them.

This evidence is built over time, beginning at the design and development stages, and continues to be accumulated for as long as the test remains operational. This volume presents the validity argument for BMAT in its current form, and does not preclude evidence being added to the overall case for BMAT in the future. Indeed, the Cambridge Assessment approach subscribes to a continuous model of test validation that continues throughout the lifetime of any test.

1.3 Structure of the volume

In the seven chapters that follow, evidence for the validity of BMAT is presented. Each of these chapters focuses on an aspect of the socio-cognitive model (see Figure 1.3) and then the final chapter draws this work together. The Appendix shows the questions that need to be considered by the test provider in gathering evidence for each of these aspects. We use these questions to develop standard quality procedures and operational analyses for a test as well as to design and conduct targeted research studies that generate empirical evidence. In this collection, therefore, we outline the quality procedures and routine analyses put in place for BMAT that relate to each of these aspects of validity, as well as presenting key evidence from research studies.

In designing a test for a particular context and purpose, we profile the intended test takers in terms of their characteristics: demographic features (such as gender), existing knowledge and prior learning experiences. The BMAT candidature has changed over the years that the test has been used and we continue to collect information in an ongoing manner during operational phases to make sure that the test is still fit for purpose. Additionally, various concerns about the composition of the medical student population have been raised by the Medical Schools Council (2014). Research studies have been conducted to ensure that BMAT is not contributing to diversity issues and these are presented as part of Chapter 2.

Chapter 3 discusses cognitive validity in the context of BMAT. Cognitive-related validity is concerned with the extent to which the cognitive processes employed by candidates are similar to those that will be needed in real-world contexts beyond the test. For BMAT, medical school represents the context of interest. This chapter focuses on the constructs assessed by BMAT sections and the work done to ensure that the skills assessed are relevant to successful study at medical school.

Chapter 4 is concerned with context validity. Discussion focuses on the conditions under which the test is performed and includes features of the tasks as well as the administration conditions. Some of the issues regarding task features examined in this chapter have a symbiotic relationship to those covered on cognitive validity, as an item's characteristics can have unintended effects on the cognitive processes used to answer the question, potentially introducing construct-irrelevant variance to test scores that should be avoided. Threats to a test's validity can also arise if administration conditions are not considered and standardised, so the operational processes that safeguard the security and integrity of BMAT are included in this chapter.

It is essential to ensure that tests are scored accurately (with no processing errors) and it is important to estimate the reliability of the results – the extent to which they are stable, consistent and free from errors of measurement. In Chapter 5, the scoring procedures for BMAT are discussed, alongside some of the psychometric procedures used to monitor and evaluate test sessions. It is also essential that tests are fair and not biased in favour of one group of test takers over another. This aspect of scoring validity links closely with the issues covered in Chapter 2; knowledge of the test taker sample informs post-test analyses of group differences and this chapter presents examples of this work.

In establishing criterion-related aspects of validity the aim is to demonstrate that test scores are systematically related to another indicator of what is being measured, or a measure of some related construct, such as another established test or a predicted outcome. Much of the research on admissions testing, particularly in the medical context, is dominated by predictive validity research focused on academic achievement. In Chapter 6, published work on how BMAT scores predict course outcomes is referred to, along with some analyses relating to other outcome variables, such as A Levels. In addition, this chapter discusses some common challenges experienced when conducting predictive validity studies. In particular, work looking at the effects of range restriction in selection situations is shared and common approaches to dealing with this phenomenon are critically discussed.

Consequential validity (or 'impact') is concerned with the effects of using a test on stakeholders (including test takers themselves) and on wider society. These consequences may be positive or negative, intended or unintended, and are particularly relevant to high-stakes tests like BMAT. Stakeholder perceptions of a test and washback effects on learning are aspects of consequential validity. Chapter 7 deals with these issues and the responsibilities of the test developer to consider BMAT's impact on society more generally.

Finally, Chapter 8 outlines the key issues raised by authors throughout the volume, in order to present some conclusions related to the use and study of admissions tests such as BMAT.

1.4 Chapter summary

This introduction chapter has highlighted the need for test developers to evaluate various aspects of validity when constructing a high-stakes admission test such as BMAT. The importance of considering various aspects of the test's candidature and administration has also been emphasised. In order to meet these requirements, we have adopted a comprehensive validation framework in the form of the socio-cognitive approach (O'Sullivan and Weir 2011, Weir 2005), and applied it to BMAT. This framework is elaborated in the following chapters to present a multi-faceted overview of BMAT, and the validity arguments that underpin the assessment. Furthermore, this collection can promote similarly comprehensive evaluations in the admissions testing literature, and potentially in other areas of educational assessment. Therefore, this volume is suitable for anybody with an interest in educational assessment.

It is hoped – and certainly intended – that those concerned with the fair, transparent, valid and reliable selection of students will find the following chapters accessible and useful. Chapter 2 addresses the importance of understanding the BMAT test taker, as the first of six components to consider from the socio-cognitive framework.

Appendix

Questions to be considered in building validity evidence for a test (adapted from Weir 2005)

Test taker characteristics	What are the characteristics of the test takers (age, gender, etc.)? Does the test make suitable accommodations for candidates with special needs? Are candidates sufficiently familiar with what they have to do in the test? Are candidates put at ease so that they are enabled to achieve their best?
Context validity	Is there any evidence that the response format is likely to affect performance? Are the marking criteria explicit for the candidates and the markers? Is the timing of each part appropriate? Is the content knowledge suitable and unbiased? Are the administration conditions satisfactorily consistent and secure?
Cognitive validity	What are the skills/cognitive processes elicited by the test tasks?
Scoring validity	Are items of appropriate difficulty and do they discriminate between candidates? Is there a sufficient level of test reliability? Is there any evidence of item bias? Are the candidates' responses their own? Are there clearly defined marking criteria that cover the construct? Are markers trained, standardised, checked and moderated? Is marking reliable and consistent?
Criterion validity	Do test scores relate to future outcomes? (predictive) Do test scores relate to other tests or measurements? (concurrent)
Consequential validity	Are actions based on test scores appropriate? Is there any evidence of differential validity? How are candidates preparing for the test? Is there a washback effect in the classroom (positive or negative)? How is the test perceived by stakeholders?

2 The biomedical school applicant: Considering the test taker in test development and research

Amy Devine

Research and Thought Leadership Group, Cambridge Assessment Admissions Testing

Lynda Taylor

Consultant, Cambridge Assessment Admissions Testing

Brenda Cross

University College London Medical School

2.1 Introduction

The test taker sits at the heart of any assessment event and ensuring that their needs are met is central to the fitness for purpose of an assessment. In this chapter we discuss the importance of the test provider having a sound understanding of the nature of the population for whom the test is intended. The BMAT test taker population is homogenous in some respects, because the majority of candidates are school leavers of a specific age range, ability level and language proficiency[1]. However, a substantial minority of those sitting the exam are referred to as 'non-traditional' applicants to medical school and test developers must be mindful not to disadvantage this subset of test takers. In other respects the candidature is more diverse. Several medical schools offer accelerated graduate-entry courses for applicants with an undergraduate degree in a scientific discipline. Also, increasing numbers of applications to medical school originate from outside the country where the medical school is based. Combined with growing use of BMAT in different locations, these factors mean that the educational backgrounds of applicants can be

1 The majority of BMAT candidates that apply to study undergraduate medicine at UK universities are home status students for whom English is their native language. Non-native English-speaking applicants to medical courses are typically required to demonstrate advanced English language proficiency (e.g. at the C1 to C2 level of the Common European Framework of Reference for Languages (CEFR), Council of Europe 2001).

quite different. An understanding of the test taker population informs meaningful evaluation of the different aspects of validity discussed in later chapters of this volume.

This chapter discusses how certain characteristics of the intended test taker population are taken into account in the overall design of the test. It also explains measures by which performance on the test is monitored and investigated to ensure fairness for different applicant groups, alongside and compared with outcomes from previous analyses.

2.2 The importance of test taker characteristics in assessment

The assessment literature often uses the term 'test taker characteristics' to describe a wide variety of features associated with the intended test taker population, which need to be taken into account when designing and administering a test. Test taker characteristics can include *physical* features (such as age and gender), *experiential* features (such as educational background or life experience) and *psychological* features (such as emotional state and motivation). Test designers need to have a clear understanding of the physical, experiential and affective features of the candidature for whom their test is intended. Test providers also need to have in place systems for investigating and monitoring test performance in relation to these factors since such features potentially influence testing outcomes. There are three main reasons for ensuring that a sound understanding and appropriate systems are in place.

First, for reasons of test validity and usefulness, it is essential that test content and format should be well matched to the intended test population (in this case applicants to medical, dental, veterinary and biomedical courses in higher education) and should be consistent with the intended purpose of the test and the scores generated. Where a test provider is informed about the nature of the target candidature for its test, and takes proper account of this in its test design, development and validation activity, the test is more likely to be fit for purpose. Combined with existing research knowledge about affective and psychological factors related to test performance, such as anxiety and risk-aversion, information about the population can support the design of constructs, tasks and scoring procedures.

Secondly, an awareness of test taker characteristics contributes significantly to test fairness. It is important to ensure that different applicant groups can access test content and formats without being unfairly disadvantaged due to demographic or background factors such as their age, gender, ethnicity or socio-economic group. In addition, any special requirements that may apply to individuals or subgroups within the intended test population, e.g. due to physical, psychological or emotional factors, need to be anticipated and addressed in an appropriate manner. Information on test taker characteristics enables test providers to offer suitably modified tests (or testing accommodations) for those test takers who have temporary or permanent disabilities (e.g. a broken wrist or visual impairment). It also informs appropriate procedures to ensure fair treatment of those test takers who encounter some difficulty prior to or during the test which risks impairing their performance (e.g. bereavement, sudden illness, electricity failure).

Thirdly, systematic monitoring and analysis of test taker characteristics over time allows test providers to observe any changing trends within the test population and its characteristics. This information can inform future review and revision cycles of the test to ensure continuing validity and fitness for purpose.

The socio-cognitive approach outlined in Chapter 1 assigns a separate component to test taker characteristics within the overall test development and validation framework, thus maintaining a 'person-oriented' view of the testing and assessment process (rather than a purely instrument-focused view). At the same time, this focus on the test taker helps to ensure that the testing instrument meets the highest possible standards as far as matters of validity and fairness are concerned. The test taker characteristics component within the validation framework can be used to pose four specific questions (adapted from Weir 2005):

- What are the background characteristics of the test takers (age, gender, etc.)?
- Does the test make suitable accommodations for candidates with special needs?
- Are candidates sufficiently familiar with what they have to do in the test?
- Are candidates put at ease so that they are enabled to achieve their best?

These four questions are used by Cambridge Assessment to develop standard quality procedures and to design operational analyses for a test. The following part of this chapter (2.3) describes the standard quality procedures and operational analyses that relate to BMAT, and addresses each of these questions in turn. The four questions also frame targeted research studies which generate empirical evidence to confirm the validity and fairness of the test, examples of which are summarised later in this chapter.

2.3 BMAT and test taker characteristics

Collection of demographic data on BMAT candidates' characteristics

Key information on test taker characteristics is routinely collected for BMAT on multiple background variables and this information is matched to other variables in a variety of ways. The current BMAT registration process captures the following candidate background information for each test taker:

- test centre details (centre number, name, address and contact details)[2]
- candidate name (family and first names)
- gender
- date of birth
- Universities and Colleges Admissions Service (UCAS) ID number
- universities applied to with course code[3]
- requests for special needs access arrangements (where applicable, and with supporting justification).

Candidate background information is linked to BMAT test results (both test-level and individual item-level) via a unique BMAT candidate number allocated at registration. To support further research, additional candidate variables collected by UCAS during the university application process (such as ethnicity and socio-economic/participation of local areas (POLAR) group) can be matched to BMAT test results via candidates' UCAS ID number, also collected at registration. It should be noted that the data is typically more diffuse or sparse for graduate-entry medicine candidates than for the undergraduate population due to the intervening period between completion of school qualifications and sitting BMAT (for example, school information may not be available). These issues, combined with smaller sample sizes for graduate-entry cohorts, limit the analysis that can be conducted with graduate-entry BMAT applicants.

The BMAT registration form captures the candidate's signed consent that the data they provide may be used by Cambridge Assessment Admissions Testing and those institutions to which the test taker is applying, not just as part of the admissions procedures but also in associated follow-up research.

Routine analyses of BMAT performance by test taker groups

Shortly after each BMAT test session, results data for the whole cohort are analysed by gender, by school type and by UK/non-UK location. This provides a useful comparison for universities that use BMAT to understand the performance of their own cohort of applicants and how it might impact on admissions decisions.

Monitoring the composition of the BMAT candidature is another way of ensuring that the test remains correctly targeted and fit for purpose. A slightly higher proportion of female (approximately 56–59%) than male candidates have taken BMAT in every year. This reflects the distribution of gender

2 Because BMAT is normally taken in the test taker's own school or college, this information identifies the test taker's school type and location, thus permitting analyses of subpopulations according to these variables.

3 Restricted to universities and courses requiring BMAT.

amongst both those applying for entry to a medical course and the successful applicants, according to a report commissioned by the Royal College of Physicians (Elston 2009). The proportion of mature applicants has remained fairly stable over time, comprising approximately 10% of BMAT test takers. Monitoring the number of mature applicants and graduate-entry medicine applicants is important because these applicants may have additional needs which should be considered. For example, the limited number of BMAT test dates may necessitate mature candidates taking time from work or university study in order to sit the test; thus, Cambridge Assessment Admissions Testing may need to add further test dates or other testing arrangements if the proportion of mature candidates were to increase in the future.

Figure 2.1 illustrates the composition of the BMAT candidature between 2003 and 2016 by location of test centre. The proportion of candidates from non-UK centres has increased from 10% to 48% over the 14-year period, showing a steady increase initially and then a steeper increase between 2011 and 2012 (coinciding with the first non-UK institution to use the test) and another increase between 2015 and 2016.

Figure 2.1 Centre location of BMAT candidates 2003 to 2016

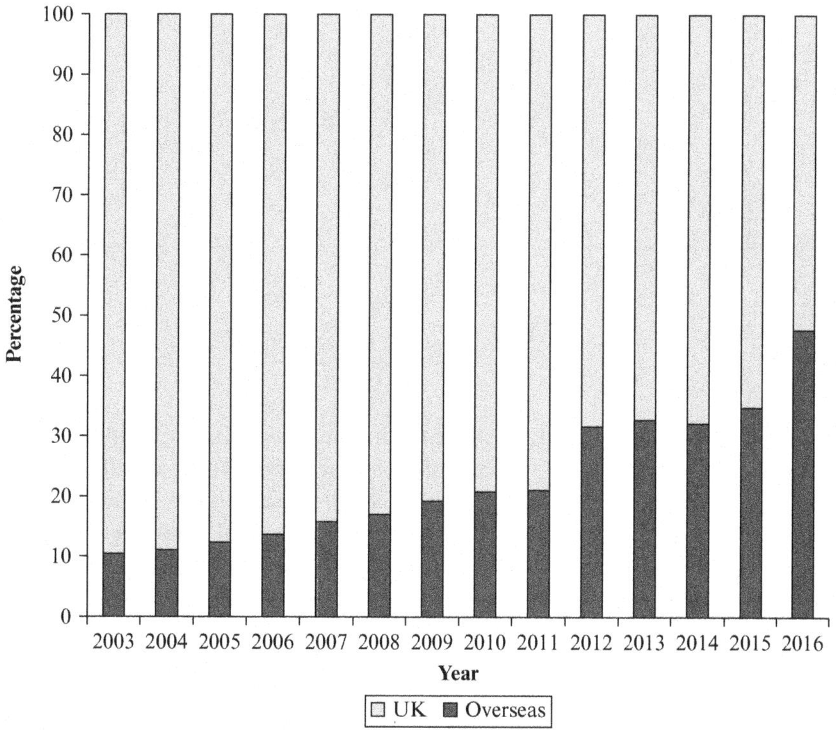

UK school types are classified for analysis as belonging to either the state (government-funded) or the independent (private, fee-paying) sector. Those within the UK state sector are categorised into further subtypes, e.g. comprehensive, selective (grammar), sixth form college.[4]

Figure 2.2 School sector of BMAT candidates 2003 to 2016 (candidates from UK centres only)

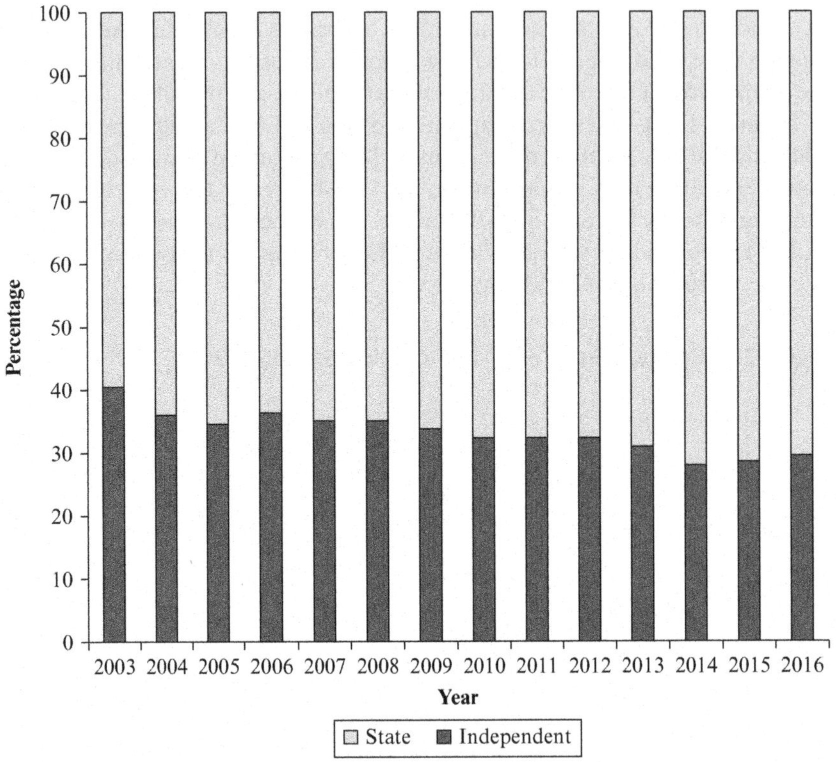

There has been a gradual decrease in the proportion of independent (fee-paying) school candidates over the 14-year period, from around 40% of the UK-based candidates in 2003 to 29% in 2016 (see Figure 2.2). This possibly suggests an encouraging increase in the numbers of state school candidates accessing BMAT over time, or may reflect changes in the universities

4 The Academies Act passed in July 2010 made it possible for all maintained primary, secondary and specialist schools to apply to become academies. By 2016, 2,075 out of 3,381 secondary schools were academies, the number growing dramatically from 203 in May 2010 (www.bbc.co.uk/news/education-13274090). Progressive reclassification of comprehensive and grammar schools to academies should be borne in mind in analysis and interpretation of data collected for subtypes of state schools post 2010.

that use BMAT[5]. Nevertheless, as with applicants to medicine in general (Medical Schools Council 2014), independent school candidates remain over-represented in BMAT cohorts and state school candidates remain under-represented with respect to the pool of UK students attaining sufficiently high A Level grades for medical study (Emery 2010a)[6]. Changing this picture requires the ongoing commitment of the medical education community.

It is important to note that, to date, analyses of the school sector of BMAT candidates have understandably focused on the school type at which the candidate is engaged in, or has had their most recent educational experience. However, the school at which a candidate is studying or has completed A Levels or International Baccalaureate® (IB) is not necessarily the same as the one at which they completed General Certificates of Secondary Education (GCSEs) (or their equivalent). Trends in school applicants do not take into account the movement that takes place between the state and independent sector post-16 years of age. Whether a pupil continues their education at a given school beyond year 11 depends on a number of factors, including the existence of a sixth form, academic performance at GCSE (or the equivalent) and the subject options available to study at A Level/IB. It also depends on financial and other considerations.

Some high-achieving state school pupils, particularly those from less advantaged backgrounds, possibly identified by schools as 'gifted and talented' or through established links between the independent and state schools sector, move to independent schools for their sixth form education, often supported by scholarships and bursaries. Some others are assisted in their move to the independent sector by parents who perceive it as an investment, to improve their chances of achieving success at A Levels and beyond. The Independent Schools Council (ISC) recently reported that the number of pupils within its schools had reached its highest levels since 1974, with one in three receiving scholarships and bursaries (Independent Schools Council 2015). Barnaby Lennon, Chairman of the ISC, noted that 'one of the interesting features [of the current figures] is that it shows parents dipping into the independent sector for crucial stages of children's education' (Garner 2015).

5 Initiatives on behalf of universities, agreed as part of their Access Agreements with the Office for Fair Access (OFFA), to raise aspirations amongst under-represented groups, may have contributed to an increase in state school candidates accessing BMAT. It is hoped that the information and preparation materials made available to prospective candidates by Cambridge Assessment Admissions Testing, especially the free, online guides (discussed in this chapter and in Chapter 4) have increased confidence and provided reassurance to state school applicants.

6 The Department for Education (DfE) 2014 survey found that 79% of academies had changed or planned to change their curriculum and, of those that had, two thirds believed that the change had improved attainment. If this improved attainment extends to A Levels amongst the increasing number of academies, one might hope to see an increasing number of state school applicants achieving sufficiently high grades to meet medical school entry requirements in the future.

The biggest expansion in numbers was reported within the sixth form, with parents 'flocking' to the independent sector for private sixth form education, possibly as a result of increased affluence and/or worries about the state sector.

From 2015, as part of the ISC census, independent schools have been asked where their pupils were educated before joining their current school. The 2016 census showed that more than one quarter of pupils new to the independent sector came from state-funded establishments (Independent Schools Council 2016). Although movement into the independent sector was shown to occur at all ages, it was most pronounced at ages 16 and above, where 15% of pupils attended an independent school compared with 6% at age 11. The rise in numbers reported within the independent sector was not confined to UK students; it was also partly attributable to an increase in international student numbers.

Movement between state and independent sector, post-GCSE, is not unidirectional. There are a number of reasons why independent school pupils transition to the state school sector for their sixth form education. Reasons include: a greater range of A Level options, the desire for a change from boarding school or single-sex school, the draw of a greater social mix and broader life experience and the desire for a new start to revitalise interest in academic work, possibly after underperformance at GCSE. The cost of fees and parental concerns about perceived 'positive discrimination' in university admissions in favour of state school applicants, to meet government targets, are cited as important reasons for students leaving the independent sector post-GCSE. Whatever the reasons, it is clear to admissions tutors that a growing number of students are leaving independent schools after GCSEs and joining local state sixth forms.

A recent study, conducted for the ISC by the Centre for Evaluation and Monitoring at Durham University, concluded that independent school pupils performed better than state school pupils at GCSE (Ndaji, Little and Coe 2016). The average of the best eight GCSEs of independent and state school pupils differed by just under two GCSE grades before deprivation, prior academic ability and school-level factors were taken into consideration. The difference was reduced to 0.64 of a GCSE grade when these factors were controlled for, but the magnitude of the difference varied by GCSE subject. Nevertheless, the results suggest that attending an independent school is associated with the equivalent of two additional years of schooling by the age of 16.

In light of the movement between the state and independent sector post-GCSE, researchers and test developers, including Cambridge Assessment Admissions Testing, may wish to consider utilising school type at year 11 (data which is included on the UCAS application form) as well as school type at the time of application in future analysis of test taker characteristics.

In addition to monitoring the BMAT candidature by gender, school type and centre location, Cambridge Assessment Admissions Testing also monitors the proportion of candidates requesting special needs access arrangements for BMAT. Since 2003, between 1.2% and 2.9% of candidates in each cohort required extra time for special needs, and this type of provision typically accounted for the majority of access arrangements made. The proportion of candidates requesting extra time does not appear to be increasing over time.

BMAT data is also monitored for evidence of test bias by gender or school type. Item-level bias analyses are carried out annually for BMAT by both gender and school sector. A technique known as Differential Item Functioning (DIF) analysis (Holland and Thayer 1988) is used for this. DIF analysis compares the performance of two candidate subgroups (e.g. male and female) on individual test items, having matched the two subgroups on their overall test score as an indicator of ability. An item is flagged as potentially biased if one subgroup has a higher likelihood of getting that item correct than another subgroup when both are matched on overall test score. For a fuller discussion of DIF analysis, please refer to the key research study in Chapter 5.

Further analyses of BMAT performance by additional test taker variables (e.g. social deprivation indicators, candidates awarded extra time versus not) are carried out as larger-scale research projects. Examples of these studies are presented later in this chapter.

Information and preparation materials available to prospective candidates

An important factor affecting test performance is knowing what to expect on the day, so that candidates can concentrate on answering the questions rather than figuring out the test format. Candidates should familiarise themselves with BMAT prior to taking the test, and Cambridge Assessment Admissions Testing is committed to making preparation materials available free of charge on the BMAT website to obviate the need for candidates to pay for additional preparation. By providing clear, accessible and transparent information, the aim is to ensure that commercial test preparation does not offer additional insights to the information available on the BMAT website. Cambridge Assessment Admissions Testing staff also attend open days of selecting institutions to answer the questions of prospective BMAT candidates and their parents.

Test takers have free access to BMAT past papers and answers on the BMAT website, including worked explanations of answers to specimen questions and model responses to the BMAT Writing Task. The test papers allow candidates to become familiar with the clear test instructions given on the front of each paper, and blank response sheets for all three test sections are provided to facilitate realistic practice.

BMAT is intended to be accessible for candidates without having to invest time learning large volumes of new material. Section 2 of BMAT ('Scientific Knowledge and Applications') is the only section that assumes subject-specific knowledge. However, it should be emphasised that BMAT Section 2 assumes core scientific knowledge in order to test the ability to *apply* that knowledge or principles to unfamiliar contexts, because this is what medical, dental and veterinary students have to do in their courses and beyond. In 2014, a review of BMAT Section 2 was undertaken to make more explicit the assumed science and mathematics knowledge, with the overarching aim of providing greater detail to test takers from a diverse range of educational and international backgrounds to support their preparation. In addition, revision guides have been created that prospective candidates can access, free of charge (*BMAT Section 2: Assumed Subject Knowledge guide*). The revision guides make clear the depth of knowledge required for each topic in a single electronic reference book (Chapter 4 of this volume gives a description of the process used to analyse core science curricula, update the BMAT specification and develop revision materials).

Published test preparation materials are also available for test takers. In 2010 (updated from the 2005 version) Cambridge Assessment, in collaboration with Heinemann, published a new set of test preparation materials entitled *Preparing for the BMAT: The Official Guide to the BioMedical Admissions Test* (Butterworth and Thwaites 2010). The book, which was authored and edited by specialists directly involved in the development and marking of BMAT, includes practice test questions and answers, together with guidance on approaching the test questions and worked examples. Its purpose is to familiarise test takers with the nature of the test, offering clear guidance about how responses will be scored so that candidates are given every opportunity to demonstrate the necessary knowledge and skills.

Understanding how candidates prepare for BMAT and the influence this has on their learning is an important consideration for the wider impact of the test. Candidates' use of the preparation materials provided by Cambridge Assessment Admissions Testing (and those from any other sources) has been the subject of BMAT research. This is described in Chapter 7. Cambridge Assessment Admissions Testing also carries out online surveys into test centres' and candidates' sources of information and preparation for our tests to better understand candidate needs, in order to guide the development of new support materials.

Access arrangements and special considerations

For test takers with special needs a range of access arrangements is available for BMAT, enabling test takers with disabilities to take the test on an equal footing as far as possible with other candidates:

- extra time (usually 25%)
- papers enlarged to A3
- supervised rest breaks
- other options on a case-by-case basis.

Access arrangements are requested in advance of the test by candidates' examinations officers (supporting evidence may be required). Where possible, Cambridge Assessment Admissions Testing adheres to the Joint Council for Qualifications (JCQ) recommendations for access arrangements and reasonable adjustments (see Joint Council for Qualifications 2016a) and BMAT candidates receive any arrangements that have been deemed necessary for their school examinations such as GCSEs.

There are also special considerations procedures in place to deal with unexpected problems that may arise immediately before or during the test, e.g. equipment failure, illness or accident on the day of the test, sudden interruption, excessive noise, etc. Requests for special consideration can be submitted by test centres on behalf of candidates within a fixed time period of the test date. An indication of the severity of the incident (as categorised by the Joint Council for Qualifications 2016b) experienced by the candidate is given to the receiving institution, so that they may take this into account, while maintaining any sensitive information about the candidate as confidential. No adjustments to candidates' marks are made by Cambridge Assessment Admissions Testing.

Psychological characteristics

One psychological factor associated with test performance is test anxiety, which is generally defined as fear and worry elicited by evaluative settings. Although there is a lack of appropriate normative data, research suggests that between 10% and 35% of school students and adults in post-secondary education are affected by test anxiety (McDonald 2001, Zeidner 1998). Moreover, females tend to report higher levels of test anxiety than males (Hembree 1988). Test anxiety is negatively correlated with test performance (Hembree 1988) and has been linked to lower performance in selection contexts (McCarthy and Goffin 2005). Item arrangement (specifically, whether test items increase or decrease in difficulty across a test) and time pressure have been associated with test anxiety and performance. Easy-to-difficult item sequences have been associated with lower levels of anxiety and better performance than other test item sequences (Hambleton and Traub 1974), whereas increased time pressure is associated with lower performance, particularly in highly test-anxious students (Kellogg, Hopko and Ashcraft 1999, Plass and Hill 1986).

Item arrangement and time pressure are considered in BMAT test construction. For example, as far as possible, BMAT items are ordered to increase in difficulty over each test section[7], in order to minimise anxiety at the outset of the test. Moreover, the number of items and the number of complex or time-consuming items in BMAT was adjusted in its first years of administration to ensure the timing of the test is sufficiently challenging but not unnecessarily stress inducing (see Chapter 4).

In addition, as mentioned above, Cambridge Assessment Admissions Testing offers BMAT preparation materials online, such as the test specification, BMAT past papers and answers. This provision potentially reduces test anxiety by enabling candidates to familiarise themselves with the test format and undertake realistic practice prior to sitting BMAT (see Chapter 7 for further discussion of BMAT candidates' use of preparation materials).

Another psychological factor which must be considered is risk aversion. There is evidence to suggest that males and females differ in the extent to which they are willing to take risks in high-stakes tests; several studies have shown that females are more likely than males to omit responses to item types in which incorrect responses are penalised (Baldiga 2014, Hirschfeld, Moore and Brown 1995, Kelly and Dennick 2009). However, there is not consistent evidence of gender bias in multiple-choice questions (MCQs) which do not employ this scoring method, particularly when it has been investigated with large-scale studies (Arthur and Everaert 2012, Bramley, Vidal Rodeiro and Vitello 2015, Buck, Kostin and Morgan 2002, Du Plessis and Du Plessis 2009). Collectively, the results suggest that negative marking may lead to gender bias in multiple-choice tests; therefore, this score-awarding method is not employed in BMAT scoring (see Chapter 5 for further details of BMAT scoring).

Small but significant group differences (including gender differences) in BMAT scores have been found (see section 2.4). However, it should be noted that group differences are fairly ubiquitous in medical admissions testing. For example, males have been found to outperform females and native English-speaking candidates have been found to outperform non-native English-speaking candidates on the United Kingdom Clinical Aptitude Test (UKCAT) (Tiffin, McLachlan, Webster and Nicholson 2014). Performance differences by gender, race/ethnicity, or socio-economic status have also been reported for the Medical College Admission Test (Association of

---

7 Note that items for each subtype are interspersed in each test section, thus there is some variation in the difficulty of items across subtypes but overall, items tend to increase in difficulty across the section.

American Medical Colleges 2016), the Erasmus MC Medical School cognitive tests (Stegers-Jager, Steyerberg, Lucieer and Themmen 2015), and the Undergraduate Medicine and Health Sciences Admission Test (Griffin and Hu 2015), used by medical schools in the US, the Netherlands and Australia respectively. Whilst the method effect (i.e., format of examination questions) is an important factor to consider when investigating the sources of these group differences, there are many other factors which may contribute to group differences in performance on medical admissions tests.

BMAT candidates are a self-selected population and tend to represent the highest performing students across a range of subjects relevant for medical study. Gender differences in science, mathematics and reading performance are more pronounced at the upper end of the performance distribution (Hyde, Lindberg, Linn, Ellis and Williams 2008, Nowell and Hedges 1998, Stoet and Geary 2013). Moreover, there are many psychological, social and cultural influences on school subject choice and performance which may contribute to self-selection into medical study (Eccles, Adler, Futterman, Goff, Kaczala, Meece and Midgley 1983, Eccles 2011). Thus, group differences in performance on BMAT may reflect factors outside of the test. Nonetheless, Cambridge Assessment Admissions Testing periodically monitors BMAT for item-level bias (see the section on item-level bias analyses in this chapter, also described in more detail in Chapter 5).

2.4 Research on test taker characteristics

Key study – Investigating the predictive equity of BMAT (Emery, Bell and Vidal Rodeiro 2011)

A key piece of research into the fairness of BMAT for selecting different test taker groups was published in 2011 by Emery, Bell and Vidal Rodeiro. This investigated the relationships between medicine applicants' background characteristics (gender, school type, neighbourhood deprivation etc.) and the following: their BMAT scores, whether they were offered a place of study or rejected, and, for those admitted, performance on their first year course examinations.

Test fairness does not require equal group performance (*Standards*, 2014). However, psychometric definitions of test bias rely on the central notion that different groups of candidates *with the same standing on the construct of interest* should attain, on average, the same test score. Group differences in test scores that reflect group differences on the construct of interest are not problematic but those that exist due to irrelevant sources of variance are.

When test scores are used to predict a future outcome, as in the case of BMAT, then scores (technically the *use of* scores) can be regarded as biased against a particular group if they *under-predict* future performance for that group (*Standards*, 2014). That is, the score implies a lower level of ability than is really the case. Scores can be regarded as biased in favour of a particular group if they *over-predict* future performance for that group (that is, the score implies a higher level of ability than is really the case). This is known as *predictive bias* (Cleary 1968) and definitions of bias or a lack of bias in the admissions testing context generally rely upon the analysis of this.

Testing for predictive bias involves using regression analysis where the criterion measure (course outcome) is regressed on the predictor variable (admissions test score), subgroup membership and an interaction term between the two. If a particular admissions test score for two groups of candidates reflects the same underlying ability on the construct of interest (i.e. potential for success on the course) then we would expect predicted course performance to be the same between them, other things being equal (Cleary 1968). Differences in the regression slope and/or intercept between different test taker groups indicate predictive bias. In Emery et al (2011), therefore, the fairness of BMAT for student selection was investigated by determining whether a particular set of BMAT scores predict the same future course performance, on average, for different groups of test takers.

Three successive years of undergraduate medicine applications data to the University of Cambridge were used for the analyses. Mature and non-UK applicants were excluded from the study so that the same admissions criteria could be assumed to have applied to all those included. Test taker characteristics included in the study were gender, school type (comprehensive versus each of the following: independent; grammar (selective); sixth form/ tertiary colleges; FE colleges) plus a range of social (neighbourhood) deprivation indicators. Neighbourhood deprivation indicators were downloaded from the Office for National Statistics (ONS) website and were matched to candidates' school postcode information (home postcode information was not available). Measures included income, employment and education deprivation indicators.

Results showed that, despite some differences in applicants' BMAT performance by background characteristics (e.g. by school type and gender), BMAT scores predicted average first year examination marks equitably for all the background variables considered. Regarding performance differences, the male applicants in these three combined Cambridge cohorts scored higher than the female applicants on BMAT Section 1 (0.19 of a BMAT point) and on Section 2 (0.23 of a BMAT point). Section 3 scores were not included in this analysis because the University of Cambridge did not use Section 3 scores in selection in these test years (2003–05), instead considering candidates' responses as a qualitative piece of evidence. The largest difference relating to BMAT scores in these cohorts was for comprehensive versus independent school applicants on BMAT Section 2, with the latter group scoring 0.34 of a BMAT point higher, on average, than the former.

Associations between BMAT scores and the neighbourhood deprivation variables were weaker or non-significant, with the largest effect found for one of the neighbourhood employment indicators (here, each 1% increase in adults on the lowest social grade in the neighbourhood was associated with only a 0.02 BMAT point decrease on Section 2).

However, and crucially for BMAT, the relationship between BMAT scores and future course performance (year 1 examination average percentage mark) did not differ for any of the test taker groups or by any of the continuous background variables. Despite differences in BMAT scores between groups, a given set of BMAT scores predicted the same medicine course examination result, on average, for all test takers regardless of group. This provides important evidence that BMAT scores mean the same for different test taker groups. That is, the empirical evidence suggests that candidates with the same BMAT scores have the same standing on the construct of interest regardless of their gender, school type or level of social deprivation.

In conclusion, differential performance on a test by different candidate groups, even if taken to be truly representative, is not a legitimate way to measure test bias (*Standards*, 2014). The real issue is whether the score differences between test taker groups reflect genuine differences between them on the construct of interest (as the analysis suggests here) or are a result of construct-irrelevant sources of variance that result in systematically higher or lower scores for certain groups. A given test score should reflect a certain level of ability regardless of group membership. For admissions tests (or any measure used in selection), scores should predict future performance equitably provided that other factors such as motivation are equal between test taker groups. Unlike bias, however, *fairness* is not a psychometric concept and views about the fairness of admissions procedures will vary even given unbiased measures. The equitable treatment of all applicants, however, is key to most definitions.

An overview of other research

In light of the importance of monitoring BMAT for fairness on an ongoing basis, a range of research studies have been carried out into both the performance of different test taker groups and the provision of suitable arrangements for candidates with disabilities.

Item-level bias analyses (Emery and Khalid 2013a)

A key research study into item bias in BMAT is discussed in detail in Chapter 5. However, to summarise the findings here, no evidence of DIF was found for any BMAT item by either gender or by school sector in the three consecutive test cohorts examined. This suggests that there is no evidence of bias in any BMAT items and therefore they do not advantage, for example, males over females or private school candidates over state school.

BMAT test taker characteristics and the performance of different groups 2003–12 (Emery 2013b)

Candidates classed as mature applicants scored lower than non-mature applicants on BMAT Section 1 in most test years (small effect sizes), on Section 2 in all test years (medium effect sizes) and on Section 3 in four years only (small effect sizes). Differences in scores between groups of applicants can be a concern to selecting institutions (particularly those that use the test as a hurdle to the interview stage) due to the possible impact on the composition of those admitted. Evidence from this research study clarifies that small but statistically significant differences in BMAT performance have been found by both gender and by school sector, with male candidates and those from independent schools performing slightly higher on the two MCQ sections of the test. Conversely, female candidates tended to perform slightly higher than male candidates on Section 3. Effect sizes often appear to be larger for Section 2 of the test (although only small to medium).

Differences in test performance do not, in themselves, equate to test bias: they may reflect genuine differences on the construct of interest between different groups of applicants. The latter has been investigated using regression techniques and the results suggest that candidate-group differences in BMAT performance reflect genuine differences in how they are likely to perform for the course of study. Additionally, DIF analyses of sets of test items can clarify whether gender and other differences are the result of item bias and whether they should therefore be regarded as a genuine cause for concern by test users (please refer to Chapter 5).

The performance of mature candidates on BMAT Section 2 is of interest to institutions using BMAT, given the longer time interval since their GCSE studies (or equivalent) at school or college. Emery (2013b) confirmed slightly lower scores for mature applicants on both Sections 1 and 2 in most years. Recent analyses comparing the BMAT performance of *graduate* applicants to the under-21s has not replicated this difference in Section 2 scores, suggesting that time out of education may be the causal factor.

Investigating BMAT for candidates with disabilities (Ramsay 2005)

A research project funded by Higher Education Funding Council for England (HEFCE) was carried out by the University of Cambridge Disability Resource Centre (Ramsay 2005). This mixed methods study looked at various admissions assessments introduced into the undergraduate admissions process by the University of Cambridge, including BMAT, and whether these appeared to disadvantage students with disabilities.

Secondary quantitative analysis of BMAT test data (originally collected by Cambridge Assessment Admissions Testing) showed that candidates with disabilities did not appear to be disadvantaged by the tests: the marks of candidates who requested access arrangements were not uniformly lower than those of other candidates, nor was there an imbalance in their success rate in being offered a place of study. Qualitative methods were used to investigate issues beyond test performance, such as the information provided to disabled candidates, the test registration process, responsibility for ensuring that access arrangements are put into place, travel to test centres, etc. Finally, a mock test of thinking skills items akin to those in BMAT Section 1 (all MCQ) was taken by a small group of admitted students with a range of disabilities, with the usual access arrangements put in place, including extra time. Participants were interviewed about their experiences with the mock test (and any actual admissions tests they had taken), such as any questions they found particularly difficult and any issues with the test format or content. Both the participants and admissions tutors were interviewed about their thoughts on whether admissions tests would aid in student selection.

Results gave no cause for concern in the access-arrangement group in terms of mock test performance, reported issues with the mock test or views of fairness regarding the introduction of admissions tests for student selection. Interview feedback was positive, with comments from the access-arrangement group typically stating that their disability had not been a problem for the (modified) test, or explaining why the extra time had been necessary for them. However, one interviewee commented that the BMAT Writing Task may be much more difficult than MCQ items for a candidate with dyslexia: 'The main part of my disability is expressing things . . . (in the MCQ format) . . . it is expressed for you.' Positive views on the utility and fairness of thinking skills tests for student selection were received from both the mock test participants and the admissions tutors. However, the author made a number of recommendations regarding issues that were 'broader than the test paper', such as the provision of information on applying for access arrangements and the accessibility of test centres for candidates with physical disabilities. The report concludes by emphasising that qualitative research into the experiences of test takers with special needs can highlight how individual the difficulties resulting from disability can be, and how it is hoped that understanding of the disability issues relevant to assessment continues to grow.

2.5 Chapter summary

In this chapter we have discussed how test taker characteristics are taken into consideration in the overall design of the test. The key study illustrated the importance of investigating the predictive equity of a test, in order to monitor any potential bias. Routine analyses of BMAT performance show that different candidate groups do not necessarily perform equally on the test, but research evidence shows that BMAT predicts course performance equitably for different test taker groups. It is also important to monitor the background characteristics of the population for whom a test is intended. Due to recent trends for movement of pupils between state and independent sectors post-GCSE, future analysis of test taker characteristics should consider utilising school type at year 11 as well as at the time of application. The procedures and research carried out on BMAT aim to ensure that the test is as fair as possible for different candidate groups, including those with special needs. This is vital given the high-stakes nature of BMAT. The test information and wealth of free preparation materials provided to BMAT candidates by Cambridge Assessment Admissions Testing aim to level the playing field for those from different backgrounds and allow all test takers to perform to the best of their ability.

Chapter 2 main points

- Monitoring the demographics of test takers can inform test development and revision.
- Information about the test taker population supports investigating various aspects of validity.
- Differences in performance between groups do not necessarily indicate bias.
- Care must be taken to understand the contexts and categorisations of different groups for a test.

3 What skills are we assessing? Cognitive validity in BMAT

Kevin Y F Cheung
Research and Thought Leadership Group, Cambridge Assessment Admissions Testing
Sarah McElwee
Research and Thought Leadership Group, Cambridge Assessment Admissions Testing

3.1 Introduction

This chapter focuses on theory-based validity (Weir 2005), which has more recently been referred to as cognitive validity (Field 2011), for the three sections of BMAT. Cognitive validity refers to the cognitive processes engaged by test takers when attempting test tasks, and the degree to which they resemble the processes engaged in non-test settings. Therefore, establishing cognitive validity requires a test developer to consider the rationale for measuring particular constructs and relevant cognitive theories of how the processes function.

Cognitive validity provides the rationale for selecting which constructs to measure and the theoretical underpinnings of these constructs; context validity is concerned with the tasks and administration conditions used to elicit these constructs; while scoring validity provides the evidence for how effectively and accurately the constructs were measured. The three together have a symbiotic relationship (O'Sullivan and Weir 2011) and can be thought of as overall construct validity (Weir 2005), which is whether the test assesses what it purports to measure, and also whether it is fit for its intended use. Terms such as aptitude, ability and skill are used to describe the constructs assessed by admissions tests, and many researchers commonly refer to admissions tests as aptitude tests (e.g. McManus, Powis, Wakeford, Ferguson, James and Richards 2005); however, this characterisation of admissions tests has been criticised and contested by others (Bell, Judge, Parks, Cross, Laycock, Yates and May 2005, Jencks and Crouse 1982), because aptitude is often interpreted as referring to innate ability. Furthermore, there have been historical changes to test specifications and theories underlying the use of particular terms, which impact on how they are used and understood by researchers. For example, the SAT, a college admissions test widely used in the US, was originally called the Scholastic Aptitude Test, but this was then changed to the Scholastic Assessment Test (Newton and Shaw 2014). These days SAT is no longer an acronym and avoids the complicated connotations associated with various terms.

To support discussions in this chapter and throughout the rest of the volume, definitions of key terms are presented in Table 3.1. These are informed by discussions in the psychometric and educational assessment literature (in particular Kaplan and Saccuzzo 2012, Newton and Shaw 2014, Stemler 2012); the definitions presented here are used by Cambridge Assessment researchers working on admissions tests, and it is acknowledged that they may not be universally accepted.

Table 3.1 Definitions of key terms

Term	Definition
Ability	The current level of performance, as contributed to by a combination of innate characteristics, academic study and individual preparation. Ability can be assessed in domain-general and domain-specific contexts.
Achievement	Competence in an area, normally subject specific, demonstrated through prior attainment of a qualification, such as A Level grades.
Aptitude	The potential for developing a skill, based on innate characteristics.
Domain-general measure	An assessment of general thinking, reasoning or problem solving skills that could be applied in a number of different contexts and subject areas.
Domain-specific measure	An assessment linked to learning information from a specific content area. The area can be explicitly defined by a curriculum or indicated by specifying a topic area.
Intelligence	Intelligence is a contested term, without a common definition. Therefore, Cambridge Assessment avoids use of the term in test specifications, which should be unambiguous. Many applications of intelligence refer to innate characteristics, although this is controversial. Cambridge Assessment researchers do sometimes refer to intelligence, and the theory of intelligence being used is explicitly referred to in such cases.
IQ (intelligence quotient)	An expression of an individual's intelligence, as measured at a particular time by a specific instrument.
Knowledge	Information about processes or topics that can be codified and learned. In particular, knowledge refers to sets of facts that can be memorised and recalled.
Potential	Having or showing the capacity to develop into something in the future.
Skill	An ability that can be progressively developed, often through learning and practice.

An important issue for discussing the cognitive validity of an admissions test is the distinction between aptitude, ability and achievement. Cambridge

Assessment researchers have previously used aptitude as a synonym for potential (Emery and Bell 2011) and BMAT Section 1 is titled Aptitude and Skills to reflect this original intended meaning. However, referring to aptitude in the test specification is currently being reviewed by Cambridge Assessment Admissions Testing in order to align the term's usage with conventions established in educational psychology. The term aptitude has historical connotations linked to assessing innate abilities, and to assessing special aptitudes as part of vocational guidance (Newton and Shaw 2014). In recognition that aptitude is not used merely as a synonym for potential by some contemporary researchers (see Box 3.1 for an example), the term is not used to describe BMAT's test construct in this volume, except where discussing Section 1's full title.

Box 3.1 Stemler (2012:11) on the distinction between aptitude, ability and achievement

For one individual, it may take a decade to learn to perform a particular piece of music, and for another individual it may take only a few days. The latter would be said to have higher *aptitude* than the former; however, both individuals share the same degree of *ability* in that they demonstrate with equal competence the mastery of a specific skill set . . . . A person with high music ability who has never participated in a concert or been evaluated by a teacher as achieving a particular "grade" level on an instrument lacks demonstrated *achievement*, even as she may possess high ability and/or aptitude. (emphasis added)

For BMAT, which focuses on combining knowledge with successful application of skills rather than mere recall, the cognitive processes targeted by the assessment form the core of the test construct. In contrast, for a test of pure knowledge, context validity would form a larger proportion of the test construct, because it includes consideration of the content knowledge required to complete tasks; whereas cognitive validity would primarily consider cognitive models of memory retrieval.

Deciding which cognitive processes to assess are key decisions made during the planning and design phases of the test development cycle (see Chapter 1 for an overview of the phases). Ongoing review of cognitive validity is also of interest for test providers, to ensure that the test assesses the skills or abilities that it is intended to measure. Questions that can be answered through trivial means, such as eliminating entirely implausible options or through unintended clues or using extraneous information, compromise the validity of an assessment. Achieving a high score on a test of thinking skill, scientific reasoning, or written communication should require candidates to engage in cognitive processes similar to those they would use in relevant real-world contexts. This illustrates that cognitive validity does not exist in isolation from the test's use; instead, consideration of how cognitive skills will be used after the test shapes the design of the assessment.

Furthermore, contextual features of a task, such as the time allocated, response format, and dependency on prior knowledge are determined by the cognitive processes that the test items and tasks are intended to assess. By outlining these issues, the present chapter demonstrates how consideration of cognitive validity and context validity is intertwined for BMAT, and argues that all test providers have a responsibility to consider both cognitive and context validity.

Researchers face specific challenges when exploring cognitive validity, partly due to the nature of standardised assessment. Generally, a test score is derived from assessing a final submission, whether a set of selected responses or a candidate-constructed response (e.g. an essay). Therefore, research based on test scores, and in fact interpretation of scores for selection purposes, rely on inferring that correct or high-scoring responses result from the cognitive processes being targeted. Similarly, a low score indicates that the test taker did not perform the targeted cognitive process to a high standard, but live test sessions rarely offer direct evidence of this inference. This means that *a posteriori* data from live test sessions can only provide limited evidence of cognitive validity; therefore, *a priori* theories about the test construct form the basis of cognitive validity (Weir and O'Sullivan 2011).

The present chapter outlines how cognitive features were considered in the development of BMAT from predecessor assessments and how the cognitive processes of test takers have been investigated with research. In order to contextualise the application of Weir's (2005) framework, the following part of the chapter focuses on cognitive validity specifically in relation to BMAT.

3.2 Cognitive validity and its importance to BMAT

Correctly answering a test task should require candidates to replicate cognitive processes which might be required in relevant non-test contexts, which in the case of BMAT are the study of medicine, dentistry and related subjects. The focus on biomedical study, rather than clinical practice, is a conscious decision that has important implications when considering the cognitive validity of BMAT. This approach recognises that universities may evaluate an applicant's suitability for the actual practice of medicine and dentistry, by employing other selection methods. Furthermore, some of the non-academic skills used in clinical settings are specific to the context and targeted for development as part of clinical training. Therefore, investigation of BMAT's cognitive validity is concerned with the relevance of the assessed skills for biomedical study, and also how these skills will be employed in the testing environment compared to the real world. In the context of high-stakes tests, a compromise is inevitably needed between considering task authenticity (i.e. the degree to which they resemble tasks faced in non-test environments) on the one hand, and safeguarding against other threats to validity on the other. Increasing the authenticity of a test at the cost of scoring validity, fairness, or security would typically not be acceptable from an overall validity argument perspective.

One approach for achieving task authenticity is to design tasks that simulate how the assessed skills will be used. For example, a speaking exam might role play situations that a test taker would expect to encounter when using the language they have learned, such as shopping or asking for directions (Galaczi and ffrench 2011). However, this is more difficult for an admissions test such as BMAT, because medical study is something that a BMAT candidate is unlikely to have experienced before sitting BMAT. Therefore, performance on an authentic and relevant task can depend on knowledge that the test taker would not reasonably be expected to have at the point of applying. An authentic task with good cognitive validity for medical study might require the test taker to complete an exam testing advanced knowledge of physiology. Alternatively, a task assessing skills used in clinical practice would ask the applicant to conduct a medical procedure or a differential diagnosis for a simulated patient. Although these would elicit relevant cognitive processes in some test takers, it is unreasonable to assume that all applicants to medical school have the necessary knowledge to complete these tasks successfully, particularly as these skills are intended to be taught as part of the course for which they are applying. In addition, more specialised tasks can be particularly difficult to prepare for, and there can be differences in the availability of preparation materials or access to work experience opportunities in the medical profession. These tasks could potentially compromise other aspects of validity, illustrating how cognitive validity is best considered alongside test taker characteristics and consequential validity, which includes issues of fairness and bias.

Given these concerns, it is clear that the cognitive processes and skills to be assessed should be the subject of careful consideration in a medical selection context. According to Weir (2005), cognitive validity poses a main research question: What are the skills/cognitive processes elicited by the test tasks? Before investigating this question however, there is another one posed by cognitive validity that is particularly relevant to BMAT: What are the skills/cognitive processes that the test **should** aim to elicit?

For BMAT, cognitive validity can be conceptualised as the extent to which test items elicit the types of mental skills required of a biomedical student during their course of study. Clearly, there are determinants of successful biomedical study that are beyond the scope of what can be validly assessed with an admissions test. For example, personal qualities and personality traits, sometimes referred to as non-cognitive skills (Patterson, Knight, Dowell, Nicholson,

Cousans and Cleland 2016), are increasingly recognised as important in the context of medical study and practice (Katz and Vinker 2014, Koenig, Parrish, Terregino, Williams, Dunleavy and Volsch 2013, Powis 2015); these might not be suitable for testing in the exam hall. Therefore, admissions tests such as BMAT should be seen as one tool in the selection process that is recommended to be used alongside other methods of assessment and evaluation (Cleland et al 2012). Standardised testing can only claim to assess a subset of the criteria that might facilitate successful medical study, and cognitive validity should inform decisions regarding all assessments that form part of this process. Part of the test developer's responsibilities for cognitive validity lie in considering the constructs and processes most relevant to the non-test setting that is being selected for. This is not a simple task in the context of biomedical study. Even if a test developer only concentrates on cognitive abilities, the constructs that might be described as relevant to biomedical study are infinite, because constructs can be broadly or narrowly defined.

A case could be made for testing numeracy, working memory capacity, knowledge of statistics, verbal reasoning, or even spelling ability. However, the strength of the theory and evidence base for the relevance of these constructs must be evaluated as part of test design. Due to the range of plausible constructs to assess, a key decision for the test developer is the selection of the ones which are most suitable. Given unlimited testing time and applicants who are immune to fatigue, a multitude of scores could be produced for various skills, but this is not a practical starting point for a test provider. Almost all of the attributes that might be tested include a cognitive component, even those referred to as non-cognitive; for example, responding to a self-report personality assessment typically requires candidates to engage reflective processes. It is these cognitive processes engaged in responding that are considered when evaluating cognitive validity.

To address both the question of what skills should be assessed and which processes are actually elicited by BMAT, the main content of this chapter is split into two parts. Firstly, in part 3.3, the original impetus for the test and its roots in predecessor assessments are described to contextualise the constructs measured by each section of BMAT, with a focus on their cognitive components. The construct of a test is what the test purports to measure, including the cognitive theory (or theories) regarding the skills being targeted by the test. Relevant literature on the cognitive processes involved in critical thinking, problem solving, scientific reasoning and written communication are briefly reviewed, alongside example BMAT tasks. The rationales for selecting these skills are discussed, presenting an argument that these are the skills that should be assessed for biomedical study. Discussion of how cognitive validity intertwines with other aspects of validity is also included throughout this part of the chapter, particularly with regard to Section 2 and context validity.

The next portion of the chapter, part 3.4, provides examples of Cambridge

Assessment research studies that evaluate how well BMAT tasks assess the identified skills. These illustrate approaches to investigating cognitive validity that can be applied to other similar tests, and how the findings can inform the overall evaluation of a test.

3.3 Selecting and defining the cognitive processes included in BMAT

Deciding on the cognitive processes to assess is an important component in the design and planning phases of a test development and validation cycle (see Chapter 1 for an overview of the cycle). It is vital that the cognitive processes targeted by a test are well defined, so that papers are constructed to capture these qualities suitably.

BMAT has its origins in a programme of collaborative research and development involving the University of Cambridge, the University of Oxford, University College London (UCL), Imperial College London and the Royal Veterinary College (RVC). The test was designed to supplement existing sources of information (such as examination results, personal statements and performance at interview) to aid the process of selection for competitive biomedical degree courses, and the kinds of reasoning assessed by BMAT reflect this.

The institutions involved in developing BMAT had a number of requirements in common:

- to differentiate between applicants with the highest prior attainment in their school examinations
- to ensure that applicants' scientific understanding is adequate for the study of biomedical sciences, and that they can cope with the demands of a rigorous science-based course
- to provide a common measure for comparing applicants from a variety of educational backgrounds and with a variety of qualifications, including overseas applicants, mature applicants, and applicants from different school types, many of whom only had predicted grades at the point of application
- to allow admissions staff to focus resources towards applicants with a realistic chance of receiving an offer.

Precursors to BMAT

Cambridge Assessment's involvement in developing tests of academic aptitude stretches back to the 1980s with the development of a Law Studies Test in collaboration with the Law Schools Admissions Services in the United States (Black 2012). This, together with further work done by Alec Fisher on a proposed test of academic aptitude for higher education (Fisher 1990a,

1990b) led to a wider project, MENO, that set out to identify, define and assess those thinking skills that are important for success in higher education (Chapman 2005). At its conclusion, the MENO project also developed standardised assessments of these skills for use in higher education selection; therefore the tests from MENO are ancestors of various admissions tests that have a domain-general thinking skills component, including the Thinking Skills Assessment (TSA) and BMAT.

The development of BMAT was influenced by the findings of the MENO project and the requirements of the various universities outlined previously. BMAT's development was also informed by two pre-existing tests that had been trialled and shown to make a positive contribution to student selection: the Cambridge Medical and Veterinary Admissions Test (MVAT) and the Oxford Medical Admissions Test (OMAT) (Emery and Bell 2009, James and Hawkins 2004).

BMAT's test construct

The rationale and construct for each of the BMAT sections, and the influence of the original MVAT and OMAT tests in the development of BMAT is outlined in the following overview. Brief descriptions of relevant theories, taxonomies and models have also been included to contextualise and promote a theory-based approach to validity (Weir 2005).

Section 1 – Aptitude and Skills

The Aptitude and Skills section is designed to assess candidates' thinking skills, which can be thought of as specific cognitive abilities. BMAT Section 1 includes three types of item: problem solving, understanding argument (sometimes known as critical thinking) and data analysis and inference. Early conceptions of the questions that now form the basis of BMAT Section 1 BMAT come from Fisher's (1992) work on the higher education aptitude tests and the MENO thinking skills project. This early work identified a number of areas that became components of overall thinking skills. For example, Fisher proposed the construct of logical reasoning as a precursor to understanding argument, which should test:

> [T]he kinds of reasoning skills which are used in everyday arguments (i.e. arguments which . . . have been actually used by authors with a view to persuading their readers). [Questions are] expressed in natural language and do not use symbolic languages (or symbolic logic). Stimulus passages contain some reasoning or they contain sufficient subject information to serve as a basis for argument. The subject matter of logical reasoning items ranges very widely and may include anything from cigarette smoking . . . or natural science to law (Fisher 1992:4).

Fisher also lists a number of core skills identified by various education and curriculum bodies as central to successful critical thinking, and representative items from the understanding argument part of BMAT Section 1 comprise:

- summarising the main conclusion of an argument
- drawing a conclusion when premises are given
- identifying assumptions
- assessing the impact of additional information
- detecting reasoning errors
- applying principles.

The MVAT pilot at University of Cambridge in 1999 drew heavily on the research and development work of the MENO project. This, in turn, influenced the content of BMAT Section 1, which includes item types developed and refined during the MENO project. The design of BMAT Section 1 was also influenced by work conducted at the University of Oxford's medical school.

James and Hawkins (2004) describe a review of selection processes at Oxford to explore the range of practices and use of test scores for the university's internal selection test for medicine. Despite a variety of selection practice across the colleges of the university, it was possible to distil key abilities that were highly rated by tutors as follows:

- understanding of written texts, particularly extracting meaning from complex work
- understanding numerical data and the representation in graphical form, including extracting meaning from datasets
- communication through the use of clear written English to express abstractions and arguments
- ability to use diagrams, graphs and text to express results and arguments
- thinking at an abstract and conceptual level, including logical and numerically based reasoning.

The resulting BMAT Section 1 specification was derived from early pilots and includes three skills considered important for successful study in higher education. As these skills are beneficial across many subject areas, some of the item types are similar to those included in more general assessments. The definitions of the skills included in the BMAT test specification are presented in Box 3.2.

The description of each item type in the test specification (problem solving, understanding argument or data analysis and inference) outlines the subskills that a test taker must employ to answer test items correctly, rather than the knowledge that they need to demonstrate; in other words, these are the cognitive processes assessed by Section 1. For each item type, the definition is restricted to aspects of the skill that are relevant for higher education study and also suitable for standardised assessment.

Box 3.2 The BMAT Section 1 test specification

Problem solving
Demands insight to determine how to encode and process numerical information so as to solve problems using simple numerical and algebraic operations. Problem solving will require the capacity to:

- select relevant information
- recognise analogous cases
- determine and apply appropriate procedures.

Understanding argument
Presents a series of logical arguments and requires respondents to:

- identify reasons, assumptions and conclusions
- detect flaws
- draw conclusions.

Data analysis and inference
Demands the use of information skills (vocabulary, comprehension, basic descriptive statistics and graphical tools), data interpretation, analysis, and scientific inference and deduction to reach appropriate conclusions from information provided in different forms, namely:

- verbal
- statistical
- graphical.

(Admissions Testing Service 2016b)

Problem solving is included in other Cambridge Assessment qualifications and examinations, such as TSA. The Cambridge International A Level in Thinking Skills provided by Cambridge International Examinations also contains a problem solving component and defines it in the syllabus as: 'a candidate's ability to analyse numerical and graphical information, which is based in real life situations, and apply the right numerical techniques to find new information or derive solutions' (Cambridge International Examinations 2016:9).

Early versions of the test task specifications that eventually became problem solving were trialled as part of MENO and described as mathematical reasoning, but this was changed to formal reasoning, referring specifically to reasoning in a mathematical context. Following a review of the trials and the cognitive processes it would be desirable to elicit, the label for the category was changed to problem solving, in order to reflect a renewed focus on dealing with novel problems presented in numerical, graphical and spatial contexts. An example problem solving item is presented in Figure 3.1.

Figure 3.1 Example problem solving (finding procedures) item from BMAT 2015

The price of a particular share varies from day to day. On Monday the price of the share was £1. Tuesday's price was 20% higher than Monday's, and Thursday's price was 25% up on Wednesday's price. By the Friday of that week the price had returned to £1.

Helen bought £1 000 worth of this share on Monday and then sold them on Thursday to make a profit of £350.

Paul bought £3 000 worth of this share on Tuesday, but had to sell them the following day.

Assuming that there are negligible costs associated with buying and selling these shares, what was the return on Paul's investment?

A He made a loss of £1 050.

B He made a loss of £750.

C He made a loss of £300.

D He broke even.

E He made a profit of £300.

F He made a profit of £750.

G He made a profit of £1 050.

To solve this problem, the candidate must evaluate the figures provided and find the procedure that will give the correct answer. It is not immediately clear what calculations need to be conducted and the test taker must think at an abstract level to discover what can be done with the information that is available. Once the correct procedure has been identified, the calculations are not difficult to carry out, because the item is not designed to assess mental arithmetic; instead, the question targets the ability to identify innovative solutions to the problem. This is supported by the incorrect response options available to the candidate, which are suitable as they are arrived at by following an incorrect procedure, rather than from making mistakes in the calculations.

Figure 3.2 shows another problem solving item, which asks the test taker to evaluate a table with over 70 cells and over 50 values. This problem requires the candidate to select the information relevant for answering the question. Identifying the correct answer as F does not require the test taker to carry out complex calculations.

Another category of items in BMAT Section 1 is the understanding argument items. Understanding argument focuses on logical reasoning and is

Figure 3.2 Example problem solving (relevant selection) item from BMAT 2016

The table below shows a record of my blood pressure and pulse readings over nine days.

Day	*Systolic*	*Diastolic*	*Pulse*
Mon am	135	98	74
Mon pm	138	94	75
Tue am	139	97	79
Tue pm	149	96	82
Wed am	146	96	68
Wed pm	133	93	77
Thu am	128	84	71
Thu pm	149	81	86
Fri am	149	97	82
Fri pm	146	97	83
Sat am	134	91	69
Sat pm	165	99	85
Sun am	141	86	87
Sun pm	139	91	77
Mon am	126	88	74
Mon pm	145	78	83
Tue am	163	96	82
Tue pm	129	90	87

What was my pulse on the occasion when I had the biggest difference between systolic and diastolic readings?

A 68

B 81

C 82

D 83

E 85

F 86

G 87

sometimes referred to as critical thinking, as in the *BMAT Section 1 Question Guide* (Admissions Testing Service 2016a). They are informed by Cambridge Assessment's extensive work on assessing and operationally defining critical thinking as part of MENO, which is summarised by Black (2012). As a result, the understanding argument items assess elements of critical thinking identified in Black's (2008) taxonomy, particularly the analysis and evaluation skills (see Table 3.2 for subskills).

Compared with the breadth of critical thinking subskills assessed in TSA, BMAT Section 1 includes a more limited set of items that focus on analysing and working with logical arguments expressed in everyday language, hence

Table 3.2 Taxonomy of critical thinking skills included in Cambridge Assessment's examinations (Black 2008)

Skill/process	Subskill/Sub-process
1 Analysis	A Recognising and using the basic terminology of reasoning
	B Recognising arguments and explanations
	C Recognising different types of reasoning
	D Dissecting an argument
	E Categorising the component parts of an argument and identifying its structure
	F Identifying unstated assumptions
	G Clarifying meaning
2 Evaluation	A Judging relevance
	B Judging sufficiency
	C Judging significance
	D Assessing credibility
	E Assessing plausibility
	F Assessing analogies
	G Detecting errors in reasoning
	H Assessing the soundness of reasoning within an argument
	I Considering the impact of further evidence upon an argument
3 Inference	A Considering the implications of claims, points of view, principles, hypotheses and suppositions
	B Drawing appropriate conclusions
4 Synthesis/ Construction	A Selecting material relevant to an argument
	B Constructing a coherent and relevant argument or counter-argument
	C Taking arguments further
	D Forming well-reasoned judgements
	E Responding to dilemmas
	F Making and justifying rational decisions
5 Self-reflection and self-correction	A Questioning one's own preconceptions
	B Careful and persistent evaluation of one's own reasoning

the label 'understanding argument'. Despite this narrower focus, the items include the core components of critical thinking and explicitly target processes involved in rational thought. This aligns the items with the Cambridge Assessment definition of critical thinking presented by Black's (2008) work using expert consensus (Box 3.3).

An example understanding argument item from BMAT 2016 is presented in Figure 3.3. This item asks the test taker to read a passage and identify the assumption underlying the argument that is presented in the text.

To identify that D is the assumption, the candidate must understand the argument made in the passage, and then evaluate the response options in relation to this understanding. Another understanding argument item is

Box 3.3 The Cambridge Assessment definition of critical thinking

Critical thinking is the analytical thinking which underlies all rational discourse and enquiry. It is characterised by a meticulous and rigorous approach. As an academic discipline, it is unique in that it explicitly focuses on the processes involved in being rational. These processes include:

- analysing arguments
- judging the relevance and significance of information
- evaluating claims, inferences, arguments and explanations
- constructing clear and coherent arguments
- forming well-reasoned judgements and decisions.

Being rational also requires an open-minded yet critical approach to one's own thinking as well as that of others.

(Black 2008)

Figure 3.3 Example understanding argument (identifying assumptions) item from BMAT 2016

Recent theories about the causes of cancer have held that most cancers are caused by internal factors, the result of inevitable mistakes in the human body rather than anything environmental. This would seem to imply that whether or not a person develops cancer is entirely out of his or her control; what that person does in terms of lifestyle choices is irrelevant. And yet the latest high-profile study has strongly challenged this. It estimates that between 70 and 90 per cent of the most widespread cancers have extrinsic causes, such as ultraviolet radiation, pollution and stress. If this study is to be believed, then whether or not you develop some cancers is no longer just something you can blame on your biology, but is to a significant extent within your own control.

Which one of the following is an assumption underlying the above argument?

A The latest study is more accurate than the previously accepted theories.

B The risk of developing cancer is simply down to extrinsic factors.

C There can be no ways of preventing the human body from making cancer-causing mistakes.

D People have some control over the influence of extrinsic factors such as stress or pollution.

presented in Figure 3.4. Again, an argument is presented in a short passage; however, this time, the question asks for the flaw in the argument.

Section 1 of BMAT and the critical thinking component in particular has been criticised in discussions on medical selection tests, which are important to address in any theoretical discussion of the test's construct. McManus et al (2005:557) argued that there is 'little agreement on what critical thinking means', and suggested that BMAT Section 1 is actually testing fluid intelligence. Whilst we concede that definitions of critical thinking are not

Figure 3.4 Example understanding argument (detecting flaws) item from BMAT 2016

When we listen to music, electrical waves in our brains tend to synchronise to the tempo. In a recent study scientists recorded the brain waves of musicians and non-musicians as they listened to music. Although the brain waves of both groups synchronised to many rhythms, those of non-musicians did not synchronise to particularly slow music. The non-musicians reported that they could not keep track of the tempo in slow music. This shows that becoming a musician requires an innate tendency for the brain to synchronise to the tempo of any speed of music.

Which one of the following identifies a flaw in the above argument?

A The tempo of slow music may be the most difficult tempo for listeners to follow.

B Musical training may develop the tendency for the brain to synchronise to music.

C Some of the non-musicians may decide to undertake musical training in the future.

D Becoming a musician may depend on a number of different abilities.

universally accepted, it is simply untrue that there is little agreement on the term's meaning among educational assessment experts. Facione (1990) conducted a Delphi study and presented a statement of expert consensus on critical thinking that informed the work of Cambridge Assessment and many other critical thinking researchers. Although several disagree on the scope of critical thinking, with some researchers conceptualising a greater number of subskills than others (e.g. Paul and Elder 2007), there is agreement that Facione's work captures the core elements of critical thinking ability, and that critical thinking skills can be developed through instruction (Halpern 1999, Sharples, Oxman, Mahtani, Chalmers, Oliver, Collins, Austvoll-Dahlgren and Hoffmann 2017). A number of assessments targeting critical thinking skills have been developed (Landrum and McCarthy 2015) and explored in higher education settings (O'Hare and McGuiness 2009). Furthermore, recent analysis using commercially available measures of critical thinking skills indicate that the construct is predictive of degree performance (O'Hare and McGuiness 2015).

The tendency by some to conceptualise BMAT as an intelligence test may be influenced by work on another admissions test used by medical schools, the United Kingdom Clinical Aptitude Test (UKCAT), which adopts a somewhat different approach to defining the construct to assess compared with BMAT (McManus, Dewberry, Nicholson and Dowell 2013). UKCAT was designed specifically to assess cognitive aptitude conceptualised as an innate construct that is intended to be independent from socio-economic factors. Therefore, UKCAT aims to assess an 'innate ability to develop professional skills and competencies' (Pearson VUE 2017:1), aligning the theoretical basis for the test with traditional IQ tests. However, critiques of BMAT describe and consider the constructs assessed by BMAT and UKCAT as interchangeable, particularly in relation to BMAT Section 1, based largely on assumptions about the degree to which BMAT scores might correlate with intelligence tests. From a cognitive validity perspective, we argue that the *a priori* approach advocated by Weir (2005) is important here, because there is little theoretical basis for treating the tests as identical.

Another critique of BMAT focuses on the fact that definitions of critical thinking often include a dispositional element. Specifically, these point out that 'critical thinking is related more to aspects of normal personality than it is to IQ' (McManus et al 2005:557). In our view, the idea that critical thinking includes dispositional aspects is not problematic. Facione (1990) clearly distinguishes between the skills and dispositional aspects of critical thinking, and BMAT Section 1 explicitly targets critical thinking skills, not dispositions, using the understanding argument items. Any comparison of BMAT Section 1 with measures designed to assess critical thinking disposition, such as Facione's (2000) California Critical Thinking Disposition Inventory (CCTDI) or Stupple, Maratos, Elander, Hunt, Cheung and Aubeeluck's (2017) Critical Thinking Toolkit (CriTT), would confirm BMAT Section 1's focus on skills.

This misinterpretation of BMAT's test construct demonstrates the importance of articulating the cognitive processes that a test is intended to assess. Given that the rationale for assessing critical thinking skills is acknowledged in discussions about admissions tests, which is that 'critical thinking skills, not dispositions, predict success in examinations' (McManus et al 2005:557), it is possible that critiques of BMAT are not based on a full understanding of the cognitive processes assessed by the test. Bell et al's (2005) response to these criticisms clarified why BMAT should not be conceptualised as an intelligence test and the present chapter prevents further confusion by providing details on the theoretical underpinnings of BMAT's test sections, particularly on critical thinking.

Section 1 also includes data analysis and inference items, which require students to apply the skills described above to handling and interpreting larger amounts of information. These typically consist of sets of between three and five items associated with an extended passage of text, graphical and/or numerical data, and closely resemble a format used in Oxford's OMAT, which itself had adopted key features from the US Medical College Admission Test (MCAT) (James and Hawkins 2004).

Figure 3.5 presents the information provided for a set of four data analysis and inference items from BMAT 2015.

As shown here, a substantial amount of data is provided in a combination of forms, such as using written text and in tables. The amount of information can impact on how easy or difficult it is to sift through the content provided. As associated items are designed to target the candidate's data interpretation skills, the density of material presented is carefully monitored and adjusted during the item authoring process. The items associated with Figure 3.5 are available in Figure 3.6.

Figure 3.5 Example information provided for a set of data analysis and inference items from BMAT 2015

According to figures published recently, 44% of criminals leaving prison will reoffend within one year of being released. So if the aim of prison (custodial) sentences is to stop people committing crimes, it really is not working. Short sentences are even worse, with 55% of offenders on short sentences reoffending within a year of leaving prison. And putting kids in prison is least effective of all – 70% of under-18s who receive prison sentences reoffend within 12 months. From a cold look at the statistics, prison does not look like a successful way to reduce crime, especially for young offenders on short-term sentences. So what are the alternatives?

Whilst they are an option only for less serious categories of offence, giving offenders community service orders has been shown to reduce reoffending rates by 6%. They may be seen as a softer option by offenders and by the public, but when people are up in the dock convicted of an indictable offence, they are less likely to end up back in trouble if the judge gives them a community service order rather than a prison sentence.

Another option, that works even better, is simply not sending someone to prison but giving them a suspended sentence instead. The figures show that people who get a suspended sentence are 9% less likely to reoffend than someone who committed a similar crime but was then sent to prison.

But the most effective way of reducing reoffending is getting offenders to meet their victims. Campaigners for restorative justice programmes, where offenders engage with the impact of their crime and often meet their victims, say it can reduce reoffending by up to 27%. However, a government analysis puts the improvement at a more conservative 14%.

The following studies contain relevant data, adapted from the November 2010 report from the Ministry of Justice, on which the above article was based:

Study 1

50 000 former prisoners were tracked for 9 years after being released in 2000, and the number of re-convictions was matched to the time since release. The figures are all cumulative:

Time elapsed following release	Re-Offending rate (%)
3 months	20.0
6 months	30.8
9 months	37.9
1 year	44.0
2 years	55.0
5 years	66.0
9 years	72.0

Study 2

126 866 convicted criminals were tracked for one year following the end of their sentence, and their reoffending rates were matched to whether they had been given a short custodial sentence (i.e. a prison sentence of less than 12 months) or a non-custodial sentence. (In this study a person was considered to be a re-offender only if he/she had been re-convicted):

	Non-custodial sentences	Short custodial sentences
Proportion of offenders who reoffended	22.0%	55.0%
Average number of reoffences per reoffender	2.49	4.11
Average number of reoffences per offender	0.55	2.26
Number of reoffences	56 181	54 835
Number of reoffenders	22 577	13 334

Figure 3.6 An example set of data analysis and inference items from BMAT 2015

Which one of the following statements is a conclusion that can reliably be drawn from the passage?

A It is a mistake to release offenders from prison after they have served only half of their sentence.

B It is a mistake to send offenders to prison when a non-custodial sentence is also appropriate for the crime.

C It is a mistake to send young offenders to prison.

D It is inevitable that an offender released from serving a prison sentence will reoffend at some point in the future.

E When a prison sentence is necessary, it should always be for a minimum period of 12 months.

In Study 1, how many former prisoners who had not reoffended within a year of release from prison then reoffended within 5 years of release?

A 2750

B 5500

C 8550

D 11000

E 22000

F 33000

Study 2 shows that 55% of offenders released from a short prison sentence reoffended within a year, whilst only 22% of offenders did so having served a non-custodial sentence. Yet the passage claims that giving offenders a community service order instead of a prison sentence "reduces reoffending rates by 6%".

Which one of the following is the best explanation for the apparent discrepancy between these figures?

A Most offences which attract a prison sentence are not eligible for consideration of a non-custodial sentence as an alternative.

B Most offenders given non-custodial sentences are first-time offenders.

C Most offenders given prison sentences are likely to have already served a non-custodial sentence.

D Suspended sentences have not been taken into account.

A politician argues that, on the basis of the report, more convicted offenders should be subjected to restorative justice, such as meeting their victims, where appropriate instead of being sent to prison, because this will reduce the likelihood of them reoffending.

Which one of the following, if true, most strengthens this argument?

A In the study which showed that restorative justice produced a 14% fall in reoffending rates, most of the offenders had also received a prison sentence.

B It is important for society that natural justice is seen to be done and that offenders are being issued with appropriate sentences for their crimes.

C Most victims do not want to meet face-to-face the person who committed a crime against them.

D Sending an offender to prison is a very expensive use of tax-payer's money.

E The study shows that subjecting an offender to restorative justice as well as issuing them with a community service order has the effect of reducing reoffending rates by 20%.

These example items demonstrate how a set of data analysis and interpretation items include some overlap with problem solving and understanding argument items. However, candidates must also employ the skills that allow them to deal with larger quantities of information, in order to successfully complete data analysis and interpretation items.

Although the cognitive processes tested in Section 1 are seen as useful for learning across a range of subjects, they are also identified as particularly relevant for university courses in medicine and biomedical sciences. In the US, the Association of American Medical Colleges (AAMC) has identified 15 core competencies for entering medical students that are organised into four categories. Four competencies are listed in the thinking and reasoning category, including critical thinking and quantitative reasoning (Association of American Medical Colleges 2016); these competencies link to the skills assessed in BMAT Section 1. However, medical training is graduate entry in the US context; therefore it is important to consider medical education in the undergraduate setting.

In relation to the skills assessed by understanding argument items, the UK Quality Assurance Agency for Higher Education (QAA) benchmark statement for medicine courses states that 'graduates should demonstrate their ability to think critically by . . . adopting reflective and inquisitive attitudes and applying rational processes' (Quality Assurance Agency for Higher Education 2002:4). Problem solving is also referred to in the benchmark statement for medicine, but the statement for biomedical science provides the clearest link with the skills in Section 1 by identifying 'analytical, data interpretation and problem solving skills' (Quality Assurance Agency for Higher Education 2015:10) as attributes developed in a typical biomedical science course. The benchmark statements are intended to inform universities about the types of skills that various subject courses should develop, and this does not necessarily mean that the skills need to feature in university selection procedures; indeed, many attributes are listed in benchmark statements and only a subset are considered for admissions decisions. However, these links explicitly suggest that the skills assessed in Section 1 are relevant to successful undergraduate biomedical study, and contribute to the cognitive validity argument for assessing these processes.

Section 2 – Scientific Knowledge and Applications

The Scientific Knowledge and Applications section of BMAT adopted item types trialled in the Cambridge MVAT, for which there was evidence of a significant positive relationship between scores on the test and performance on the Cambridge Medical and Veterinary Science Tripos (Emery and Bell 2009). When deciding what might be assessed in Section 2, the key considerations were to develop a test of applicants' scientific understanding that would be accessible to candidates from a range of educational backgrounds, and would require candidates to do minimal additional new learning or preparation. Scientific knowledge is acknowledged as an important aspect of medical study, but there has been some debate about how best to assess science ability in the selection context. For example, McManus et al (2005:559) suggested commissioning a new test of 'high grade scientific knowledge and understanding' as a possible way of supporting medical selection. BMAT's Section 2 is a test of scientific knowledge and understanding, but it is unclear what would be needed to meet the criterion of 'high grade' for a test specification.

One important decision when developing BMAT Section 2 was that it should assess not only that a candidate has certain core scientific knowledge, but that they can apply it in a way that demonstrates an understanding of the scientific principles that underpin their knowledge, to distinguish a range of ability within a group of students with near-perfect grades or predicted grades in their school examinations. Therefore, Section 2 has an explicit focus on the cognitive processes involved in applying scientific knowledge to novel problems. This differentiates BMAT Section 2 from other science assessments administered as part of school qualifications, which typically include some questions testing recall of factual knowledge. Having access to a range of scientific knowledge is recognised as important for medical study; however, BMAT Section 2 is intended to complement school science qualifications rather than to serve as an alternative, hence the focus on applying school-level science knowledge to novel contexts.

There is some overlap between BMAT Section 2 and problem solving in Section 1; however, Section 2 items require problem solving skills to be applied to subject-specific knowledge. The current BMAT specification defines the skills and knowledge assessed by the BMAT Scientific Knowledge and Applications section as follows:

Box 3.4 The BMAT Section 2 test specification

This element tests whether candidates have the core knowledge and the capacity to apply it which is a pre-requisite for high level study in biomedical sciences. Questions will be restricted to material typically included in non-specialist school Science and Mathematics courses. They will however require a level of understanding appropriate for such an able target group.

(Admissions Testing Service 2016b)

The design of BMAT Section 2 draws on a large body of research that conceptualises scientific thinking and reasoning as a form of problem solving (Dunbar and Fugelsang 2005). In this approach, scientific thinking is characterised as a search, or searches, in problem space (Simon and Newell 1971). BMAT Section 2 tasks can therefore be thought of as problems where the solution requires application of core science knowledge. This definition underpins guidance for item writers, who submit a description of the problem solution, which includes an account of the reasoning that a test taker needs to employ in order to solve the item. The solution for each item is analysed to make sure it involves a combination of both science knowledge and application. The nature of this analysis and the checks involved are described in Chapter 4.

A BMAT Section 2 item from 2016 is presented in Figure 3.7. This biology question requires a candidate to draw upon their knowledge of the anatomy of the kidney, their knowledge of the role of the kidney in the excretion of urea, and their knowledge of the structure and function of blood vessels. Candidates would not be able to answer this question by recall of this biological knowledge alone; instead, they must combine multiple aspects of their understanding to deduce the correct answer.

Figure 3.7 Example biology item from BMAT Section 2

The diagram shows a kidney and its associated vessels from a healthy individual.

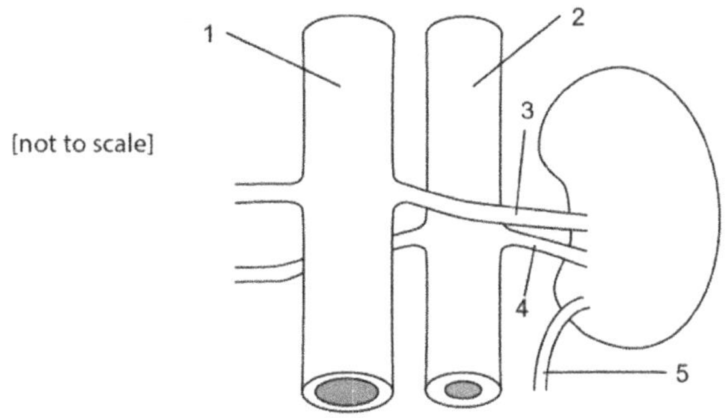

Which row correctly identifies the vessels along with the concentration of urea they contain?

	lowest concentration of urea	*highest concentration of urea*
A	1 is the aorta	2 is the vena cava
B	1 is the vena cava	2 is the aorta
C	3 is the renal artery	5 is the urethra
D	3 is the renal vein	5 is the ureter
E	4 is the renal vein	5 is the ureter
F	4 is the renal artery	5 is the urethra

Using their knowledge of the structure and function of blood vessels, a candidate should identify that vessel 2, which has thicker walls, carries blood away from the heart, and that vessel 1 carries blood returning to the heart. Using this information, and their knowledge of the anatomy of the kidney, they should be able to identify 3 as the renal vein and 4 as the renal artery.

A candidate should know that blood enters the kidney via the renal artery and leaves through the renal vein, and that a primary function of the kidney is to remove urea from the blood. This results in the production of urine, which leaves the kidney via the ureter, vessel 5. This information can then be used to deduce that the lowest concentration of urea will be in the renal vein (3) and that the highest concentration is in the ureter (5), so the correct answer is D. The incorrect options are based on candidates lacking knowledge of the function of the kidneys (A and B) or failing to correctly identify the vessels (C, E and F).

Figure 3.8 Example chemistry item from BMAT Section 2

Calcium carbonate reacts with hydrochloric acid. The reaction gives off carbon dioxide gas.

Line **X** on the graph shows the volume of carbon dioxide formed against time when 100 cm^3 of 1.0 $mol\,dm^{-3}$ of hydrochloric acid reacts with calcium carbonate chips at 20 °C. There was an excess of calcium carbonate chips.

$$CaCO_3 + 2HCl \rightarrow CaCl_2 + CO_2 + H_2O(l)$$

Which line best represents the volume of carbon dioxide formed against time when the reaction is repeated with 50 cm^3 of 2.0 $mol\,dm^{-3}$ of hydrochloric acid reacting with excess calcium carbonate chips at 20 °C?

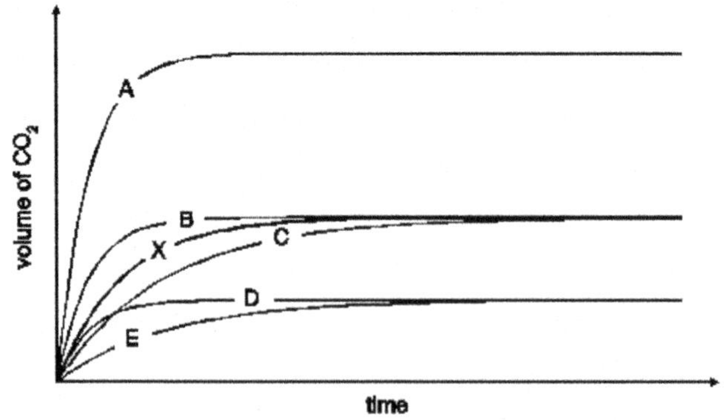

A line A
B line B
C line C
D line D
E line E

An example chemistry item is presented in Figure 3.8. The chemistry knowledge needed by the test taker includes understanding of a balanced chemical equation and familiarity with a formula for calculating the amount of substance (in moles) from a known volume and concentration of a solution. Knowledge of the specific reaction itself has not been assumed and the chemical equation is given to remove the need to construct it otherwise.

Using this subject-specific knowledge to successfully answer the question with B requires the test taker to recognise that as the calcium carbonate is in excess, the amount of carbon dioxide generated (proportional to volume measured at a given temperature and pressure) is only dependent on the amount of hydrochloric acid used. Using the given numbers, the amount of hydrochloric acid is the same in each experiment, and this observation narrows the choice of options down to line B or C. The gradient of line B is steeper than line X at the start of the second experiment, and the candidate needs to understand that in the second experiment, the initial rate of the reaction will be higher as the acid is more concentrated. The other response options are based on a misinterpretation of the gradients of the curves and/or mistaken use of the 2:1 ratio of hydrochloric acid to carbon dioxide in the chemical equation.

Another example of a BMAT Section 2 item is provided in Figure 3.9. This mathematics question requires the candidate to draw upon both their knowledge of how a mean is calculated and their facility with basic algebraic manipulation. The calculation of means is something students will have met early in their secondary mathematics education, and the algebraic manipulation needed in this question is straightforward. The candidate is required to assess the information given in the question and then to devise a strategy to move from that information to an answer. Any successful strategy adopted requires the candidate to possess a conceptual understanding of mean that reaches beyond rote learning; as such the question requires both the recall of elementary mathematical knowledge and the ability to assimilate given information whilst building a strategy that draws on a conceptual understanding of the relevant knowledge. The item's distractors are constructed to identify candidates who do not bring the conceptual understanding to their approach; for instance, E would appeal to candidates who fail to account for three extra people joining the group when they assimilate 78 into their strategy.

The physics item in Figure 3.10 requires the candidates to apply their knowledge of the relationship between mass, density and volume, alongside their facility with interpreting diagrams, extracting relevant information, and devising a strategy to solve the problem. Specifically, the test taker needs to know that density is equal to mass divided by volume; however, they must also have a conceptual understanding that the density of the material from which

Figure 3.9 Example mathematics item from BMAT Section 2

The mean mass of a group of N people is 75 kg.

Jim, Karen and Leroy join this group, without anyone leaving; the new mean mass is 78 kg.

The mean mass of Jim, Karen and Leroy is 90 kg.

What is the value of N?

A 4

B 12

C 15

D 30

E 48

F 90

Figure 3.10 Example physics item from BMAT Section 2

A student carries out an experiment to determine the density of the material from which two identical solid objects are made. She uses a balance and a measuring cylinder containing a fixed volume of liquid. The diagrams show different stages of her experiment, with some of the readings on the balance and some on the measuring cylinder.

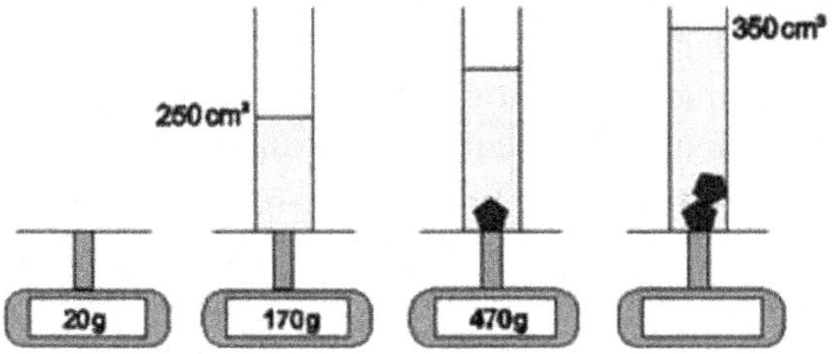

Which calculation should be used to determine the density of the material from which the objects are made?

A $\frac{280}{50}$ g/cm³

B $\frac{280}{300}$ g/cm³

C $\frac{280}{350}$ g/cm³

D $\frac{300}{50}$ g/cm³

E $\frac{300}{100}$ g/cm³

F $\frac{600}{350}$ g/cm³

G $\frac{750}{350}$ g/cm³

H $\frac{770}{350}$ g/cm³

the objects are made could be the mass of one object divided by the volume of one object or it could be the mass of two objects divided by the volume of two objects.

In order to solve the problem, these concepts must be applied to the information given, and the test taker must identify and ignore irrelevant information. The distractors are used to assess misconceptions in physics concepts or incorrect applications of skills and knowledge in devising a strategy. For example, distractor A would appeal to those who incorrectly use the initial reading on the balance to correct the final mass.

Including both knowledge and application in the specification of Section 2 recognises that scientific reasoning is sometimes understood as subject-specific conceptual knowledge and at other times as domain-general reasoning (Zimmerman 2000). Although we distinguish between task features that assess knowledge and those that are more related to reasoning, the approach employed for BMAT recognises that attempting to separate knowledge and strategy completely when operationalising scientific reasoning is highly artificial (Klahr and Dunbar 1988). For clarity, the knowledge and cognitive process elements of Section 2 are discussed separately in the present volume, as work defining the knowledge specification is described in Chapter 4. However, the theoretical perspective adopted for Section 2 acknowledges that they are often intertwined.

The UK General Medical Council's report on outcomes and standards for undergraduate medical education, *Tomorrow's Doctors* (2009), discusses the role of the 'doctor as a scientist' making explicit reference to the ability of the doctor to apply biomedical scientific principles and the scientific method to the practice of medicine. The AAMC (2014) also identifies scientific enquiry as a core thinking and reasoning competency for entering medical study in the US.

BMAT's Section 2 recognises the important role of scientific problem solving in undergraduate medical education. However, BMAT does not assess all of the scientific knowledge and reasoning needed to fulfil the role of 'doctor as scientist'; instead, the section is designed to address the needs of admissions tutors by ensuring that applicants' scientific understanding is adequate for the study of biomedical sciences, and that they can cope with the demands of a rigorous science-based course. BMAT Section 2 focuses on the application of basic science knowledge, which can be regarded as a pre-requisite for developing more advanced clinical reasoning. It is acknowledged that other perspectives on scientific reasoning are potentially important in the development of doctors, such as conceptualisation of scientific thinking as hypothesis formation and testing (Dunbar and Fugelsang 2005). The skills tested by BMAT Section 2 facilitate the development of further cognitive processes and skills, which are targeted in medical school and foundation-level training. Patel, Arocha and Zhang (2005:734) explain how basic science knowledge is inexorably linked to clinical problem solving (clinical reasoning):

> Basic science or biomedical knowledge is supposed to provide a scientific foundation for clinical reasoning. The conventional view is that basic science knowledge can be seamlessly integrated into clinical knowledge, analogous to the way that learning the rules of the road can contribute to one's mastery of driving a car.

The cognitive skills assessed by BMAT Section 2 focus on applying science knowledge to novel problems, as a precursor to extending this application to more complex decision-making scenarios specific to clinical contexts. Indeed the ability to apply science knowledge can be viewed as a set of skills that will improve with further training in clinical schools. This conceptualises them as abilities that can be developed, in line with the findings of research on scientific thinking skills and metacognition conducted with children (Zimmerman 2007, Zohar and Peled 2008). Furthermore, the ability to apply scientific knowledge to novel problems depends on use of cognitive and metacognitive strategies that are not assumed to routinely develop as part of childhood development (Morris, Croker, Masnick and Zimmerman 2012); indeed, the skills assessed in BMAT Section 2 are recognised as important skills to practise and develop.

Section 3 – Writing Task

It was noted in Cambridge Assessment's early work on admissions tests that while multiple-choice questions (MCQs) provided an objectively marked assessment which could address many of the elements of critical thinking, a test of students' 'productive' reasoning capacities – that is, the ability of candidates to produce a reasoned argument of their own – would also be welcomed by universities (Fisher 1992). These early observations of Cambridge Assessment researchers fit with more contemporary views on assessing higher order thinking skills expressed by international test providers, which advocate using multiple item formats in tests (Butler 2012, Ku 2009, Liu, Frankel and Roohr 2014). The recently revised MCAT dropped the writing task component based on limited evidence of predictive validity and an understanding that medical schools did not use the scores as extensively as other sections when ranking (Schwartzstein, Rosenfeld, Hilborn, Oyewole and Mitchell 2013). This decision was made despite the AAMC (2014) identifying written communication as a core thinking and reasoning competency for students entering medical study in the US. Removal of the writing task from MCAT prompted researchers at the Australian Council for Educational Research (ACER) to outline a cognitive validity argument for writing tasks that described how MCQs 'cannot reach into the cognitive recesses where a generative written task can' (McCurry and Chiavaroli 2013:570). Similarly, Cambridge Assessment's rationale for including a writing task in BMAT emphasises cognitive validity and the theoretical arguments for assessing written communication.

Communicating clearly in writing is a crucial skill that is sometimes underappreciated and regarded as secondary to clinical knowledge in medical contexts (Goodman and Edwards 2014). Oxford's OMAT test, as a precursor to BMAT, included a structured writing task based on the desire to examine 'communication through the use of clear written English to express abstractions and arguments' (James and Hawkins 2004:250). BMAT's Section 3 Writing Task requires candidates to produce a short piece of communicative writing on a topic of biomedical, general or scientific interest. It assesses the ability to select, develop and organise ideas, conveying them concisely and effectively.

The Writing Task is intended to complement the other BMAT sections, allowing demonstration of analytical reasoning skills and the ability to develop an argument, which extends the evaluation of these skills in a structured multiple-choice context in Section 1. In particular, the Section 3 task is designed to assess test takers' ability to construct clear and coherent arguments, which is an important part of Cambridge Assessment's definition of critical thinking (Black 2008). The current BMAT specification for Section 3 is in Box 3.5.

Box 3.5 The BMAT Section 3 test specification

Questions will provide a short proposition and may require candidates to:

- explain or discuss the proposition's implications
- suggest a counter proposition or argument
- suggest a (method for) resolution.

The Writing Task provides an opportunity for candidates to demonstrate the capacity to consider different aspects of a proposition, and to communicate them effectively in writing. Skills to be assessed include those concerning communication, described above. All specified skills may be assessed.

(Admissions Testing Service 2016b)

The approach to task design for Section 3 is informed by cognitive models of writing developed in psychology (Scardamalia and Bereiter 1987), which distinguish between knowledge-telling and knowledge-transforming strategies when writing. Knowledge-telling focuses on the topics and genres of a writing task to generate content. Knowledge-transforming, on the other hand, conceptualises a writing task as a rhetorical problem with goals and problems to overcome. Teaching English to Speakers of Other Languages

(TESOL) also target knowledge transforming in their writing components, but only at higher levels because it is an aspect of processing that can place great demands on non-native speakers of English. An example Section 3 question and response from BMAT 2014 is provided in Figure 3.11.

Figure 3.11 Example response to BMAT Section 3 that achieved a 4.5A

There is no such thing as dangerous speech; it is up to people to choose how they react. Explain the reasoning behind this statement. Argue to the contrary that there can be instances of dangerous speech. To what extent should a society put limitations on speech or text that it considers threatening?

The statement here is arguing from an extremely liberal viewpoint - they believe that people should be completely free to say what they want to and that when they do, other individuals or groups do not have the right to be offended or react harshly. Essentially they are saying that free speech is acceptable, even if it comes at the expense of others in society.

However, I strongly believe that while in theory, free speech and saying what you believe is to be condoned, that there are multitude of occassions and instances where it is inappropriate or unresponsible. For example, if a doctor has promised to provide a confidential service to their patient but goes on to release the information publicly, this is ethically unjustifiable and the patient has it within their rights to react negatively. Furthermore, where text or speech is used to promote violence, hate or prejudice, I feel that society should do more to stand up to it as it is known that incitement of violence and hate almost inevitably leads to negative consequences. Free speech used in this way can not only provoke individuals but can have large scale devastating effects on the security and welfare of different communities and groups.

Therefore, as there is a myriad of ways in which speech used carelessly and thoughtlessly can be threatening and provoke negativity, there should, to some extent, be controls on how far free speech can go. The main aim here is not to silence groups or communities, but to promote equality and empathy for others opinions and views. The main example here would be with groups inciting hate or prejudice against other groups, be that for their culture, gender, political beliefs, etc. Here, careful considered measures should be taken to ensure that speech and text are not used in a derogatory way which undoubtedly would provoke a negative response, but that it is used to promote equality, dialogue and reasoned debate. Therefore, it is not honesty that should be limited, but inappropriate and out of date agenda which should be reduced. While it is difficult to control, in an equal society promoting values such as respect for one another and placing value on reasonable discussion, people should be careful what they say and consider the long-term effect it could have.

The response in Figure 3.11 demonstrates knowledge transformation in the opening paragraph by expanding on the statement from the question to reach a broader conclusion. Importantly, the response does not merely describe the statement. Instead, the candidate infers arguments from the statement and extends the reasoning to comment on societal issues. The response also uses examples to develop and present a logical argument. As a result, it received a high score, as shown by the examiner's comments associated with this particular writing sample (see Box 3.6).

Box 3.6 Examiner comments for a BMAT Section 3 response that achieved a 4.5A

This response follows a clear plan; it is obviously structured by the components of the question. It begins with a clear definition and also explains the reasoning behind the statement (rather than just stating what it means), which shows that the writer has carefully read the question.
It uses a simple but relevant example to make its point and comes to a definite conclusion that society should monitor speech but not directly control it.
All aspects of the question are addressed effectively, providing a good counter-proposition. The argument is expressed in a clear and rational form, drawing things together into a balanced consideration of both sides.

Marks: 4.5A

The examiner comments for this response demonstrate BMAT Section 3's focus on argument and task completion. A response that exclusively used knowledge-telling strategies would not be able to achieve a high score, because knowledge transformation is needed to extend the opening statement from the question prompt (see Chapter 5 for details of the scoring criteria). According to Shaw and Weir (2007), careful task specification is needed to promote a writer's use of appropriate writing stages for English language tests. This observation also applies to the Writing Task in BMAT Section 3, which is structured to elicit the cognitive processes required to produce a well-structured argument; these processes include macro-planning, organising and monitoring one's text. The specific features of the BMAT Writing Task that support this are discussed in Chapter 4; however, it is clear from the examiner comments above that planning and organisation are needed for a Section 3 response to be scored highly. Another example Writing Task and response illustrates how a weaker answer tends to rely more heavily on knowledge-telling (Figure 3.12).

This response includes a number of relevant statements that are presented in isolation, but not joined together into a cohesive argument. Stating that many animals live in the wild is an example of knowledge-telling that does not extend the observation to make an overarching argument. The examiner comments (Box 3.7) associated with this response highlight that the counter-argument and conclusion fail to justify the response; they also omit any mention of planning or organisation.

Figure 3.12 Example response to BMAT Section 3 that achieved a 2A

Modern veterinary medicine is more for the benefit of humans than the animals under its care. Explain what you understand by this statement. Argue to the contrary that veterinary medicine is concerned more with the benefit of non-human animals. How might human and non-human interests diverge within the practice of veterinary medicine?

The statement suggests that vetinary medicine is available for the 'selfish' nature of humans who wish for their animals to undergo medical proceedures for their own benefit with no benefit understood, or felt, by the animals.
I wholely disagree. Not least on the grounds that at the most simple level, animals may be in pain and their suffering may be easily stopped by a dose of pain killers or a simple operation. In addition, the statement disregards the fact that one of the fundamental instincts of animals is to stay alive and to live the most successful lives possible. This is no different from ourselves. If treatment is available, then an animal would take it - even in the wild, grooming is practiced amongst some primates to avoid bites and infections. How is this different? From another angle, many animals (including dogs) live in the wild in packs - as families. Many a time, people have said that a pet may be 'one of the family'. When another in the pack is unwell, others help them out and in this, domestic, situation the owners are the others in the pack - the pet would expect help.
Although I understand that occasionally, the emotional attachement of an owner to a pet may affect judgement and that sometimes (as with humans) palliative care may be more appropriate, on the whole, vetinary medicine is primarily there for the good of the animal.

Box 3.7 Examiner comments for a BMAT Section 3 response that achieved a 2A

There is a simple and concise explanation of what is understood by the statement. The response clearly addresses all aspects of the question, although presenting the counter-argument as the candidate's own disagreement diminishes the force of the argument. The relief of an animal's pain could still be done purely for the benefit of humans. However, making the point that there is more similarity of interests between humans and animals than divergence is a good point. The counter-argument and conclusion are unconvincing – they fail to reasonably justify the response or to consider the whole of the argument around this topic.

Marks: 2A

Cambridge English writing exams that target knowledge transformation tend to include substantial stimulus materials for the writer to use, whereas BMAT Section 3 relies on a much shorter opening statement and the writer's own knowledge. This means that there are fewer opportunities to manipulate ideas when there is a limited pool of knowledge available to include in the response. Figure 3.13 shows a slightly stronger response to the same question answered in Figure 3.12. This example has a more

Figure 3.13 Example response to BMAT Section 3 that achieved a 3.5A

The relationship between humans and animals has evolved and changed over time. However, it is unequivocal that the current 'status-quo' of the owner-pet relationship results in a modern veterinary medicine which is tailored to the needs of the owner, more so than the pet. As humans, we have developed connections with animals that, in many ways, means that our well-being mentally, physically and psychologically is greatly impacted by the health of not only others of our kind, but also others who are non-human animals. Even in instances where the non-human animal is not a pet and not domesticated, our instincts are to further our knowledge by treating it and also gaining a sense of satisfaction, that we have been helpful.

Nonetheless, veterinary medicine involves animals, so it consequently benefits the non-human animals more. Treating animals ensures their survival or increases the longevity of their lives; therefore, the population of the species is more likely to survive, which is intrinsically more of a benefit for the animal than for humans. Animals are living beings as well, so to treat animals differently than what we would expect from health care for ourselves is unfair; the patient's needs must be the main priority.

On the surface, it appears that modern veterinary medicine has focussed more on humans and our expectations, but it impacts both animals and humans; to claim that only one is targetted would not be justifiable and certainly not something that can be judged or quantified. Both human and non-human interests diverge in veterinary medicine as the underlying basis of treatment is for the welfare of the animal, but the reasons are different. Humans own animals as pets for their pleasure and as a result of this, decisions made in relation to the animals will be based upon personal gain. If medicine only valued the well-being of animals, then treatment would be free, which would avoid the vast numbers of animals left untreated due to financial constraints. Although veterinary medicine is about animals, the reasons behind treatments vary.

sophisticated explanation of the statement from the prompt that extends beyond describing it. By developing points that build on each other in the opening paragraph, this response demonstrates knowledge transformation early on, but this opportunity could be easily missed. Therefore, it is possible that knowledge transformation is more difficult to achieve with Section 3 Writing Tasks when compared with writing papers designed specifically to assess language proficiency.

Although the opening argument of the response in Figure 3.13 is well structured, the rest of the response is not as organised. In addition, the examiner comments (Box 3.8) pointed out that some relevant areas were not considered, which may result from a lack of macro-planning. The example responses we have reviewed suggest that BMAT Section 3's Writing Task elicits use of knowledge transformation strategies by candidates. However, we should acknowledge that inferring activation of these strategies from reviews of written submissions is limited, due to the retrospective nature of this approach.

Box 3.8 Examiner comments for a BMAT Section 3 response that achieved a 3.5A

This has a strong start; it is well phrased and immediately engages with the candidate's understanding of the statement. It uses an interesting approach, taking the benefit to animals to be as a benefit to the species rather than to individual animals, but does not explain why veterinary care targeting only one of either animals or humans 'would not be justifiable and certainly not something that can be judged or quantified'. This is a good response, which is reasonably well argued but concentrates on pet owners with no consideration of livestock care or working animals. So it does not quite get into the marks for a good answer that makes effective use of material.

Marks: 3.5A

Compared with the writing components of Cambridge English's language examinations, BMAT Section 3 is a relatively short writing assessment. *Cambridge English: Advanced (CAE)* and *Cambridge English: Proficiency (CPE)* both include a Writing paper that is 1 hour and 30 minutes long, and each paper includes two separate tasks. The 30 minutes allowed for BMAT Section 3 might not provide the same opportunity for macro-planning and organisation that is given by longer tasks, because test takers may be more inclined to start writing without preparing a plan, despite the advice and instructions provided by Cambridge Assessment (see Chapter 4 for examples). However, it is important to acknowledge that many BMAT candidates are native speakers of English and all of them should have a high level of English language proficiency (see Chapter 2). This means that the majority of BMAT test takers are capable of engaging in knowledge transformation more quickly than typical test takers in a language testing context.

Writing samples, examiner comments and grade distributions indicate that the majority of candidates plan and organise their responses to Section 3. Nevertheless, it would be useful to directly investigate the degree to which macro-planning, organisation and monitoring are activated for individuals completing BMAT Section 3. Recent investigations of cognitive validity in language testing make use of verbal protocols (e.g. Bridges 2010), eye tracking (e.g. Yu, He and Isaacs 2017) and keystroke logging (Leijten and Van Waes 2013). So far, these techniques have not been used to investigate BMAT; employing these approaches with BMAT Section 3 could provide additional evidence of the test's cognitive validity.

Another area to investigate is the cognitive process of writing revision, which is not currently targeted by BMAT Section 3. The short time available for the Writing Task makes it unlikely that test takers have the opportunity to revise their responses. Further work could identify the impact that having more time for the written component of BMAT would have, because this potentially allows the task to assess candidates' abilities to revise their writing, which may fit with the applicant's potential to succeed at written tasks in biomedical study.

Although the cognitive validity of BMAT Section 3 draws on Cambridge English Language Assessment's work on writing assessment, the skills targeted by BMAT's Writing Task do differ slightly from those assessed in language tests. Notably, Section 3 focuses on the ability to organise and construct a cohesive argument. This means that aspects of critical thinking categorised as synthesis in Black's (2008) taxonomy (see Table 3.2) are being targeted. In particular, the skills targeted by BMAT Section 3 are the ability to construct a coherent, relevant argument or counter-argument and the ability to make and justify rational decisions.

Not only is it important to elicit the targeted cognitive skills, it is also crucial to reward successful use of these skills appropriately. Importantly, performance on a BMAT Section 3 task largely depends on the cogency and clarity of the argument in the response, so the criteria are aligned with skills from Black's (2008) taxonomy (see Chapter 5 for details of the grading criteria). Two scores are given to ensure that aspects relating to argument are given sufficient weight in the quality of content grade, which is considered separately to a quality of English grade. The quality of English grades tend to be negatively skewed, whereas the quality of content grades are more normally distributed, indicating that many, but not all, demonstrate the planning and organisation of ideas that are crucial for making strong arguments.

The use of two scores allows medical schools to primarily consider the quality of content score, unless the candidate has an unusually low quality of English score. Prior to 2010 a single score was awarded for Section 3, but institutions using BMAT requested that Cambridge Assessment distinguish a written response's argument quality from the quality of English demonstrated by the candidate. Assessment managers also noted that markers could be influenced by linguistic features and writing style in the response, which was not the main focus of BMAT Section 3. Scripts impacted by this were more likely to be identified for marking a third time by a senior examiner and the changes were made to respond to the ways that Section 3 was being used. The change in marking system made it easier for examiners to focus on construction of the argument when awarding the quality of content grade, which is the cognitive process that the task is designed to assess.

The first part of this chapter has focused on selecting and defining the cognitive processes that BMAT should assess, and the theories that underpin Cambridge Assessment's conceptualisation of these skills. The next portion of the chapter turns to research investigating how successful BMAT tasks are at targeting these skills.

3.4 Research on cognitive validity

Cognitive processes are difficult to investigate because they cannot be directly observed; instead their influence is inferred from indirect measures. In cognitive psychology, experimental methods have been used to uncover much of what is known about the way that individuals reason. A person's reaction time (Wilhelm and Oberauer 2006), where they are looking (Ball 2014) and even their brain activity (Goel, Navarrete, Noveck and Prado 2017) have been used to construct theories about the cognitive processes they are engaging. These methods and cognitive paradigms have been used to examine reasoning in a wide range of areas, such as problem solving (Gilhooly, Fioratou and Henretty 2010), hypothesis testing (Gale and Ball 2008) and deductive reasoning (Evans and Ball 2010).

Think-aloud studies

The kinds of data collected in experimental settings are rarely available in formal testing contexts, although developments in computer-based (CB) testing have encouraged some limited investigation with eye-tracking studies, particularly for tests of scientific problem solving (Tai, Loehr and Brigham 2006, Tsai, Hou, Lai, Liu and Yang 2012) and reading performance (Bax 2013). In educational assessment it is more common to collect data on cognitive processes by conducting think-aloud studies, which are sometimes referred to as 'cognitive labs', such as in the *Standards* (2014:82). Data from these studies is then interpreted using verbal protocol analysis, which is an established technique for gaining insight into the cognitive processes of candidates that would otherwise remain covert (Norris 1990). In this method, candidates (or research participants) are asked to 'think aloud', usually at the same time as they work through test items. The resulting information (the 'verbal protocol') is recorded, transcribed and then its content analysed according to a coding scheme.

Verbal protocols can be an account of how one *would* solve a problem, of how one *is currently* solving a problem or a retrospective account of how one *did* solve a problem. If performed concurrently with the task, candidates are asked to say out loud everything that goes through their head as they work through the task: to verbalise all their thoughts in the present tense. Retrospective reports from candidates of how they went about solving a problem have the advantage of lower interference with the task in hand but have the disadvantage of short-term memory decay. The nature of the test items may influence which method is the most suitable, for example, whether speed of processing is an aspect of the cognitive skill being assessed.

Early research by Cambridge Assessment on admissions tests for entry to higher education used verbal protocols to evaluate the cognitive validity of question types. The understanding argument and problem solving item types used in BMAT Section 1 have been investigated in this way with in-depth studies by Thomson and Fisher (1992) and Green (1992). These informed further development of thinking skills and reasoning tests including BMAT, and the findings were used to refine and improve the processes by which test questions are produced.

Green (1992) focused on questions similar to the problem solving items included in BMAT today. The analysis indicated that most items functioned well and that students did not approach them in a routine manner. Errors relating to routine execution and computational slips were low, suggesting that the items did not merely require the application of routine procedural methods. Green used a taxonomy by Mayer, Larkin and Kadane (1984) to plot phases of problem solving including understanding, method finding, planning and execution, and the associated knowledge that might be invoked such as linguistic and factual, schematic, strategic and algorithmic. Green's research overall found that the problem solving questions examined were appropriate but pointed to some areas for improvement. Notably, the findings highlighted two key features of items that can impact on the cognitive processes used by test takers:

- the language used in the item must be straightforward to ensure errors do not arise from problems with linguistic encoding, translation or understanding of the problem itself
- problems should not require reasoning that is counter-intuitive to real-life situations.

These findings informed guidelines for item writers which are used in authoring of BMAT questions today. In addition, reviews explicitly check linguistic features of items, and how the reasoning in each item relates to real-life situations. This ensures that construct-irrelevant variance is not introduced due to belief bias (Evans, Barston and Pollard 1983), which is the tendency to endorse arguments or solutions based on their believability in real-life settings rather than on their logical validity (Ball and Stupple 2016). The operational checks on BMAT items are designed to safeguard cognitive validity by checking the task features of items; some of these checks are described by Shannon, Crump and Wilson in Chapter 4 of this volume, which focuses on context validity.

Thomson and Fisher's (1992) research investigated questions similar to the understanding argument items in BMAT Section 1 using verbal protocol analysis. This work is presented in more detail below as a key study, to illustrate the research methods employed by Cambridge Assessment in these contexts.

Key study – A validation study of informal reasoning items (Thomson and Fisher 1992)

Main findings

- Think-aloud accounts of reasoning confirmed that test takers use targeted cognitive processes when answering the majority of tested MCQs.
- Complex wording and the design of options can result in items that assess reading comprehension rather than critical thinking.
- Minor changes and edits can reduce ambiguity and improve how well an item elicits the targeted skills.
- Terms used in MCQs assessing critical thinking are appropriate and understandable by test takers.

Introduction and context

Thomson and Fisher's (1992) study employed a similar approach to Green's (1992) investigation of formal reasoning items by using verbal protocols to examine informal reasoning items. This item type eventually became the critical thinking items in TSA and the understanding argument items in BMAT Section 1. The study was conducted as part of a larger pilot project (MENO) that trialled tests of six skills considered generally relevant to selection for university study (Willmott 2005). As part of evaluating the tests, the cognitive processes assessed by items were investigated using think-aloud studies. These were used to explore the theoretical underpinnings of the skills targeted using Cambridge Assessment's tests.

Research questions

The study explored types of items that now commonly appear in BMAT Section 1 and posed the following three questions:

- Do the items function as intended in the sense that candidates must reason correctly in order to answer the question correctly?
- What factors determine the difficulty of items (e.g. complexity of reasoning, language level, nature of distractors)?
- Do any items present obstacles which prevent candidates from demonstrating their reasoning ability? Do candidates understand terms such as 'main conclusion', 'assumption' etc.?

Data collection and analyses

Ten undergraduate participants (five each male and female, including two mature students) were interviewed individually, and after practice attempts, were asked to think aloud as they worked through 30 questions. Prompts to keep talking were given following long pauses. Most were able to tackle the questions and comment on their thinking as they progressed to a solution, although one participant found it particularly challenging. At the end, they were asked to reflect on what may have made particular questions difficult.

To facilitate coding of the transcripts, the test questions were analysed before the interviews took place to identify the reasoning intended to be necessary for correctly answering each item. The entire process, including the reflective interviews at the end, were transcribed verbatim and analysed by Cambridge Assessment researchers involved in the MENO thinking skills project.

Results

The percentage of correct answers given was calculated and participants' responses were categorised as 'reasoned well', 'no reasons given' or 'reasoned badly', by comparing the protocols with the reasoning process identified in analysis of the items. Instances where a correct answer was attained by poor reasoning were flagged for concern. Overall, the participants found the questions easier than expected, consistent with the fact they were undergraduates, rather than university applicants. Additionally, the standard time constraints were not imposed so more time was available to candidates to consider their answer.

In total 20 questions were judged to work well and test the intended reasoning processes. It was suggested that a minor change to wording in three further questions would ensure they worked as intended – this was to clarify confusion by one or two participants only, so overall the questions were successful (see Figure 3.14 for an example). It was recommended that two items needed a replacement for one distractor, and two items were functioning badly and should be rejected, based on the complexity of the question text or weaknesses in the arguments or answer options.

This study provided valuable insight into the processes that candidates use when completing items similar to the understanding argument questions in BMAT Section 1. Several recommendations from this study were proposed and adopted for the development of future test items. The researchers recommended avoiding complicated wording, less common or technical words and convoluted sentences. They also flagged that some items appeared to be measuring reading comprehension rather than reasoning, and so recommended that where candidates are asked to identify main conclusions of a stimulus passage, the distractors should be components of the argument (e.g. reasons or intermediate conclusions); originally some questions had distractors that were not asserted in the stimulus passage, making it possible to answer the question by merely noticing that the correct answer is included in the passage whereas the other options were not, rather than through reasoning.

Overall, participants understood terminology related to critical thinking and could explain terms like 'conclusion', 'assumption', and 'flaw in an argument'. Regarding a definition of conclusion, a number of participants referred to the 'main message' or 'theme, idea, what it's driving at' in their response, which led to a recommendation that the main conclusion of an item needed to be the most interesting or focal point of the argument, rather than a more trivial but related point. Based on the participants' verbalisations, all question subtypes functioned well and did not pose problems, provided that the stimulus passages and distractors were appropriately crafted.

The following example illustrates the in-depth process of analysing candidates' verbalisations and using these to interpret the cognitive processes employed in responding to the question.

Figure 3.14 An example question analysed in the study

In order to succeed in academic examinations it is necessary to study. Therefore if a student studies hard in a particular subject, that student should succeed in examinations in that subject.

A major flaw in the argument above is that it:

A Assumes that it is necessary to study in order to succeed.
B Overestimates the value of studying in preparing for examinations.
C Ignores the fact that some examinations are more difficult than others.
D Assumes that studying hard is a sufficient condition for academic success.
E Ignores the fact that some students do not need to study very much in order to succeed.

In order to recognise D as the flaw in the argument, participants needed to see that the fact that something will not occur without a particular antecedent condition does not guarantee that this same something WILL occur if the antecedent condition is met. Those who gave the right answer reasoned as above ('The problem is that a student could study hard and still fail the exam') and their comments about the distractors did not indicate misunderstanding. One person rejected D because it talked about 'academic success' which he thought was more general than success in exams. Overall, six participants gave the right answer and reasoned well, while three reasoned poorly and gave an incorrect answer (choosing distractors A, C and E), and one candidate chose incorrect answer E but gave no reason. The results suggest the question is relatively difficult and that the distractors work well in tempting some candidates. However, the researchers also recommended that the wording of D should be amended for clarity.

Discussion

Cognitive validity studies such as Fisher and Thomson's (1992) demonstrate the complexity of developing questions that tap the relevant cognitive processes identified in test specifications. This research provided information to test developers about the structure and function of the types of questions that appear in BMAT Section 1, their capacity to measure the intended reasoning appropriately, and areas that could be targeted for improvement by question writers and editors. Findings from studies such as this inform the process through which questions are commissioned, reviewed and used in papers to ensure the best measurement performance of the questions, and the construct relevance of the test. The checks and reviews relevant to cognitive validity are outlined in a description of the question paper production process in Chapter 4.

Although useful for informing operational processes, there are specific drawbacks to these types of think-aloud studies and, as in the case of this particular research, the participants did not work under the same time constraints as in a real test; therefore their performances may be somewhat different from those elicited under exam conditions. In addition, there are some practical limitations to these studies that should be acknowledged. Data collection for think-aloud studies takes a large amount of participant time, so it is often only possible to conduct the study with a small number of participants, or a small number of items. There is also substantial time commitment needed on the part of the researcher. Whilst the richness of data captured by think-aloud studies is a strength, transcription and detailed analysis are painstaking processes that preclude these studies from being conducted regularly as part of operational processes. These issues mean that, whilst informative, generalisations from these kinds of studies need to be supported with other research into cognitive validity. One of the other approaches to cognitive validity is outlined in the following part of the chapter.

Latent constructs as cognitive processes

Some data from live test administrations is available to researchers interested in cognitive validity, such as candidate performances on each separate task or item. At an individual level, this information is not particularly useful; however, data from large cohorts can reveal if a test taker getting one item correct is more likely to get other particular questions correct. Statistical techniques known as factor analysis (FA) are used to examine performances on items and the relationships between them. These analyses can help a researcher understand whether the items in a test are all assessing one latent construct or whether subsets of items are testing separate constructs. Latent constructs are any variables that are not directly observable, which are often conceptualised as different cognitive skills or bodies of knowledge. In educational assessment, exploratory factor analysis (EFA) and confirmatory factor analysis (CFA) are used to investigate the number of latent constructs being assessed by a test, which is commonly referred to as test dimensionality.

Investigating dimensionality has traditionally been considered as a problem for mathematical modelling that involves the application of various psychometric theories (McDonald 1981). EFA is used to indicate the number of latent constructs that can be theorised as present in the dataset. In addition to how many latent constructs might be present, the EFA identifies which items group together. It is then up to the researcher to interpret what is represented by each cluster of items *post-hoc*. CFA is a form of Structural Equation Modelling that is used when there are already ideas about which constructs might be observable in the dataset. In this approach the researcher specifies which items will group together to represent a latent construct or separate constructs. Essentially, CFA examines how well the data fits with previously determined models by examining the structure of item performances and the relationships between them. These statistical approaches to investigating cognitive processes are powerful tools, but Weir (2005:18) cautions against relying on these types of analysis too heavily:

> There is a need for validation at the *a priori* stage of test development. The more fully we are able to describe the construct we are attempting to measure at the *a priori* stage, the more meaningful might be the statistical approaches that can subsequently be applied to results of the test. Statistical data do not in themselves generate conceptual labels. We can never escape from the need to define what is being measured.

In light of these warnings, admissions tests developed by Cambridge Assessment are designed with an *a priori* definition of the skills and knowledge being assessed, and CFA studies are preferred over EFA ones, although they can be more technically challenging to conduct and interpret. A CFA study conducted by Cambridge Assessment researchers is presented as a key study here, after a brief note on dimensionality that highlights important issues to consider when investigating this aspect of a test.

A note on dimensionality

The dimensionality of a test relates to cognitive validity because dimensions identified using statistical methods can be interpreted as skills or cognitive abilities that are underlying an assessment. For example, data from a maths test might be analysed to show that it is assessing two latent constructs, which can be thought of as two aspects of mathematical ability, or two cognitive skills. The results indicate that the test is assessing two dimensions, but caution should be exercised when referring to a test as unidimensional or multidimensional. Like many other psychometric concepts, such as internal consistency, dimensionality is sometimes misleadingly attributed to a test. The statistical indicators used to make these claims actually reflect a dataset. Claims of dimensionality based on analyses are not strictly referring to a characteristic of the test *per se*, but rather to the performance of a particular group in a specific testing context.

This distinction is best illustrated by returning to our example. Consider the aforementioned maths test administered to primary school children. The results of the analysis indicate two dimensions and provide information on which questions, or items, relate to each dimension. All of the items for one dimension feature multiplication whereas those linked to the other dimension require addition. One can conclude that multiplication and addition are two separate abilities in the test. Now consider another administration of the same test to secondary school children who have had more maths teaching. In this cohort, you might expect those who have successfully mastered multiplication to have also learned addition, whereas low performers are likely to have general issues with their arithmetic skills. Analysis of this data is more likely to indicate that a single dimension is being assessed, even though the same test is being used.

Aside from the candidature, other aspects of the testing context might also impact analyses of dimensionality. For example, consider a result showing that the same test is assessing three dimensions, where the third dimension includes a mixture of multiplication and addition questions, but all of them require multiple steps. This finding could be difficult to interpret based on a review of the test in isolation, but an understanding of the test administration can be revealing. A low-stakes administration could explain the result if test takers did not complete questions requiring multiple steps due to the effort needed. This would suggest that the third dimension can be interpreted as motivation. Alternatively, if the test is administered under strict time limits, or if test takers were prohibited from writing down their calculations, this third dimension might be conceptualised as working memory capacity. In summary, the following points should be noted about dimensionality:

- dimensionality is not a property of the test alone
- claims about a test's dimensionality may not hold if the test is administered in different cohorts
- contextual factors such as motivation can impact on dimensionality
- most descriptions of test dimensionality are based on *post-hoc* statistical analyses of test sessions.

These issues should be considered when investigating dimensionality in the context of a test or test section. For brevity, the rest of the chapter refers to BMAT and BMAT sections as unidimensional or multidimensional, in line with conventions in the psychometric literature. However, the nuanced issues outlined here are considered by Cambridge Assessment researchers when conducting and reporting FA analyses, such as in the following key study.

Key study – Confirming the theoretical structure of BMAT using Structural Equation Modelling (Emery and Khalid 2013b)

Main findings

- It is valid to interpret Section 1 as measuring a unified construct of thinking skills.
- It is valid to interpret Section 2 as measuring a unified construct of scientific reasoning.
- There is some evidence that an aggregate score for BMAT Section 1 and 2 is appropriate.
- The MCQs in BMAT assess the intended constructs as defined in the test specifications.

Introduction

Cambridge Assessment Admissions Testing conducted the study described here to investigate the cognitive validity of BMAT through analysis of test performance data. Factor analysis was used to investigate the underlying factor structure of BMAT in its earliest years, following changes made to the structure of MVAT that resulted in the introduction of BMAT. More recently, research has been carried out to verify the theoretical structure of BMAT (Emery and Khalid 2013b) using CFA. Each of the three sections of BMAT theoretically measures a different construct, or set of cognitive skills, and each of these sections is assumed to be unidimensional. That is, each section is designed to measure a single construct. Candidates receive a single score for each BMAT section on this basis.

However, Sections 1 and 2 of the test each contain items belonging to various subtypes. BMAT Section 1 contains three item subtypes: problem solving, understanding argument, and data analysis and inference. BMAT Section 2 contains four item subtypes: biology, chemistry, physics and maths. We therefore wished to test the assumption that BMAT Section 1 and BMAT Section 2 are each unidimensional, rather than multidimensional, in nature.

Methods and models tested

As Section 3, the Writing Task, consists of a single item, only the dimensionality of Sections 1 and 2 were investigated. The item-level response data of a BMAT test cohort was analysed (BMAT 2011, N = 6,230 candidates). BMAT Sections 1 and 2 consist of 62 items in total: 35 items in Section 1 and 27 items in Section 2. LISREL software was used to conduct the CFA. Initial exploratory analyses (in SPSS Version 20) indicated that a single factor was suitable for all 62 test items. CFA models were therefore constructed on theoretical (i.e. test specification) grounds. For each section, a single-factor model (i.e. a model assuming unidimensionality) and a multi-factor model were specified. For Section 1, the multi-factor model tested was a three-factor model, with items specified as belonging to problem solving (13 items), understanding argument (10 items) or data analysis and inference factors (12 items). For Section 2, the multi-factor model tested was a four-factor model, with items specified as belonging to biology (seven items), chemistry (seven items), physics (seven items) or maths factors (six items).

Models were compared using five model-fit indices. Model-fit adequacy was judged against common reference values for these indices (Hu and Bentler 1999).

Results

For BMAT Section 1, model fit statistics were similar and indicated adequate fit for both the single-factor 'Aptitude and Skills' model and the three-factor 'problem solving, understanding argument, data analysis and inference' model. In the three-factor CFA model, the problem solving, understanding argument, data analysis and inference factors were highly correlated, supporting the notion that items in Section 1 are measuring a unidimensional construct. For BMAT Section 2, model fit statistics were similar and adequate for both the single-factor Scientific Knowledge and Applications model and the four-factor 'biology, chemistry, physics and maths' model. Again, the multidimensional four-factor model included strong correlations between the biology, chemistry, physics and maths factors, supporting the conceptualisation of Section 2 items as collective measures of a unidimensional construct. A final, two-factor model of all 62 BMAT items, with items specified as belonging to either Section 1 (35 items) or Section 2 (27 items), again showed adequate model fit.

These analyses provide evidence that the multiple-choice BMAT sections are assessing the intended cognitive skills. Weir (2005) cautions against over-interpreting *post-hoc* analyses of test scores as evidence of validity and presents FA studies as an example of this; however, the CFA approach for this study used *a priori* theorisations of the skills and their relationships with each other. Therefore, the results can be seen as confirmation of theories developed during test design, rather than a post-test model of the skills underlying BMAT. Note that the results do not completely rule out conceptualising each of BMAT sections 1 and 2 as multidimensional. However, using this alternative approach would potentially compromise scoring validity as shorter subtests would have low internal consistency (discussed in Chapter 5 of this volume). Combined with the theoretical basis for the two sections, the CFA provides evidence that Sections 1 and 2 are assessing two separate, but related, processes.

3.5 Chapter summary

This chapter has focused on the cognitive processes assessed by each section of BMAT. In accordance with Weir's (2005) original emphasis on theory-based validity as cognitive validity, the discussion has included relevant models from educational assessment, science education and writing assessment. These have informed the theoretical basis for assessing thinking skills, scientific problem solving and written communication in BMAT. Additionally, some of the difficulties facing researchers interested in cognitive validity were outlined. While acknowledging the limitations in conducting research on cognitive validity, Cambridge Assessment Admissions Testing has conducted significant research in this area and two examples are presented in the chapter as key studies. These represent some of the more common approaches to investigating cognitive processing in educational assessment. The descriptions of these studies are potentially useful for researchers who are interested in the concept of cognitive validity, but are unfamiliar with methods used more widely in educational assessment. It is hoped that this encourages consideration of cognitive validity, both in the design and the evaluation of assessments, particularly in smaller scale contexts where bespoke tests or methods are being used.

On the other hand, considering relevant educational and psychological theory is no doubt a familiar practice for the seasoned test developer. Despite it being a core issue in educational assessment, test providers do not always describe the theoretical bases for their assessments, possibly under the impression that few individuals outside of testing fields will be interested. We see the presentation of theory underlying a test as an important responsibility of the test provider, because it allows the cognitive processes targeted by an assessment to be interrogated and challenged, particularly by users of the test. In the case of BMAT, it is important that medical schools are able to evaluate the reasons for including the constructs present in the test, even if only to support their communication with prospective applicants.

Although the discussion of cognitive processes assessed by BMAT in the current chapter has been detailed in comparison to the approaches adopted for some other assessments, they are still not as extensive as they might be. In particular, our understanding of the interaction between subject-specific knowledge and domain-general reasoning could be investigated further for BMAT Section 2 items. Also, the possible limitations of BMAT Section 3 should be considered in light of its short length and reliance on a single task.

Eye-tracking, key-logging and CB-testing technologies present greater opportunities for investigating these areas and others. They can complement traditional methods such as think-aloud studies, to potentially further our understanding of the cognitive processes elicited by educational assessments, which can inform the theory and practice of assessing all kinds of learning. In addition, investigating these issues in educational assessment could improve models and frameworks used in other fields, such as cognitive psychology. Collaboration between psychologists, medical educators and assessment experts is likely to support these endeavours, and multidisciplinary approaches should be encouraged in research and practice. Perhaps this recommendation is unsurprising, given the authors contributing to the present volume; however, we should point out that other disciplines have plenty to offer. Early indications and collaborations suggest that machine learning could have paradigm-changing impacts on our understandings and models of educational assessment.

The role of theory in informing assessment is not limited to future development. The opportunities afforded by cross-disciplinary collaboration and technologies are potential, whereas current test construction practices are actively informed by understandings of theory. Weir (2005) recognised that the interaction between theory-based and context-related aspects of validity is crucially important when considering overall construct validity. The present chapter has touched upon the relationship of cognitive validity with context-related validity, and with scoring validity. In the following chapters, these relationships are explored in greater detail, starting with the ways that context validity is informed by cognitive theories underlying an assessment. The next chapter details how decisions taken on item design and task setting affect the cognitive processing required to successfully complete test items in BMAT.

Chapter 3 main points

- Explicitly identifying the cognitive processes targeted by a test such as BMAT allows linking to relevant theories.
- Cognitive validity has been investigated in BMAT using verbal analysis protocols and factor analysis studies.
- Eye-tracking and computer-based testing present other opportunities for better understanding cognitive validity, particularly for Sections 2 and 3.
- Understanding the theoretical basis for any assessment can improve the design and production processes.

4 Building fairness and appropriacy into testing contexts: Tasks and administrations

Mark Shannon
Cambridge Assessment Admissions Testing
Paul Crump
Cambridge Assessment Admissions Testing
Juliet Wilson
Cambridge English Language Assessment

4.1 Introduction

In Chapter 3 of this volume, Cheung and McElwee focus on the theoretical basis for the cognitive processes assessed by BMAT sections. They point out that designing test tasks is necessarily intertwined with the cognitive processes targeted by items. The aim of the present chapter is to closely examine context validity, which includes the task design considerations that can influence whether BMAT tasks are assessing what they are intended to measure. Similarly, features of the test administration can also impact candidates' cognitive processes and threaten the validity of an examination. Context validity is concerned with the conditions under which a test is taken. It asks whether, and to what extent, the characteristics of the test tasks and their administration are fair and appropriate for candidates (Weir 2005). Principles of fairness dictate that all candidates should have the same experience wherever in the world they take a test.

As mentioned in the previous chapter, context validity exists in a close relationship with cognitive validity, in that it includes the representativeness and authenticity of the test tasks to the wider domain. Task design decisions regarding the response format, method of marking and number of tasks in a section also impact on the ways that a test can be scored, so context validity affects scoring validity.

Features of the task can impact on the testing situation in many ways. For example, the length of time allowed to complete a task or tasks must consider the impact on the cognitive processing of candidates, particularly if there is not sufficient time to complete the items. A key research study on time pressure is presented in this chapter to illustrate how this issue can be investigated, and how analysis of test data can inform the quality assurance procedures used in paper production. These procedures include a range of checks for each section that ensure tasks elicit the cognitive processes outlined in Chapter 3.

Context validity also encompasses questions concerning test administration conditions. Some of these impact on the security and uniformity of testing conditions, which are key issues when considering high-stakes exams. The present chapter describes how Cambridge Assessment deals with this wide range of context validity issues, both in terms of research and operational practice. In part 4.3, the key considerations in task design are outlined, along with the checking procedures that are used to ensure design decisions are maintained in practice. Following this, Cambridge Assessment's approach to standardising administration conditions is presented, along with examples of the inspection process that is used to monitor test centres. Firstly, in the next part of this chapter, we examine context validity as outlined in the socio-cognitive framework (O'Sullivan and Weir 2011, Weir 2005) and situate it in relation to BMAT.

4.2 Context validity and BMAT

Aspects of context validity are generally classified as features of the task or features of the administration conditions. Under the task aspect come considerations such as the authenticity of the types of tasks, response format and rubric. Also included are considerations that apply to an entire test or test sections, which can include multiple tasks. Examples of these are the time constraints for completion, the weighting and order of items, and candidates' knowledge of the marking criteria. For Sections 1 and 2 of BMAT, these issues are monitored in the item authoring and paper production procedures used to construct versions of the test. Writing tasks for Section 3 undergo similarly rigorous production procedures, but equally important are the rubrics and processes that ensure valid assigning of marks, which are discussed in Chapter 5. The 'administration conditions' aspect includes a consideration of the uniformity and the security of the testing conditions. The logistics of ensuring security should not be underestimated for large-scale examinations, and BMAT's increasing use internationally presents challenges to maintaining standardised test administrations.

Any of these factors, unrelated to the candidate's ability on the construct of interest, could impact test performance. In ensuring test validity it is essential that the test provider understands the effects of such features on performance and ensures that they are controlled and standardised as far as practically possible, both between test papers and between testing situations.

The context validity component within the socio-cognitive validation framework can be used to pose specific questions as follows: Is there any evidence that the response format is likely to affect performance? Are the marking criteria explicit for the candidates and the markers? Is the timing of each part appropriate? Is the content knowledge suitable and unbiased? Are the administration conditions satisfactorily consistent and secure?

The representativeness, appropriateness and authenticity of the tasks in a test are what give us faith in the generalisability of test results to what we are trying to measure. Response format (e.g. multiple-choice questions (MCQs) versus constructed response) is often constrained by considerations such as scoring validity (e.g. the desire to have items that are marked objectively) and practicality (e.g. the speed and lower cost of marking MCQ items). These issues are considered carefully in language testing, where it is common to use a mixture of response formats across the four skills commonly evaluated in a test (Elliott and Wilson 2013, Galaczi and ffrench 2011, Khalifa and Weir 2009, Shaw and Weir 2007). It is also considered good practice to use more than a single response format in a test when assessing higher-order reasoning (Liu et al 2014), as each response format has its advantages and disadvantages. The timing of the test is an important consideration but one that is also often constrained by practicalities. Speededness[1] may be a part of the test construct but the time pressure should not be such that candidates are unable to complete the test within the time allocated or are unduly stressed. Candidates should be made aware of the timing, number of items, weightings, marking criteria and any penalties for incorrect responses. The task rubric must be explicit, unambiguous, simple and brief yet comprehensive. No candidate should be able to misinterpret the test tasks.

A crucial threat to the context validity of a test (and the reputation of the test provider) is the potential for malpractice on the part of the candidate or the test centre (Cizek 1999). The higher the stakes of the test, the more of an issue cheating is likely to be. For this reason, the security of administration conditions is a vital concern of both the test provider and stakeholders, including test takers themselves who must perceive the test as fair. The increasingly sophisticated technology available for cheating in examination conditions means that detection (post-test), as well as prevention, is a responsibility of the test provider. Admissions tests for biomedical and dentistry study are certainly high stakes and a summary of the statistical approaches used with BMAT for malpractice detection is available in Chapter 5 of this volume. For those interested in the more technical aspects of statistical malpractice detection, our approach in this area is informed by work

1 Speededness refers to 'the situation where the time limits on tests do not allow substantial numbers of examinees to *fully* consider all test items' (Lu and Sireci 2007:29, emphasis added). In contrast, a 'power test' is one where the correctness of the answers is key, regardless of how long test completion takes.

on Cambridge English exams, as outlined by Bell (2015) and discussed by Geranpayeh (2013). The present chapter focuses on the standardised procedures and security checks used by centres administering BMAT, and the centre inspections used to ensure that the test is administered according to Cambridge Assessment's standards.

The following part of this chapter, part 4.3, addresses the aspects of context validity that focus on BMAT tasks. This includes a case study of work conducted to revise and define the content knowledge examined in Section 2 and a key research study into the appropriateness of the time constraints in BMAT.

4.3 Cambridge Assessment practice: Task features

Response format and task design

Two types of response format are used in BMAT and this is a fixed feature of the test, as is the number of items per section. Sections 1 and 2 of BMAT are multiple-choice format (with each item weighted equally) whereas Section 3, the Writing Task, requires candidates to construct a brief essay response to a structured prompt. These two response types, both of which are likely to be encountered in the future course examinations of successful applicants, can be seen as representing each end of the response-type continuum. There are advantages and disadvantages to both formats. Here we discuss the context validity considerations related to each response format.

Multiple-choice questions/items

MCQs are a popular form of standardised assessment because they are objective, low cost and it is possible to mark them quickly after the test session. Liu et al (2014) point out that MCQs typically cost more in assessment development than constructed-response items, but are cheaper overall due to the cost of marking constructed-response tasks. This observation applies to BMAT MCQ items, which go through multiple stages of checks in the question paper production process (these are outlined later in the chapter under test content). Responses to these are then objectively marked using optical scanners. Compared with constructed-response tasks, MCQs fit better with psychometric models used to investigate internal consistency and reliability, because a greater number of MCQs can be included in a test with limited time (see Chapter 5 for details). Also, quality assurance processes can be automated to evaluate test sections based on the responses in a session and this post-test evidence of validity is available to the test providers before results are released. Given that medical schools using BMAT work to tight timescales when making selection decisions, these are substantial advantages over constructed-response items, which take longer to mark reliably and quality assure. However, there are some criticisms of MCQs that need to be considered by test providers. Chiefly among these are observations that the reasoning used to answer an MCQ is different from the reasoning employed in non-test settings, because test takers rarely select from a defined set of options. This is often raised in relation to listening and reading exams (Field 2013, Khalifa and Weir 2009); for example, Field points out that MCQs in listening exams often require candidates to engage processes that fall outside of a real-world listening event, such as disconfirming available response options.

Similarly, answering MCQs can require BMAT candidates to engage reasoning that is somewhat different from the reasoning involved in clinical practice. Indeed, Sam, Hameed, Harris and Meeran (2016) observe that clinical medicine is often nuanced, which runs counter to the idea of a single correct answer as assumed by MCQ formats. However, it should be noted that BMAT targets the potential for biomedical study rather than practice in a clinical environment, and MCQs are used as an assessment tool in undergraduate studies. Their use is an established method in medical education contexts (Downing 2002), where MCQs are used to evaluate both factual recall and higher-order cognition (Palmer and Devitt 2007).

Furthermore, there is evidence that constructed-response items correlate positively with MCQs (Klein, Liu, Sconing, Bolus, Bridgeman, Kugelmass and Steedle 2009, Rodriguez 2003), indicating that MCQs can be valid assessment tools when constructed appropriately. In reference to the medical education setting, Downing (2002:240) points out that in order to produce valid MCQs, 'item writers must have the willingness to invest considerable time and effort into creating effective MCQs'. Cambridge Assessment invests a great deal of time not only authoring items, but also in reviewing, editing and vetting them. A process-driven approach is used to review items and consider the plausibility of the incorrect response options (distractors), the cognitive processes needed to reach the correct answer and the number of response options available to candidates.

Another issue to consider is whether particular formats might advantage or disadvantage particular groups of test takers, and this question has been raised in relation to MCQs, particularly in terms of gender differences. However, evidence of gender bias in MCQs is mixed. Large studies and meta-analyses conducted by Arthur and Everaert (2012), Buck et al (2002) and Du Plessis and Du Plessis (2009) did not find any systematic bias in MCQs. Similarly, a study conducted by Cambridge Assessment researchers on General Certificate of Secondary Education (GCSE) data did not show that MCQs advantage a particular group over others (Bramley, Vidal Rodeiro and Vitello 2015). However, a clear bias exists in MCQs which penalise test takers for incorrect responses, as this is linked with differential response rates between males and females. Baldiga (2014), Kelly and Dennick (2009) and Hirschfeld, Moore and Brown (1995) found that a male advantage exists for MCQs which use negative marking in diverse disciplines including history, medicine and accounting. Baldiga (2014) argues that it is the high-stakes nature of the environment, coupled with score-awarding that exacerbates a socialised (rather than cognitive) difference between males and females. Therefore, negative marking should not be encouraged in high-stakes testing and BMAT does not penalise incorrect responses in MCQ sections of the test.

Due to their efficiency, reliability and objectivity, the majority of testing time in a BMAT session is allocated to MCQs in the form of Section 1 (60 minutes) and Section 2 (30 minutes). However, an essay task (for which 30 minutes is allowed) is also used to assess productive reasoning in Section 3, which requires a constructed response.

Constructed-response essay task

Developing and producing a written argument is a key skill for higher education study that is not possible to assess with MCQs. This provides a strong theoretical rationale for including a constructed-response test section that complements the MCQ sections of BMAT. For a discussion of these theoretical issues, see the cognitive validity arguments outlined by Cheung and McElwee (this volume).

The essay task for Section 3 was originally modelled on the US Medical College Admission Test (MCAT) in use at the time, and in the early years of BMAT the structure and wording from the original Oxford Medical Admissions Test (OMAT) was followed. This has been modified in order to make the rubric clearer and more accessible. For example, early questions asked candidates to produce a 'unified essay', meaning a structured and coherent argument rather than unconnected statements. This phrasing was discontinued in case it should prove confusing or unfamiliar for candidates. In other words, the instructions were improved to better elicit the targeted cognitive processes from candidates.

The BMAT Writing Task prompts are highly structured in order to guide test takers through the task, ensuring that even weaker candidates are supported to produce a script that can be scored. On each Section 3 paper, candidates are presented with three questions, from which they must choose one; in broad terms, the three questions will cover a general, a scientific and a medical topic. Topics are carefully chosen and the questions are vetted by two independent consultants to ensure that they are accessible to a diverse international candidature. Each Writing Task question presents a statement and asks the candidate to explain what it means. The candidate is then asked to argue to the contrary and finally to summarise or conclude with reference to the wider context of the statement. An example question is available in Box 4.1.

Box 4.1 Sample question from BMAT Writing Task

When treating an individual patient, a physician must also think of the wider society.
Explain the reasoning behind this statement. Argue that a doctor should only consider the individual that he or she is treating at the time. With respect to medical treatment, to what extent can a patient's interests differ from those of the wider population?

The prompt used in BMAT Section 3 encourages the use of knowledge-transforming strategies and processes (Scardamalia and Bereiter 1987), which produce more advanced writing, by providing an explicit argument for the test taker to conceptualise as a rhetorical goal. This encourages writers to form mental representations of their main points, which is essential to producing a cogent argument. Shaw and Weir (2007) argue that a writing task should be designed to elicit a response with a clear purpose and the prompt should make this explicit to the test taker. According to Weigle's (2002) categorisation of written discourse, there are six purposes, or dominant intentions, that can be specified for a piece of writing (Box 4.2).

Box 4.2 Categories of dominant intention from Weigle (2002:10)

Metalingual mathetic (intended to learn)
Referential (intended to inform)
Conative (intended to persuade or convince)
Emotive (intended to convey feelings or emotions)
Poetic (intended to entertain)
Phatic (intended to keep in touch)

By focusing BMAT's Section 3 prompt on argument, it is made clear that the dominant intention of the written response should be conative (intended to persuade or convince). In addition to specifying an argument, the structured prompt provides questions that should be addressed as part of the written response. Answering these questions requires a candidate to generate ideas on the topic area, as source material is not provided for candidates to reorganise or reproduce. Instead candidates are expected to draw on relevant general knowledge and develop ideas from these to construct an argument.

The answer sheet provided to candidates is also designed to encourage planning before writing a structured argument. Only one side of A4 is provided for the actual essay and candidates are told that no additional answer sheets may be used. Test takers with permission to use a word processor are instructed not to exceed 550 words. This limitation on the length of the response means that candidates need to plan and structure an essay that will fit in the space available. Whilst a single side of A4 is enough to produce an example of extended writing, it is also intended to be easily manageable for BMAT candidates in the 30 minutes provided for Section 3, even when accounting for the time needed to select a question; therefore, there should be time that is allocated to planning, and space is provided for this on the question paper.

The design considerations required for MCQ and constructed-response tasks have been discussed here, focusing on matters relevant to the tasks included in BMAT. These issues are monitored in early stages of the question paper production process, which focus on evaluating items and tasks in isolation. Also monitored are issues that apply across entire test sections, such as the time allocated to complete all of the items in Section 1 or Section 2.

Test timing

Speededness is a feature of BMAT and a part of its test construct because test takers are expected to engage reasoning processes efficiently to complete questions. However, it is important that the time pressure is not excessive, so that the majority of test takers attempt every item, particularly for the MCQ sections.

In the first year of BMAT, 2003, there were slightly higher numbers of items in the two MCQ sections than in the years that followed: 40 items in Section 1 (Aptitude and Skills) and 30 items in Section 2 (Scientific Knowledge and Applications). The time allowance was the same as in the current test: 60 minutes for Section 1 and 30 minutes for Section 2. Due to finding higher than expected omit rates in the 2003 test, the numbers of items were reduced (for the 2004 test) to 35 for Section 1 and to 27 for Section 2.

Shannon (2005) conducted statistical investigation of the BMAT 2004 test items and again found potential evidence of excessive time pressure for Section 2, with omit rates rising towards the end of the section. As a result of these findings, the number of test items was not reduced any further but the recommendation was made to limit the number of time-consuming or complex items (e.g. those requiring candidates to answer a number of parts in order to gain a single mark). The number of BMAT items has therefore remained at 35 (in 60 minutes) for Section 1 and at 27 (in 30 minutes) for Section 2 since 2004.

These studies also informed guidelines for authoring items that consider the length of time required to read a question fully, carry out necessary calculations or apply reasoning. More recent studies have been used to monitor the time pressure of BMAT items and investigate hypothesised group differences about their impact. An example of this work is presented below as a key study.

Key study: Are the time constraints of BMAT appropriate? (Emery 2013a)

Introduction

One aspect of context validity is whether the time limits of a test are appropriate or overly pressured. Here we summarise aspects of a study investigating this issue in BMAT (Emery 2013a). Time pressure is an intended feature of BMAT but the time pressure of a test should not be such that the bulk of candidates are unable to finish the items or be forced to guess response options by the time pressure. Each of the three BMAT sections has its own, separate time allowance and all items in the two MCQ sections (Sections 1 and 2) are scored equally. Items in BMAT Sections 1 and 2 are intended to increase in difficulty throughout the paper (based on the judgement of the item writers). Items of each subtype (e.g. biology, chemistry, physics, mathematics) are interspersed throughout Section 2, but within each item subtype, the items judged to be easier are positioned earlier in the paper. An upward trend in guessing is therefore expected with item position in the paper.

Omit rates (the proportion of candidates that do not respond to an item) in excess of around 5% of candidates may be a cause for concern in non-MCQ examinations (Elliot and Johnson 2005), possibly indicating an unclear or difficult question. Given that BMAT is MCQ and it is advisable for candidates to guess items they do not know, omit rates for BMAT items are expected to be very low, and high omission of items might be suggestive of excessive time pressure.

The appropriateness of the BMAT time constraints was investigated using item-level response data from 2010 to 2012. The study also investigated whether the impact of the adverse effects of time pressure differed by gender. This is of particular interest given observations that male candidates have tended to score slightly higher on the MCQ sections of BMAT, as discussed in Chapter 2. The analysis for this study assumes that candidates work through the test in the order the items are presented in the paper, therefore if time pressure is excessive one would expect higher omit rates at the end of sections. The summary here focuses on omit rates, although the full report by Emery (2013a) also looked at other statistical indicators that may indicate guessing, such as item facility, item difficulty and item fit. As these largely confirmed the findings from analysis of the omit rates, these additional statistics are not discussed in the present summary; however, descriptions of these statistics and their application in test validation are available in Chapter 5.

Research questions

Is there evidence of excessive time pressure in BMAT Sections 1 and 2? Is there any evidence that females are affected more adversely by the time constraints in the test?

Data collection

Six item-level response datasets from BMAT Sections 1 and 2 were analysed (test years 2010, 2011 and 2012, whole cohort data). Candidate gender was captured at the time of test registration. All items were in MCQ format, apart from a single item that required a numerical response in BMAT 2010. Since 2011, all Section 1 and 2 items have been in MCQ format.

Datasets contained candidate gender and responses to each of the items (A/B/C/ . . . or 'omitted'). Candidate numbers in each cohort were as follows:

- BMAT 2010 N = 6,225 (57% female)
- BMAT 2011 N = 6,230 (57% female)
- BMAT 2012 N = 7,046 (56% female).

Results

Figure 4.1 and Figure 4.2 plot the omit rates for BMAT Section 1 and 2 by gender, for the 2012 administration. Charts for all years were originally reported by Emery (2013a) and the results showed a similar pattern in each, with the largest difference in 2012.

Figure 4.1 Omit rates for BMAT Section 1 items (2012)

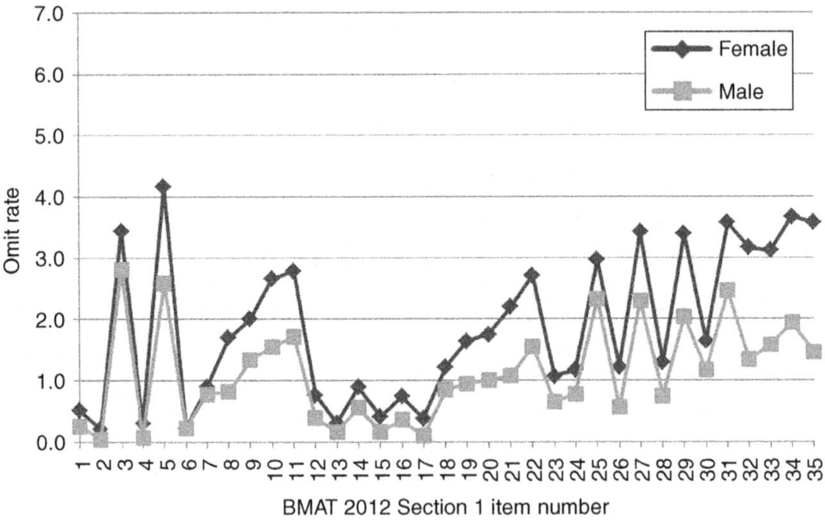

As shown in Figure 4.1 and Figure 4.2, a slight increase in omit rates specifically towards the ends of BMAT Sections 1 and 2 was evident for all three of these test years. Omit rates in all three years were low, however, with the values for items at the ends of the test sections amounting to less than 5% of the candidates failing to respond. There was also a trend for a higher

Figure 4.2 Omit rates for BMAT Section 2 items (2012)

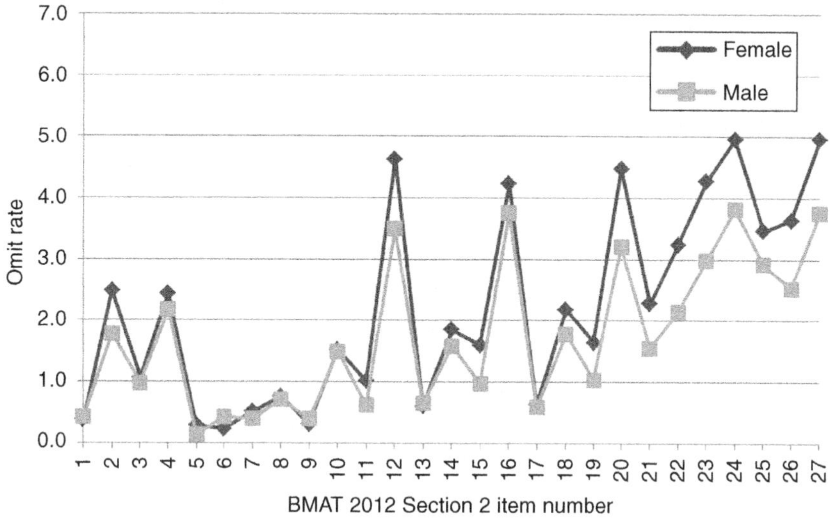

proportion of females than males to omit items towards the end of the sections, and this was most markedly the case in Section 1 of BMAT in the 2011 and 2012 administrations. However, it is important to note that the gender differences in omit rates are very small; in cases with the largest differences this was 4–5% of females versus 2–3% of males. Other statistics indicated similar item fit for the later items in a section when compared to earlier items in a section. This suggests that the candidates who filled in a response for these end-of-section questions (i.e. the vast majority of candidates) were not guessing disproportionately at these compared to earlier items.

Discussion

The time pressure in BMAT was not excessive for most candidates based on the statistical evidence in this study. Both the Classical and Rasch item statistics did not suggest an unexpected decrease in candidate performance for items specifically towards the end of the test sections that would indicate their running out of time. Nor was there evidence that female candidates performed worse than male candidates on items towards the ends of the test sections. This latter finding is supported by Differential Item Functioning (DIF) analyses of BMAT items by gender (Emery and Khalid 2013a; see Chapter 5 for an outline of this study).

Omit rates *did* appear to show a clear increase towards the end of both test sections and this was more apparent for the female candidates. However, even in the years with the greatest number of omissions, the omit rate for females was only around 4–5% of candidates (compared to around 2–3%

of the male candidates). This indicates that relatively few candidates were unable to complete their responses within the time allowance, albeit a very slightly higher proportion of females than males. The slight difference in omit rates for males and females towards the test section ends did not translate into differences in the average number of correct responses for males and females on these items. It therefore seems unlikely that time pressure effects could explain the slightly lower performance of females on Sections 1 and 2 of BMAT overall in these years. This finding reflects that of Ben-Shakhar and Sinai (1991), who found a consistent pattern of greater omission rates among females in a battery of aptitude and selection tests but concluded that gender differences in guessing tendencies account for only a small fraction of the observed gender differences in multiple-choice tests.

The obvious caveat of this study is that candidates may answer items within BMAT Section 1 and within BMAT Section 2 in any order they wish because the test is paper-based (PB). The assumption was made for the purpose of these analyses that candidates tend to work through items in the order they appear in the test. It is possible, though, that the adverse effects of excessive time pressure could be manifest *throughout* the test sections rather than affecting only those items towards their ends, resulting in increased guessing (i.e. higher item difficulty and lower discrimination) throughout the test than might be obtained with a greater time allowance. Indeed it could be argued that the existence of omit rates at all is suggestive of time pressure given that there is no penalty for guessing.

Further research may therefore be warranted on the timing of BMAT. Manipulating the time allowance in experimental participants to assess its impact on item functioning is one potential method. Observational, interview and questionnaire data from live BMAT candidates would provide a valuable source of evidence. It will be particularly important to investigate the timing of BMAT should any changes be made to the test in future years. Omission of item responses seen in the BMAT data (albeit very minor) is a peculiarity given that there are no penalties for incorrect guessing. Cambridge Assessment is currently enhancing the free resources and support for BMAT preparation available on its website, and emphasising to candidates the advantage of attempting all questions is key. These observations also apply to Section 3, where the timing of the test has not been investigated as systematically as it has for the MCQ sections. Although responses submitted for the Writing Task are generally similar in length, it might be the case that time pressure has an impact on how candidates engage the cognitive processes involved in writing.

This study highlights the importance of considering the time available to complete a test as part of context validity and the value of investigating this issue with research. Earlier studies resulted in changes to the number of items included in BMAT sections, whereas the findings of this study confirm the suitability of BMAT's format, and inform the processes that check the appropriateness of test items.

Test content – knowledge, suitability and freedom from bias

Ensuring that the content of BMAT is of a suitable level of difficulty targeted to the intended test takers is a central aspect of context validity. Another issue relevant to context validity is the knowledge related to answering items and the topic areas associated with test tasks. For test sections that do not specifically include bodies of knowledge (Sections 1 and 3), task content must be checked carefully to confirm that the context used to present an argument or problem would be encountered in everyday settings. They are also reviewed to ensure that answering an MCQ correctly or composing a suitable written argument does not rely on subject-specific knowledge.

Across Cambridge Assessment, guidelines are used to ensure that exam questions do not include emotive topics that can influence the performance of candidates, or particular subsets of test takers. These guidelines are used in the design of admissions tests; however, it is acknowledged that topics used in BMAT Section 3 might include more sensitive issues than normally considered acceptable throughout Cambridge Assessment, in order to authentically represent the issues that biomedical students will need to consider in their studies. Due to this relaxation of the guidelines, all Section 3 questions are scrutinised carefully by an assessment manager to evaluate potential for bias against specific groups. Topics that might evoke a different emotional response from subsets of candidates are avoided, even if they would be encountered in medical study. For example, medical issues more likely to seriously affect one sex over another, such as fertility or abortion, are avoided. Similarly, content for all sections avoids referring to religious or ethnic issues in their context.

An appropriate coverage of topics should be maintained for test sections that include subject-specific knowledge, such as Section 2. Because candidates are expected to be familiar with scientific knowledge and apply it to novel problems, it is important to define the scope of the topics that might be included in BMAT Section 2. To illustrate Cambridge Assessment's approach to specifying the science knowledge that underpins Section 2, a case study of a recent specification revision is presented in the next part.

Case study – Revising the BMAT Section 2 knowledge specification

In 2014 a revision of BMAT Section 2 Scientific Knowledge and Applications was undertaken by Cambridge Assessment Admissions Testing, with the aim of updating the syllabus and maintaining its relevance for biomedical education. This case study details the circumstances that prompted the revision and the intended outcomes, as well as the work carried out to shape and develop the new Section 2 specification.

An important consideration in BMAT's development was that preparation should not require students to invest large amounts of time or money and should complement a student's school study. As BMAT is typically taken early in students' final year at school it was decided that the specification should cover topics that students would have been expected to study up to the age of 16 by the end of their GCSE examinations in the UK (approximately 18 months prior to BMAT).

When BMAT was developed it was used initially by universities in England, and therefore the National Curriculum for England, Wales and Northern Ireland, which outlined the compulsory science curriculum in state schools up to age 16, was an appropriate basis for the test content of Section 2. The intended message to test takers was that the core knowledge required for BMAT was already familiar to them through their compulsory schooling and significant amounts of new learning should not be required; it should instead be a matter of revision to refresh their understanding. At the time, the National Curriculum specified in detail the content to be covered, and this was reflected in the GCSE specifications from the major UK examination boards and textbooks, so there was plenty of information available to students preparing for the test, including those from overseas. On this basis, the content specification for BMAT itself was relatively brief, giving a broad overview of the test and topics that might be examined but referring students to the National Curriculum documents for further information.

Changes to the National Curriculum resulted in a less detailed programme of study and an increased diversification of curricular pathways to achieving GCSEs in Science and Mathematics. The changes made the task of ensuring that BMAT Section 2 contained only content covered in state schools by age 16 more difficult. Therefore, it was decided that a review of BMAT Section 2 content and the creation of a more detailed test specification was necessary to ensure candidates were supported, which comprised three main phases:

1. Compilation of draft specification.
2. Consultation with university stakeholders.
3. Trial by BMAT item writers and international experts.

Compilation of the draft specification

The first stage in establishing the basis for the new content specification was to conduct a review of major GCSE double-award Science and Mathematics syllabuses across five major UK examination boards to establish the breadth of topics that were encountered by potential BMAT test takers.

Senior examiners evaluated the specifications to identify the areas and specific topics that were common across several examination boards, to derive the core material that would form the revised BMAT curriculum. Examiners identified the general topic areas, the details of the sub-topics that were covered in common, and commented on the overlaps in specifications (e.g. the depth of knowledge expected on the topic, diversity of exemplars used by the exam boards, and which boards did not include the topic).

The examiners were permitted to recommend the inclusion of some additional topics, provided they were accessible and easy for able students to learn independently. In these cases, one or more of the following justifications were required:

- topics judged to be essential to a core understanding of the particular science, even if there was less commonality in their appearance on the various exam board specifications
- relevant scientific principles taught earlier than GCSE that should be included for completeness (for students' reference)
- details or examples that draw links between topics to promote understanding of the inter-relatedness of science as a discipline
- topics of particular relevance to the study of medical/biomedical sciences.

Consultation with university stakeholders

A round-table discussion with senior academics involved in student selection and medical or biomedical education at the universities using BMAT was organised to refine the draft specification. Thirty-nine broad topic areas had been distilled from the examiners' initial review of GCSE curricula, comprising over 500 sub-topics. Each topic and associated sub-topics were discussed in turn and three questions were used to guide the discussion: Are the knowledge and concepts important for biomedical study? Is the context provided for the underlying principles relevant? Is the type of thinking that a topic affords important or useful in studying medicine, dentistry and veterinary medicine?

The first two questions are central to the construct validity of BMAT Section 2 and assuring its relevance for students who are preparing to study medicine or biomedical sciences. Two specific examples outline how the draft specification was amended to meet these principles. Electricity was identified by the senior examiner for physics as a core area common across multiple GCSE syllabuses. The academic panel agreed that the topic should be retained on the BMAT specification for its relevance to biomedical topics such as nerve impulses, but indicated that the sub-topic of domestic electricity be excluded. Cosmology was also excluded from the BMAT draft specification for physics, despite frequent representation on GCSE programmes, but relevant concepts such as the Doppler effect and line absorption spectra were retained and categorised under the topic areas of waves and wave behaviour, and the electromagnetic spectrum respectively, as medical tutors argued they were of central relevance to undergraduate study. In line with the objective of BMAT to test students' understanding of scientific principles rather than specific facts, this categorisation both ensured that candidates would not invest time revising topics that are not relevant to medical study, and encourages the abstraction and generalisation of principles beyond the initial context in which they were encountered, which is a key feature of advanced scientific reasoning.

Specific examples for core topics that would appear in the BMAT specification were also agreed. For example, homeostasis featured on most GCSE biology syllabuses but a variety of examples were used to teach the principle (e.g. regulation of blood glucose, temperature, or water content). Prior to revising the specification, only very general questions on homeostasis could be used in BMAT to avoid disadvantaging students who had encountered different examples. By including a core set of examples in the revision of the BMAT specification, a wider range of high-quality test questions could be generated.

Trial by BMAT question writers and international experts

The revised specification was shared with BMAT item writers, who assessed it again for omissions based on their experiences of writing test questions. In particular, they were asked to check that it afforded enough coverage to allow creation of high-quality questions. Feedback was very positive, and the overall opinion was that as the new specification was more explicit on the topics that could be examined, it presented new opportunities to devise challenging high-quality questions in subject areas that were previously not possible.

One aim of the revision was to support overseas students' preparation. Science and mathematics curricula internationally may place different emphasis on certain topics or techniques. Variation in question difficulty on the basis of candidate nationality presents a type of construct-irrelevant variance that test providers should seek to limit. Education professionals with a background in biomedical sciences, including teachers and university faculty staff from the Netherlands, Malaysia and Singapore reviewed the new specification to confirm that content was targeted at the level expected of students in their final year of school study in their respective countries. Creating a more detailed specification for BMAT Section 2 and defining the expected content knowledge for the test supported international students by allowing them to identify specifically where they may need to focus revision and highlighting particular areas for study.

Development of an Assumed Subject Knowledge guide

Creating a more detailed specification for BMAT also had other potential benefits for test takers. Updating and expanding the detail of the content specification provided opportunities for producing free revision materials for BMAT, because a blueprint of the content knowledge examined by BMAT Section 2 had been developed.

As the revisions to the Section 2 specification proceeded, Cambridge Assessment Admissions Testing approached Coordination Group Publications (CGP), a well-known publisher of GCSE revision guides, to collaborate on a BMAT guide, based specifically on the new specification. CGP was chosen as the preferred partner for this work as their books are visual with a minimum of text, and well known to many students and schools already, to reinforce the idea that this section of BMAT requires *revision* but not significant commitment to new learning for test takers. BMAT assessment managers reviewed CGP guides for GCSE subjects and selected pages relevant to the BMAT specification, before editing their selections to remove duplication or superfluous material. CGP commissioned their authors to produce some text and illustrations for BMAT topics that did not appear in their current books. The revision guide was compiled and made available as an online e-book, which prospective candidates can access by registering online for free.

Discussion

This case study demonstrates some of the steps that can be taken to specify a body of knowledge examined by a test, which may inform the work of others designing assessments with a knowledge component. Of course, the approach adopted for any assessment must consider the context and candidature that is being assessed. For example, a lecturer designing the assessment for a specific course they teach may find that a process similar to the one above is overly laborious. However, the principles guiding the case study should be considered in most assessment contexts. For example, consulting with colleagues responsible for more advanced courses, or even clinical placement supervisors, would help to identify crucial topics and distinguish them from those that might be considered less relevant. Simply listing the topics and sub-topics that might be included will give an idea of the scope of knowledge being assessed, which can influence decisions about the most suitable form of assessment.

Once established, a content specification can be used to consider various aspects of context validity. Although many issues that impact on BMAT's validity have been investigated using trials and research studies, some of which have been presented in previous chapters, it is also important to evaluate them when producing papers. The processes and checks involved in checking test content are presented in the following section, including the checks that compare items to the Section 2 specification.

Question paper production process

Constructing a BMAT paper is a multi-stage, iterative process which ensures that items are high quality and that each element of the test construct is represented appropriately. From the time that questions are commissioned to their appearance on the exam paper, each question goes through a rigorous process of checking and editing to ensure it is appropriately targeted to the ability of the candidates, that the topic maps to the content specification, that there are no flaws in the logic or reasoning of the question or the answer options, and that it reflects the types of general or subject-specific thinking skills stated as important by the BMAT specification.

These checks are conducted by subject matter experts (SMEs) and co-ordinated by assessment managers, who are typically recruited by Cambridge Assessment Admissions Testing for a combination of their subject area expertise and experience of educational contexts. A number of these assessment managers hold higher research degrees in relevant subject areas, and have experience of teaching their subject in school or university settings. On joining the organisation, they are then trained on assessment principles and interpretation of psychometric indices. Therefore, assessment managers working on admissions tests are regarded as another layer of SMEs that add to the reviews conducted by assessment experts working as consultants.

Review by SMEs has traditionally been described as a method of ensuring content validity in occupational test settings (Lawshe 1975). Content validity is concerned with the relevance of the assessment, and its items, to the targeted construct, and the degree to which it is adequately representative of the construct (Haynes, Richard and Kubany 1995); however, the term has been controversial and Fitzpatrick (1983:3) argued that 'content validity is not a useful term for test specialists to retain in their vocabulary'. Due to the focus of this volume, the technical and historical debate on content validity is not discussed fully here. Instead, we align the checks performed by SMEs on BMAT with context validity as conceptualised in the socio-cognitive framework, which includes content validity when discussing features of the task (Weir 2005).

A range of SMEs review tasks during the question paper production process. The checks focus on specific features of the task, such as the length of text input, the linguistic complexity of instructions and the time expected to be available for completing the item. Importantly, the knowledge needed to answer the task is also considered as part of the checks. For Sections 1 and 3 this is considered against a standard of everyday knowledge, whereas Section 2 items are checked against a detailed maths and science specification.

The outlines in the next sections present processes as they currently stand. Efficient and rigorous procedures have taken a great deal of time and experience to develop, so it should be noted that the sequence of reviews and checklists of issues to consider have been honed over a decade, and will continue to be improved over time. The number of experts available for carrying out the checks considered important by Cambridge Assessment has also varied. Where necessary, item writers, vetters and academic subject experts have been recruited from educational settings and trained in the specialist skills required for reviewing test items and papers. Therefore, no claims are being made about how long the procedures described here have been in place and whether they remain a blueprint for producing future BMAT papers. There are four main phases to the preparation of a BMAT paper for Sections 1 and 3, which are item commissioning, item editing, paper construction and paper vetting. Section 2 uses a similar process but includes an additional layer of item vetting prior to the paper construction process, which is sometimes referred to as science vetting. There are some differences in the precise checks conducted for each section due to their content, and flowcharts representing each separate process are available in Figure 4.3, Figure 4.4 and Figure 4.5. However, the main focus of each stage of review is similar across the sections; these are outlined in the next parts of the chapter.

Item commissioning

A store of items, referred to as an item bank, is maintained for each subject area and thinking skill domain. This storage is used to manage the items and any associated metadata relating to them, including whether they have been used in previous tests. This allows assessment managers to monitor the number of secure items available for upcoming tests. Additional question development for BMAT begins approximately 18 months before the test. Item writers are commissioned to submit questions in their area of expertise for review and eventual inclusion in the relevant item bank. Typically, item writers are experienced teachers and question writers for school-based qualifications. Because BMAT items target constructs and reasoning that are somewhat different from those examined in GCSEs and A Levels, item writers new to the test are trained to author items targeting the skills and knowledge specified for BMAT. Training is conducted using group workshops facilitated by assessment managers.

Items submitted by less experienced item writers are scrutinised carefully by assessment managers, who provide substantive feedback. In addition, the item writers are provided with guidance on good question writing, and checklists to ensure the quality and standard of the items, which are developed from research and operational analysis. All item writers are also given feedback regularly on how certain items have performed in recent tests (e.g. the proportion of candidates getting them correct, and how well they discriminated between candidates of different levels of ability) in order to encourage reflection on the questions they develop and anticipate problems or weakness.

Item editing

Submitted items are reviewed by BMAT assessment managers to ensure the language and formatting is appropriate and to identify any obvious flaws or concerns. Typically, assessment managers for Sections 1 and 2 check the correct answers and the solution for each item submitted by the item writer. At this stage, items that are not assessing the relevant cognitive processes are identified. For example, Section 2 assessment managers identify items that can be answered correctly without knowledge of scientific processes or principles. Similarly, items that only require a test taker to recall specific scientific knowledge or facts are rejected. Assessment managers for Section 1 check the solutions submitted by item writers to ensure they match the skills defined in the test specification, and that the correct response is not ambiguous once suitable reasoning has been applied.

A senior educationalist is recruited to act as the chair for each subject (maths, physics, biology, chemistry) or thinking skills domain (understanding argument, problem solving, data analysis and inference). For BMAT Section 3, a single chair is recruited to review submitted writing tasks. Chairs are typically teachers or lecturers with extensive experience of educational contexts, and who have held or currently hold leadership roles in education. The chair reviews each item for their area, making suggestions for changes if they believe items are too easy or difficult, or that phrasing is unclear or repetitive. Items are amended and re-submitted by item writers, and then scrutinised at an editing meeting by a team of experienced item writers. Each question is critically reviewed by every group member according to a checklist of features to ensure that they are clear, solvable in the allocated time, and if destined for the Scientific Knowledge and Applications section, that the topic is relevant to the specification and the item is scientifically sound.

Due to the multiple-choice response format of Section 1 and 2 items, the cognitive processes that might lead a test taker to select each incorrect answer can be described in terms of the miscalculations or misapplication of certain processes, for further analysis. Considering this ensures that the incorrect options, referred to as distractors, are plausible answers. Furthermore, these analyses ensure that arriving at an incorrect answer can result from a failure to successfully employ the cognitive processes targeted by each section (of course they might also be selected through guessing or misreading the question). Distractors attractive to test takers for other reasons are reviewed critically to make sure that they are not contributing to construct-irrelevant variance. For example, a Section 2 question with complicated phrasing might have a distractor that would be commonly selected by those with poor language ability. This would need to be revised, because incorrect responses on Section 2 items should indicate deficiencies in science knowledge, or ability to apply this knowledge, rather than low linguistic ability. The response option specified as correct is then subject to further scrutiny to ensure that it is not an answer that might be arrived at by accident using poor reasoning. This is done by completing the items whilst applying common flaws in reasoning, misunderstandings of scientific concepts and miscalculations.

During the editing meeting, the assessment managers also carry out checks related to English language proficiency. Although this is conducted across all sections of BMAT, it is reviewed particularly closely with Section 1 items to ensure that:

- difficulty does not come from the way the item is expressed
- difficulty does not come from the reading load
- difficulty does not come from unfamiliar cultural assumptions.

Where an editing panel or vetter considers that the level of language is too high, there are a number of remedies that can be applied. In-text glosses or paraphrases of unfamiliar terms can be provided (if such terms cannot be avoided altogether). The tone of a passage or question can be made more neutral, or the register less formal. The length of a passage can be shortened, the syntax simplified or the density of information presented can be reduced. UK-centric names, institutions or customs can be replaced with generic equivalents. All of these measures help to ensure that construct-irrelevant variance is minimised.

Item vetting (Section 2 only)

After editing meetings, Section 2 items are submitted to an extra layer of vetting at the item level that focuses on science and maths concepts, because candidates are expected to apply subject-specific knowledge when answering them. This is completed with the support of academic subject specialists, who are active research scientists in relevant fields of science and maths. These SMEs scrutinise the knowledge underpinning each Section 2 item. In particular, they check that items:

- do not rely on scientific principles taught in secondary schools that are contradicted when a more advanced model of the phenomenon is understood
- do not become ambiguous or more difficult when one considers scientific advances beyond the scope of secondary school level science
- are not answered correctly by merely recalling advanced scientific knowledge that sits outside of the BMAT Section 2 specification.

Paper construction

After editing and vetting conducted at the item level, questions are selected from available items in the bank by the chairs, taking into account how well the questions cover the test specification and the difficulty of the paper. For

Sections 1 and 2, they also estimate the difficulty of each item and then arrange the items in order of ascending estimated difficulty. The Section 3 chair selects the tasks and judges whether they are equally difficult. All chairs also select reserve items that can be substituted if later stages of review identify material to be rejected. The first draft is reviewed by an assessment manager for each subject or subskill, who also consults other assessment managers working on that section of the test to check for repetitions between topics submitted by chairs for different subjects. The assessment managers for Sections 1 and 2 also review the overall coverage and content of the section, along with the orders proposed by the chairs. The materials across the three thinking skills domains (Section 1) or four subject areas (Section 2) are collected together to form a first draft of each paper.

Paper vetting

The draft papers are then subject to paper vetting, which differs from item vetting in its focus on an entire section together. Paper vetters are typically teachers and educationalists who have worked in general educational settings. Although they come from subject specialist areas, they tend to have a broad knowledge of educational contexts that extends beyond subject-specific education. These SMEs are trained to review the entire paper in detail to check that the items conform to the specification, that there are no errors in the wording, that the keys are correct, and that the questions and any diagrams are correctly formatted. The paper is proofread for language and conformity with Cambridge Assessment's internal style guidelines. At each stage suggested changes are referred back to the chairs for checking and amendments made before the paper progresses to the next stage of checks.

A final version of the paper is scrutinised by academics from the institutions that use BMAT, who take the paper under timed conditions, and attend an extended meeting to discuss the test content and communicate any observations or issues from their experience. This engagement with the university academics is an important step in ensuring that the using institutions can give feedback on how the current paper aligns with the test construct and in maintaining the face validity of BMAT for test takers. Following this, papers are sent to externally contracted proofreaders who have not been involved in item writing or paper construction so far. Comments from this process are reviewed by Assessment Managers, who decide whether changes are made to the paper, before finalising the sections for print.

Figure 4.3 Question paper production process for Section 1

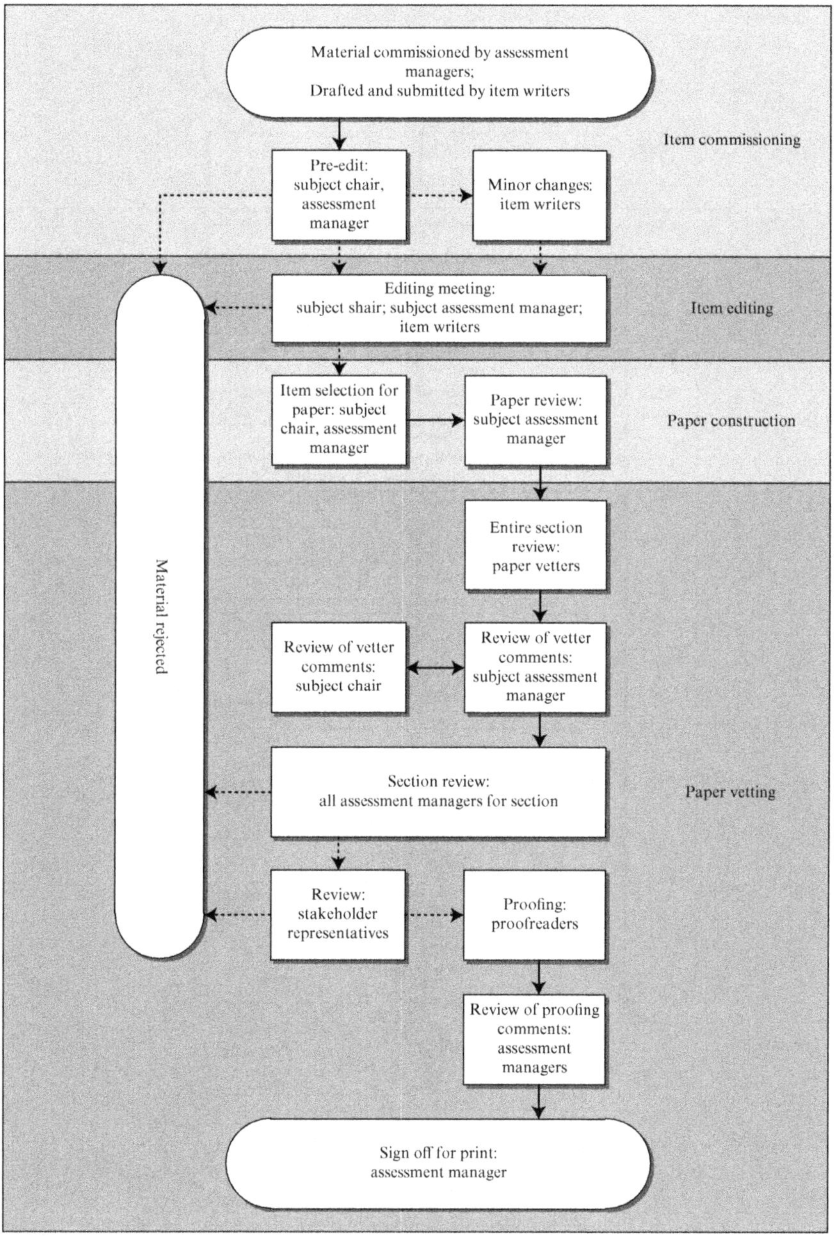
Material commissioned by assessment managers;
Drafted and submitted by item writers
Item commissioning
Pre-edit: subject chair, assessment manager
Minor changes: item writers
Editing meeting: subject shair; subject assessment manager; item writers
Item editing
Material rejected
Item selection for paper: subject chair, assessment manager
Paper review: subject assessment manager
Paper construction
Entire section review: paper vetters
Review of vetter comments: subject chair
Review of vetter comments: subject assessment manager
Section review: all assessment managers for section
Paper vetting
Review: stakeholder representatives
Proofing: proofreaders
Review of proofing comments: assessment managers
Sign off for print: assessment manager

Figure 4.4 Question paper production process for Section 2

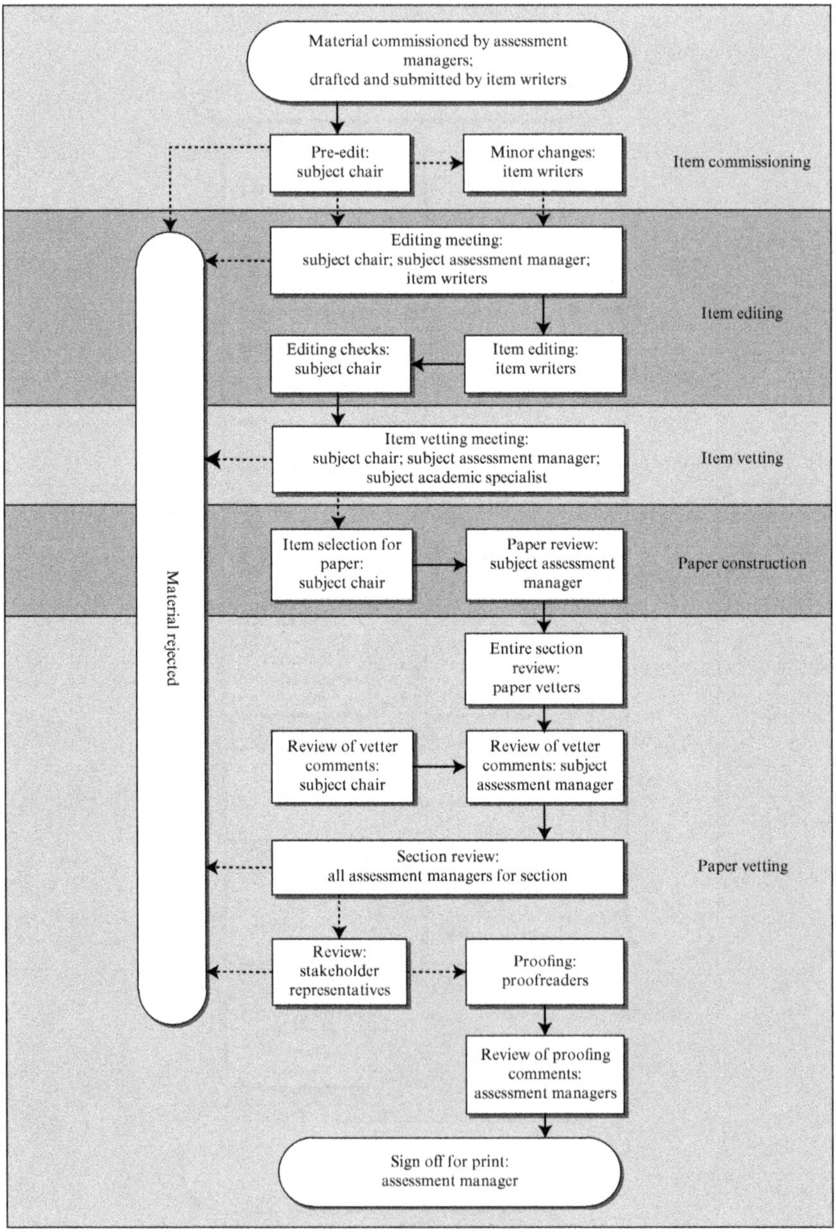

Figure 4.5 Question paper production process for Section 3

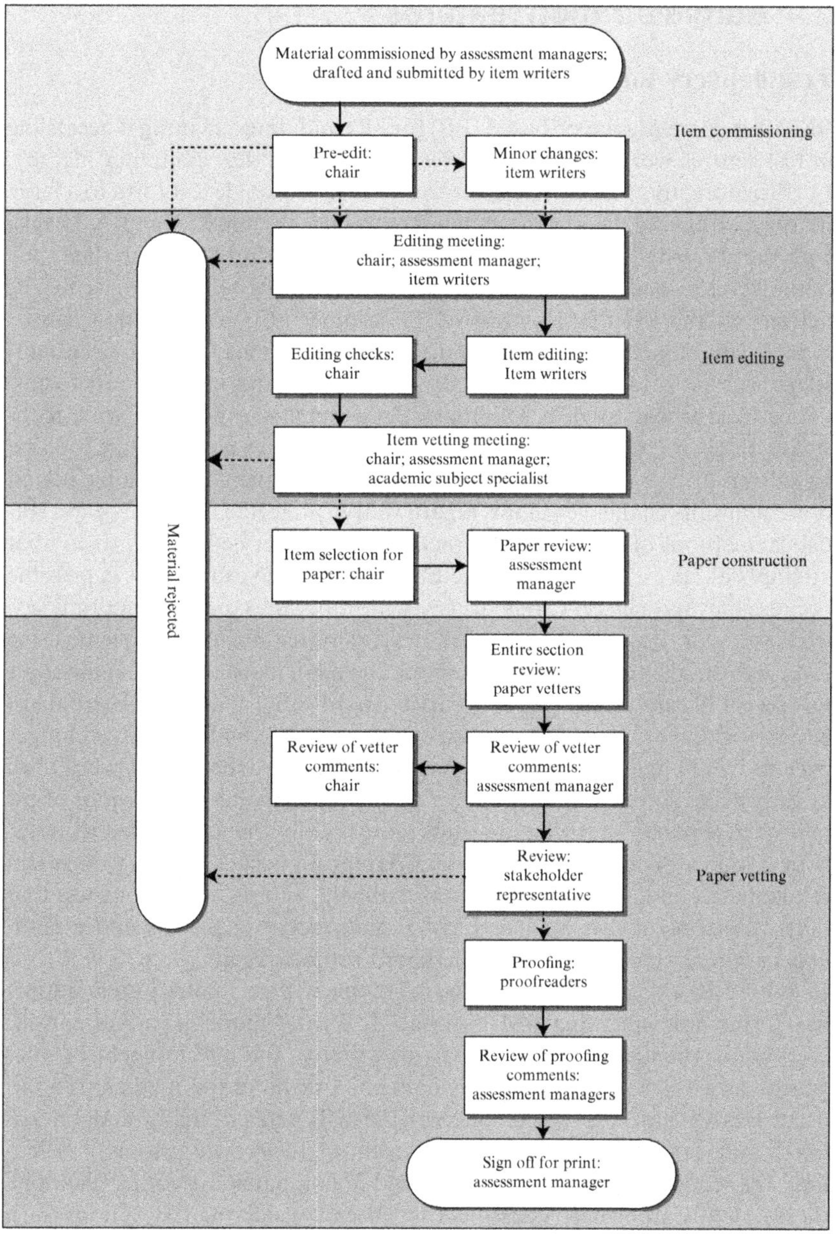
Material commissioned by assessment managers; drafted and submitted by item writers
Pre-edit: chair
Minor changes: item writers
Item commissioning
Editing meeting: chair; assessment manager; item writers
Editing checks: chair
Item editing: Item writers
Item editing
Item vetting meeting: chair; assessment manager; academic subject specialist
Material rejected
Item selection for paper: chair
Paper review: assessment manager
Paper construction
Entire section review: paper vetters
Review of vetter comments: chair
Review of vetter comments: assessment manager
Review: stakeholder representative
Paper vetting
Proofing: proofreaders
Review of proofing comments: assessment managers
Sign off for print: assessment manager

4.4 Cambridge Assessment practice: Administration features

Test delivery format

BMAT is currently paper-based (PB) for all candidates, making it accessible in test centres worldwide and unaffected by candidates' computer literacy. Furthermore, this makes it possible to administer a single test form to a large number of candidates on the same date, much like GCSEs and A Levels, with the majority of school-aged test takers completing BMAT in their own schools. At present, this would not be possible with computer-based (CB) delivery of the test due to limits in the number of computers that can be made available at the exact same time. CB would instead have to be administered across a longer time period, potentially using multiple test forms. From Cambridge English Language Assessment's experience with high-stakes English exams, we know that there are always some people looking to subvert the system. Testing windows that are open over a long period present unique challenges in this regard. Large pretested item banks and statistical methods of detecting malpractice are used very effectively to combat attempts at cheating in Cambridge English language exams; this is possible because they have larger candidatures than admissions tests and multiple sessions per year. Because these procedures are more difficult to implement for tests with smaller candidatures, it should be recognised that CB admissions testing could raise challenges to security. Specifically, a CB model would not allow every candidate to take the test on the same day, and testing over longer periods would require several test versions to be constructed as a precaution against malpractice. Furthermore, multiple language testing sessions allow malpractice panels to withhold results more readily when presented with statistical indicators of malpractice (see Chapter 5), because the test taker can retake the assessment when a result is withheld. For an admissions test that takes place once a year, such as BMAT, malpractice panels are understandably cautious when considering whether to withold results.

Whilst these security issues can be overcome with technology and multiple test forms, implementing BMAT in a CB format requires careful consideration of potential risks and threats to validity, and development of safeguards against malpractice in this context. Furthermore, medical schools using BMAT have expressed concerns that CB delivery might make it less likely that candidates could take the exam at their own schools, particularly for schools that are under-resourced in comparison to others. Despite these issues, Cambridge Assessment has been considering CB options for a number of years and consulted with BMAT stakeholders on the issue extensively. This is because CB testing has a range of advantages over PB delivery that should be recognised.

Firstly, the cost and logistical complexity of sending test papers is reduced using a CB format, and responses can be made available for operational analysis immediately. Currently with PB testing, secure delivery and return of test materials is a major undertaking that requires constant monitoring by operational teams. Secondly, contrary to the issues posed by item exposure discussed with CB admissions tests, some security issues are actually reduced when the testing organisation can control the timing of when test materials are made available more precisely, which can be achieved using technology. Currently, schools and test centres support examination boards by conforming to strict regulations governing the exam hall. Centres are instructed precisely about when packs of secure materials can be opened, to reduce the possibility that papers are exposed before a test session. Therefore, it is necessary for Cambridge Assessment to maintain a network of centre inspectors to quality assure the locations where BMAT is administered in PB form. Although CB testing would not eliminate the potential for institutional malpractice, it would likely reduce the risk from this particular threat.

The considerations outlined here are important for anyone involved in developing and delivering assessments, who might be interested in the advantages and disadvantages of PB and CB testing. It should be noted that the discussion presented here adopts the perspective of Cambridge Assessment, which is a large examining organisation that administers English exams and school-level qualifications around the world. This makes it possible to maintain inspection processes worldwide, whereas other organisations would find it difficult to accommodate this. Therefore, decisions on PB and CB assessment should include consideration of the resources available for supporting a programme of testing; this may include the financial, technological and technical assets that can be accessed readily.

Instructions to candidates

It is important that candidates can familiarise themselves with the structure of BMAT in advance so that on the test day itself their efforts are directed at performing well on the questions, rather than figuring out the format of the paper. The BMAT website provides candidates with all necessary information on the test timing, number of items, weighting of items and mark schemes, and provides sample test papers and response sheets for each test section. The mark scheme for the Writing Task is given on the BMAT website and is the same as that used by the markers themselves. This information also appears in the BMAT test specification document, which is available to candidates on the BMAT website.

In the testing situation itself, the test paper for each separate BMAT section has a front cover of instructions to candidates. The instructions state, in clear and concise terms, what candidates are required to do, the time limit, the number of items and the marks for each item (one mark for each MCQ item). For the Section 1 and 2 test papers, candidates are instructed to work quickly (in bold), that there are no penalties for incorrect responses and (therefore) that they should attempt all questions.

For the Section 3 test paper, the instructions encourage the development of ideas, macro-planning and organising. They indicate that candidates should develop, organise and communicate their ideas, and explicitly instruct test takers to spend time thinking carefully about what they need to say (see Box 4.3).

Box 4.3 Extract from instructions on BMAT Section 3 front cover

The tasks each provide an opportunity for you to show how well you can select, develop and organise ideas and communicate them effectively in writing.

Before you begin writing, take time to think carefully about what you need to say and the ways in which the organisation and layout of your response might help convey your message. Diagrams etc. may be used if they enhance communication.

Take care to show how well you can write and be concise, clear and accurate.

These instructions are designed to support context validity by explicitly providing guidance on test-taking behaviours that give test takers the best opportunities to perform well. Providing a reminder of these in the exam hall acknowledges that candidates can forget these considerations in the pressure of a high-stakes testing environment, even if they have prepared extensively for the test.

Consistency and security of testing conditions

Cambridge Assessment provides an extensive network of test centres offering BMAT to ensure that candidates should not have to travel long distances to take the test. By guaranteeing a high degree of access to the test, institutions using BMAT can extend their own commitment to ensuring equity in access to their courses.

All candidates worldwide take BMAT under strict examination conditions. For UK-based candidates the test centre is typically in their own school or college, which is usually already a registered Cambridge Assessment examination centre running regulated examinations such as GCSEs and A Levels. This is possible because Cambridge Assessment Group includes

Oxford Cambridge and RSA Examinations (OCR), which is one of the main awarding bodies for school-level qualifications in the UK. Overseas candidates can sit BMAT in their own school or college if it has been approved by Cambridge Assessment as a suitable centre for administering high-stakes tests; applications are accepted for the approval process throughout the year. In some cases, overseas schools will already be approved by Cambridge Assessment to administer qualifications provided by Cambridge International Examinations or Cambridge English Language Assessment. Alternatively candidates may sit the test at an 'open' centre, which accepts external candidates.

Centre approval and quality assurance processes

Institutions that apply to run BMAT go through a number of checks on their suitability including storage arrangements at the premises, the availability of suitably trained invigilators and supervisors to run the tests and the centre's experience of running high-stakes international assessments. Pre-approval checks are carried out using photographic evidence, face-to-face inspections or, for some applicant centres, a 'remote' inspection using video technology may be deployed. Each application is reviewed by a number of senior managers before a decision is taken as to whether or not to authorise the institution as a centre. If there are any concerns, the centre application is declined and the candidate is directed to an alternative centre.

All Cambridge Assessment centres are provided with standardised test administration regulations. The regulations for BMAT administration are stringent and intended to ensure the highest quality in the delivery of the test, covering the secure storage, checking and return of test materials. Seating plans are also mandatory for test sessions; these record where candidates were seated in the room and in relation to each other. They are used when investigating any suspected malpractice, particularly if statistical procedures identify unusual strings of matching responses (see Chapter 5 for details). Timetable clashes, access arrangements, special considerations and the reporting of suspected malpractice are also detailed in regulations. Centres must adhere to these regulations and centre inspections are carried out to ensure their compliance. Some examples of the issues covered by regulations are described in the next parts of this chapter.

Regulations for secure storage of test materials

The centre regulations set out in detail how to transport materials securely, how to check them when received, store them safely before the test date and when exactly it is permitted to open packets of test materials. The regulations include a clear instruction to centre staff that any breach of these conditions is treated extremely seriously. An extract from the regulations is presented in Box 4.4.

Box 4.4 Extract from the Instructions for Secure Administration of Admissions Tests

Test materials should be stored in a safe; however if that is not available, a non-portable, reinforced metal cabinet with a secure lock must be used. The safe or container must be situated in a locked room, preferably windowless and on an upper floor.

The availability of secure storage is checked as part of the centre approval process and also during centre inspections. This is important because materials sometimes arrive two to three days in advance of the test date. These materials are packed so that it is not possible to remove individual papers without substantial breaches to the packaging. Exams officers at centres are instructed to store the materials securely, without opening this packaging. Centre inspectors also check that these instructions are followed and a failure to do so would be considered a serious breach of regulations.

Checking the identity of candidates

Confirming that the person who takes the test is the same one who is registered for it and who receives the result is central to safeguarding the validity of test results. Stringent identity checks are also detailed as part of Cambridge Assessment's regulation documents, which specify that candidates need to produce 'an original photographic ID, for example, a passport, national identity card, photographic driving licence etc.'. These precautions are used to avoid the possibility of imposters taking a test in place of the genuine candidate.

Monitoring centres' compliance with regulations

Test centres are regularly monitored on the quality and compliance of test delivery. These inspections are carried out by trained inspectors who visit a test venue on the test day and observe the secure storage arrangements, checking of IDs and invigilation of the test, with the aim of ensuring compliance with the regulations in the *Instructions for Secure Administration of Admissions Tests* (Cambridge English 2014). Reports detailing the centres' performance, including recommendations for improvements, are produced after each inspection. An example report extract from a centre inspection is given in Box 4.5. The inspector visited the centre and observed the secure storage and invigilation arrangements, rating them as 'Fully compliant' (i.e. no faults).

Inspections do occasionally identify centres that do not meet the standards set by Cambridge Assessment Admissions Testing. Another example report extract from a centre inspection is given in Box 4.6, but this time, the centre was rated 'Unsatisfactory'. As shown in the extract, reports provide

Box 4.5 Report from an inspection of a UK centre – November 2013

Security arrangements at the school are excellent. The [storage] room has no windows, a solid and lockable door and a security 'grill' on the outside of the door. The room is also alarmed and exam/test materials are stored in locked metal containers that are bolted to the wall. There is also an area where papers can be sorted and processed on arrival and packaged up prior to being returned to exam boards.

The Exams Officer and her team are meticulous in the planning for each exam/test.

I was with the Exams Officer when she removed the papers from the security room and transported them to the invigilator. At no time during the whole session were the papers left unattended and they were opened in front of the candidates. When materials arrive at the centre they are checked immediately and locked away in the security room.

After the exams/tests have been completed they are stored according to the ATS instruction booklet.

The room had excellent light and was warm, well ventilated and quiet, very conducive to doing an exam.

feedback for the exam centre to act upon. Whilst inspections that identify unsatisfactory centres happen rarely, instances are taken seriously. Centres receiving this rating are referred for inspection again at the earliest opportunity, and failure to address concerns can result in withdrawal of a centre's eligibility to administer exams.

Cambridge Assessment is continually looking for ways to enhance the security and quality of examination delivery. Regulations are used to ensure BMAT is delivered as uniformly as possible around the world, and centre inspections are used to maintain these standards. While costly to maintain, these measures are essential for ensuring that candidates and other test users can have complete confidence in the consistency and fairness of the assessment.

These measures are proportionate to the scale and stakes involved in taking BMAT. For individuals designing bespoke assessments or class tests, the level of scrutiny outlined here might be considered excessive. However, even small-scale examinations can have very high stakes; in these contexts those designing assessments are advised to consider the security of their administration conditions carefully. In addition, the environment for administering any assessment should be evaluated, because this is easily overlooked even though it can impact on candidates' performances. For example, the

Box 4.6 Extracts from an inspection report – November 2016

After the test the exam scripts from the test room were transported to another exam room unsealed. The inspector also noticed that the materials were left in an office briefly before being transported for packing in another room. Please ensure that test materials are always sealed before leaving the test room; this is to ensure the materials cannot be tampered with or become lost or damaged in transit.

In an exam room, the invigilator was using a mobile phone to send messages, a tablet and a laptop during the test. The invigilator also briefly left the test room unsupervised whilst going out into the corridor to monitor noise levels. Invigilators must be attentive throughout the test and must not do any other activity in the test room, for example, reading a book or working on a laptop. Candidates should also never be left unsupervised, even for a brief period of time. Where there is only one invigilator present they must be able to get help easily, without leaving the test room.

temperature in a room and its dimensions can influence the comfort of test takers, particularly if the assessment is a long one.

4.5 Chapter summary

In this chapter we have outlined the factors that constitute the context validity of a test, focusing on the tasks and administration conditions that are considered when providing an admissions test such as BMAT. Many decisions related to the initial design of BMAT were informed by research evidence, such as the inclusion of both MCQs and constructed-response tasks in the test. Studies have also been conducted by Cambridge Assessment researchers to investigate specific aspects of BMAT, such as timing allocated to sections. Importantly, this research informed improvements to BMAT's specification and also to the processes that consider context validity in item production.

The processes used to govern BMAT item writing and test administration have also been described in detail as part of the present chapter. Our practice in this area strives to safeguard cognitive validity and make the experience of sitting BMAT as fair as possible to candidates, wherever in the world they may be taking it. Worldwide access to BMAT means that there are no exemptions to taking the test, and this is an important consideration for selecting institutions that wish to have a common measure on which to compare *all* their applicants. It is important for Cambridge Assessment to demonstrate the rigour of our processes to universities using BMAT and also to test takers, who should be confident that the testing conditions they face are controlled as far as practically possible. However, the detail included in this chapter also serves a second purpose. By outlining our approach and the issues we consider as a large examinations organisation, we hope to share experiences that are useful for those designing their own assessments. In many cases the resources available to smaller organisations will prevent the level of scrutiny outlined in the present chapter, but the examples should serve to demonstrate how context validity principles and questions posed by Weir (2005) can be applied in practice.

The present chapter has highlighted the emphasis on item and paper production that underlies BMAT, which can be considered part of *a priori* validation in Weir's (2005) framework, along with cognitive validity. Both context and cognitive validity are used to ensure that test design and production supports the ultimate goal of providing BMAT scores that are meaningful for the medical, veterinary and dentistry schools using the test to select applicants. The next chapter on scoring validity focuses more specifically on the meaningfulness of scores, and represents the first stage of *a posteriori* validation (Weir 2005).

Chapter 4 main points

- Context validity focuses on features of the tasks and features of the administration.
- For BMAT, Cambridge Assessment considers a wide range of issues that relate to task design, task construction and test administration.
- Different response formats have varying strengths and weaknesses; this can be addressed in assessments by including both MCQs and tasks requiring constructed responses.
- The exact processes used can differ depending on format, focus and scale of the test, but the underlying issues to consider can be applied to many assessment contexts.

5 Making scores meaningful: Evaluation and maintenance of scoring validity in BMAT

Mark Elliott

Cambridge Assessment Admissions Testing

Tom Gallacher

Research and Thought Leadership Group, Cambridge Assessment Admissions Testing

5.1 Introduction

Previous chapters have considered test taker characteristics, cognitive validity and context validity in relation to BMAT. This chapter concentrates on how aspects of scoring a candidate's responses to BMAT contribute to the test's validity, for both the multiple-choice Sections 1 and 2, and the constructed response marked for Section 3. We outline how 'reliability' is reconceptualised in Weir's (2005) socio-cognitive framework into scoring validity and applied to BMAT. Scoring validity is a wider evaluation of scoring issues than traditional approaches, which separate reliability from validity.

Careful examination of scoring validity sheds light on the operational analyses that are used to monitor BMAT sessions and the steps taken to ensure the integrity of results that are released to universities. Statistical methods are used in the monitoring of BMAT scores, which rely on psychometric models and established forms of evaluation. In particular, data from the sections containing multiple-choice questions (MCQs) is used to calculate statistics that inform test development and evaluation. As psychometric theories underlie the statistics presented and the scoring of MCQ items in BMAT, overviews of Classical Test Theory (CTT) and Rasch analysis are presented to contextualise the discussion of scoring validity in BMAT Sections 1 and 2. Although the issues discussed throughout this chapter necessitate use of statistical terminology, we have kept this to a minimum by describing theories conceptually rather than in technical detail. A more critical examination of these concepts is beyond the scope of this volume and there are many seminal texts that include more nuanced evaluations of these theories (e.g. Andrich 2004, DeVellis 2012, Lord and Novick 1968, Mellenbergh 2011, Rasch 1960/1980).

Instead, the focus of this chapter is on answering questions posed by scoring validity. BMAT's MCQ sections and scoring of BMAT Section 3 are addressed separately, as many of the questions are specific to the scoring of responses in each format. First, we will outline scoring validity as conceptualised by Weir (2005) and further developed by others in language testing (e.g. Geranpayeh 2013, O'Sullivan and Weir 2011), before applying this concept to BMAT.

5.2 Scoring validity and its importance in assessment

Scoring validity 'concerns the extent to which test results are *stable over time, consistent in terms of the content sampling,* and *free from bias*' (Weir 2005:23, emphasis in original) – in other words, do the measurement properties and scoring make the candidate's results useful in decision making? Some of these aspects are traditionally (e.g. Lado 1961:31) referred to as 'reliability', and are often discussed alongside a narrow conceptualisation of validity that deals with the aspects covered in other chapters of this volume. Departing from this traditional model, the socio-cognitive framework follows the arguments made by Messick (1989), and conceptualises reliability as part of scoring validity, which is a facet of overall validity. Validity is a property of the inferences drawn from test scores, not a property of the testing instrument in isolation. Therefore, anything that impacts upon the inferences that can be made with a test affects its validity. Scores have limited use when a test is not reliable, while it is equally difficult to draw meaningful inferences from a test that is reliable but does not sample the theorised construct adequately. Within this modern paradigm of validity, a test must demonstrate acceptable levels of 'reliability' as a component of its validity argument. By conceptualising reliability as part of validity rather than a separate characteristic of the assessment, it is not acceptable to argue that a test's shortcomings in either validity or reliability are a consequence of a focus on the other aspect.

Weir's (2005) original conceptualisation of the socio-cognitive framework presented scoring validity as an alternative term for reliability, by extending the traditional approach focused on internal consistency and statistical coefficients, to include marker reliability. Weir included aspects such as rater selection, rater characteristics, the development of criteria/rating scales, the rating process, rating conditions, rater training, rater standardisation and moderation, grading and awarding in the scoring part of his validity framework (see also Shaw and Weir (2007), which presents a fuller treatment of these). In addition to the reliability of the test, scoring validity has thus been expanded to cover other scoring-related test aspects which affect the usefulness of inferences drawn from test scores. For example, Geranpayeh (2013) includes the topics of test difficulty, item discrimination and item bias in discussion of scoring validity in Cambridge English Listening exams. These are key issues to consider when evaluating how MCQs, such as those in BMAT Sections 1 and 2, are scored. The scoring validity component within the socio-cognitive validation framework can be used to pose specific questions for Sections 1 and 2 of BMAT, as follows:

- Are items of appropriate difficulty and do they discriminate between candidates?
- Is there a sufficient level of test reliability?
- Is there any evidence of item bias?
- Do the responses being scored come from the candidate?

For the scoring of written tasks, such as those in BMAT Section 3, a range of other issues must be considered as part of scoring validity, to ensure that examiner marking is free from error (Shaw and Weir 2007):

- Are there clearly defined marking criteria that cover the construct?
- Are markers trained, standardised, checked and moderated?
- Is marking reliable and consistent?

We will now consider each of these questions in turn, in terms of why the question is important for test validity arguments, how they can be answered, and the degree to which BMAT answers that question, before summarising the key issues and concerns. In the following discussion, we consider the scoring validity issues relevant to MCQ sections of BMAT.

5.3 Scoring validity in MCQ sections of BMAT

Psychometric theories such as Classical Test Theory (CTT) and Rasch modelling are commonly used for scoring tests with MCQ items. These theories also provide the basis for statistics that are used to evaluate the performance of tests and items. An outline of these theories is presented in the next two sections to contextualise the statistical coefficients presented later in the chapter, and to provide a summary of how Sections 1 and 2 are scored.

Classical Test Theory

CTT is a psychometric theory widely used across most, if not all, areas of applied scale development, evaluation and assessment research (Devellis 2012). While the technical details of CTT will be familiar to many working in test development and validation, a conceptual summary is useful for those less familiar with the theory. The following overview of CTT is adapted from an unpublished doctoral thesis (Cheung 2014); therefore, portions are similar to the conceptual descriptions provided in that text.

CTT conceptually defines the way that a test response for any item or set of items should be interpreted; this response is known as an observed score, which can be the score for a single item, combined items, or an entire test. Novick (1966:1) specifies CTT as the theory that 'postulates the existence of a true score, that error scores are uncorrelated with each other and with true scores and that observed, true and error scores are linearly related'. This definition specifies that any observed item score is composed of the true score, which represents their ability in the trait being tested, and measurement error, which represents the combination of all non-trait related elements which can affect a candidate's test score (for example fatigue, carelessness and lucky guesses). Mathematically presented this refers to the premise that for each item:

$$X = T + \varepsilon$$

(Where X = the candidate's observed score, T = the candidate's true score and ε = error.)

In its strictest form, CTT assumes that error scores are random across items and not correlated with each other, so the error associated with each individual item has a mean of zero across a large sample of responses (DeVellis 2012). In addition, the errors are not correlated with the observed score or the latent true score. By definition, this latent score is unobservable; therefore, the degree of error associated with item responses is estimated using the concept of parallel tests, by treating each item, or set of items, as a mathematically equivalent measure of the same trait. These concepts are particularly important for calculating estimates of reliability, and they also underpin indicators of difficulty and discrimination (how well the item differentiates between test takers of low and high ability). CTT analysis is conducted immediately after a BMAT session; often on a number of occasions as increasing volumes of test data become available.

However, CTT has some limitations when applied to test data. One issue arises from the assumption of equal errors across items and respondents. This is unlikely for any test or given testing situation, because the error associated with each item will be different for each respondent (Hambleton, Swaminathan and Rogers 1991). For example, a test administered to a specified sample would include multiple items that vary in difficulty. Taking two items from a test, we could describe one of them as easy to answer correctly and the other one comparatively difficult. Each of these items has associated error that is not fixed across all of the test takers, because the degree of error varies dependent on the ability of the respondent. The easier question will be more useful for discriminating between those of low and mid ability, whereas the more difficult question would more accurately discriminate between those of mid and high ability. Therefore, the amount of error due to guessing is not randomly distributed. Many CTT-based coefficients do not account for these differences and conceptualise error using assumptions that are unlikely to be met precisely in applied testing situations.

Another shortcoming of CTT analyses is that statistics from this framework are descriptive and sample dependent. Therefore they only provide information on how a particular cohort of candidates performed on a particular occasion. The theoretical and practical limitations of CTT have been overcome by complementing CTT analysis with statistics based on a different test theory, known as Item Response Theory (IRT). Cambridge Assessment Admissions Testing uses a specific version of IRT known as Rasch modelling (Rasch, 1960/1980) to score BMAT Sections 1 and 2.

Rasch analysis

The Rasch model (Rasch 1960/1980) is a probabilistic model in which the likelihood of a candidate responding correctly to an item is a function of the difference between the candidate's ability and the *item difficulty*; ability and difficulty are placed on the same scale in units called *logits*. The relationship between ability and the probability of a correct response to a dichotomous item is shown in Figure 5.1, which depicts an *item characteristic curve* (ICC). All Rasch ICCs are parallel, with ICCs for more difficult items located higher (i.e. to the right) along the x axis.

Figure 5.1 Rasch item characteristic curve (ICC)

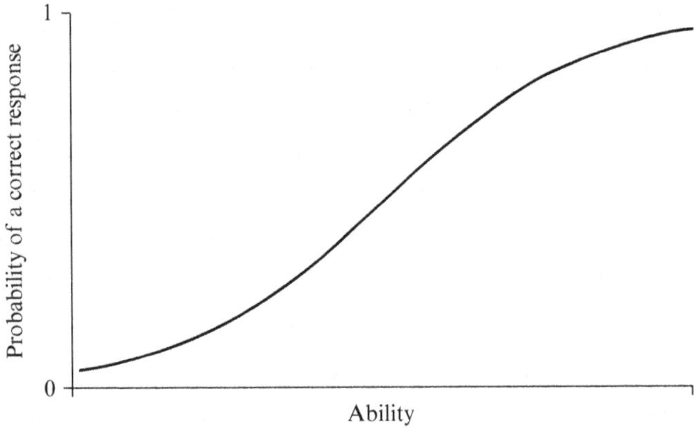

The Rasch model represents an idealised measurement model which carries the properties of fundamental measurement in the physical sciences, in particular that 'a comparison between two individuals should be independent of which particular stimuli within the class considered were instrumental for the comparison; and it should also be independent of which other individuals were also compared, on the same or some other occasion' (Rasch 1961:332); in other words, unlike CTT, the Rasch model is sample independent within the parameters of a specified class of items and a specified population – a property known as *specific invariance*. A mathematical feature of the model is that it is possible to condition out person abilities when calculating item difficulty estimates, and vice versa – there is separation of persons and items.

Whereas CTT operates at test level, Rasch analysis focuses at item level, and generates a linear measurement scale. Rasch has advantages over CTT because its results are generalisable beyond the specific test administration, due to the separation of persons and items within the model. Therefore, Rasch-based indicators of item performance, unlike CTT statistics, are not tied to the specific administration of the test from which they were calculated. However, Rasch-based statistics do not supersede CTT ones in operational analysis of BMAT; instead, Rasch- and CTT-based figures are evaluated by data analysts and validation managers as providing complementary information on test performance.

Scoring BMAT MCQ sections

Scores for BMAT Sections 1 and 2 are calculated using the Rasch model. The reported scores are Rasch candidate ability estimates scaled via a linear transformation and reported to one decimal place on a scale that goes from 1.0 to 9.0.

When reporting scores, test providers are concerned with maintaining standards across different versions of the test. For high-stakes testing, using the same test repeatedly is not an option and the test provider must create different forms of the test that are as similar to each other as possible. In language testing, assessments are often benchmarked against external descriptors of language proficiency, such as the Common European Framework of Reference for Languages (CEFR, Council of Europe 2001). In contrast, admissions tests are primarily used to make comparisons within a single cohort of test takers, so the equivalence of BMAT scores between different test years is not a primary concern for selecting institutions. However, it is still necessary to maintain a relatively stable standard from one year to the next for an admissions test. Also, successful applicants may defer their university place for a year and so candidates from two consecutive BMAT test cohorts could be found in a particular *entry* cohort.

Comparability of BMAT scores from consecutive test years is therefore necessary for carrying out predictive validity work within a particular entrant cohort. This comparability is achieved by calibrating scores on the live test cohort using Rasch analysis and then benchmarking them to a subset of the cohort that is regarded as stable in ability. The scaling sets an approximate mean of 5.0 for the subset; scores are capped upwards at 9 and downwards at 1. The scaling ensures that reported test results are comparable within a cohort, with equal intervals in BMAT scale scores representing equal differences in candidate ability. Benchmarking against a stable applicant group allows scores from different sessions to be treated as approximately comparable. However, more precise comparability of test scores is desirable to allow BMAT scores to be used across different test sessions; therefore, Cambridge Assessment Admissions Testing researchers are actively investigating methods of test equating suitable for a high-stakes medical admissions test such as BMAT. This work draws on Cambridge English Language Assessment's expertise in item banking and applying Rasch analysis for test-equating procedures. In addition, relevant experts across Cambridge Assessment's group of exam boards have advised on developments related to scoring; some of the investigations are discussed in the next part.

Developments in scoring BMAT Sections 1 and 2

Recent trials conducted by Cambridge Assessment researchers have explored methods of statistical equating and methods that use expert judgement (e.g. Bramley and Oates 2011) for MCQ sections of BMAT. Rigorous equating methods that allow precise comparability, such as those used with Cambridge English exams, can be achieved by including pretested items when constructing live papers, or by sharing items across sessions. The Cambridge Assessment approach to English language item banking includes anchored pretesting of items, which harnesses the properties of the Rasch model to equate items. Pretesting is a step where candidates that represent the live cohort complete items of known difficulty, referred to as anchor items, along with items whose difficulty is not known; the new items are calibrated through Rasch analysis, using the anchor items to place them on a standardised scale. This produces a bank of pretested items that are available for test construction.

Cambridge English's pretesting model relies on administering items to appropriate cohorts outside of live testing situations. This model has not been applied to BMAT, and while it would provide benefits to test equating across live administrations (contributing to 'parallel forms reliability'), these methods have associated logistical challenges and security issues that need careful consideration before operational deployment. There are some differences between the language testing and admissions testing contexts that influence the viability of pretesting, particularly for a narrowly defined group, such as applicants to study medicine and dentistry. Given these considerations, a range of approaches have been trialled and a number of robust options have been identified. Initially, more than one method will be introduced so that they can be evaluated in parallel. Although this may not be sustainable in the long term, it will provide an evidence base that will allow reliance on a single method of calibrating BMAT scores in the future.

In addition to equating tests and producing scores, psychometric principles are used to analyse test sections that include MCQs. These analyses are employed to evaluate scoring validity of BMAT as part of operational processes, and are outlined throughout the rest of the chapter.

Are items of appropriate difficulty and do they discriminate between candidates?

A test comprised of items which are too difficult or too easy for a candidature will not function well in differentiating between candidates since the scores will be too similar – nearly all correct for an easy test and nearly all incorrect for a hard test. Items need to be of an appropriate difficulty to give a range of scores that reflect the range of abilities within a candidature. If BMAT gave a pass/fail criterion mark based on demonstrating or not demonstrating a fixed level of ability, the most appropriate range of difficulties would be narrowly centred around this level of ability. But since BMAT scores are used by multiple institutions with interests in a range of ability estimates, BMAT questions need to reflect a range of difficulties.

BMAT item writers consider the intended level of test taker abilities when they author items but can naturally never be certain of how difficult their items are until they are taken by real candidates. Basic summary statistics that describe the distribution of scores – the mean and standard deviation – can show whether the overall difficulty of the test was appropriate. If the mean number of items correct is low, it indicates a paper that is too difficult for the candidature and vice versa if the mean is too high. If the standard deviation of scores is too small, then a suitable range of abilities has not been captured.

From a CTT perspective, *item facility* is a statistic that reflects simply the proportion of a candidature that gets an item correct; the higher this value, the easier the item.

$$Item\ facility = \frac{N_{correct}}{N_{total}}$$

(Where $N_{correct}$ is the number of candidates getting the item correct, and N_{total} is the total number of candidates attempting the item.)

Item writers generally intend that 50–60% of their target candidates will get each item correct. As a general rule, items with facility values below 0.1 and above 0.9 are deemed too difficult and too easy respectively to add scoring validity to a test. That is, items cannot discriminate well among candidates if either a very low or very high proportion of candidates get that item correct.

Two items or fewer out of the 62 used in BMAT November 2016, 2015 and 2014 live administrations were outside of the ranges of 0.1 to 0.9, with mean item facilities of 0.47, 0.48 and 0.52 respectively. This indicates how BMAT items are consistently set at appropriate difficulty levels for the cohorts.

From a Rasch perspective, item difficulties need to map reasonably closely to candidate abilities in order to maximise precision of the test for the candidature. By plotting histograms of the distributions of candidate ability estimates and contrasting these with histograms of the distributions of item difficulty estimates, one can visually inspect the appropriateness of a set of items for a set of candidate abilities. Figure 5.2 and Figure 5.3 illustrate the spread of abilities of candidates ('PERSONS': above the line), and the difficulties of the items ('ITEMS': below the line) drawn from a Rasch analysis of BMAT Sections 1 and 2 from November 2016. These confirm that the items were set at appropriate difficulty levels for the cohort. CTT and Rasch analyses of difficulty are routinely used to train item writers in estimating the difficulty of newly authored items.

Figure 5.2 Item difficulty and person ability estimates from BMAT Section 1, November 2016

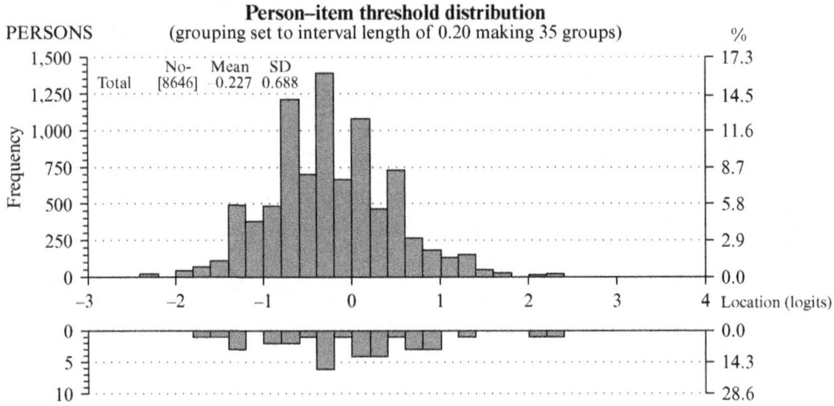

Figure 5.3 Item difficulty and person ability estimates from BMAT Section 2, November 2016

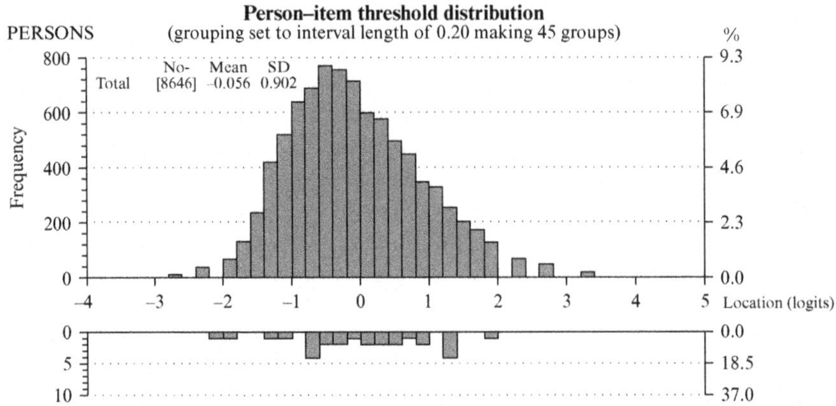

Having covered difficulty, we now turn to *discrimination* of the test items, which refers to how well the items differentiate between test takers with high ability and those with low ability. One simple CTT measure, the *discrimination index*, involves dividing the cohort into three groups (high performers, medium performers and low performers) based on their total score on that paper, then calculating the difference between the facility of each item for the high-scoring group and the low-scoring group. Discrimination index values range from 1 (perfect discrimination) to -1 (perfect negative discrimination). If the discrimination index is too low, it indicates that the item does not discriminate well between candidates among the cohort. Typically, discrimination index values should be 0.3 or higher.

A more sophisticated CTT index, the *point-biserial correlation*, represents the correlation between a candidate's overall test score, and the likelihood of choosing one of the responses. This approach conceptualises the overall test score as an indicator of the candidate's ability. Candidates with higher overall scores will be expected to choose the correct response more often and the incorrect distractor responses less often, compared with those test takers who have lower abilities. The most important point-biserial correlation is therefore the correct response, for which point-biserial values less than 0.25 generally indicate poorly discriminating items. Poor discrimination can be a result of extreme facility values – items which are answered correctly or incorrectly by nearly all candidates naturally cannot discriminate effectively – but can also occur if an item does not assess the same ability as the other items in the set.

As well as a test of the quality of the items in a test, the point-biserial index also forms a key part of the quality assurance process during BMAT marking as a means of checking the correctness of the answer key. All items in BMAT Sections 1 and 2 are multiple-choice format, and any distractor options that have a higher point-biserial correlation than the correct option are flagged for scrutiny, since this may indicate that the given key is incorrect (the flagged option is chosen more often as ability increases, and more so than the given key).

Discrimination is treated somewhat differently in a Rasch analysis; one starts with the premise that all items discriminate, and tests this assumption against the data. Therefore, discrimination is conceptualised as an issue of how well the observed data fits the Rasch model. Figure 5.4 demonstrates the principles of an item where the Rasch model fits the data well. Along the x axis is the 'person' ability estimate in logits, and along the y axis is the expected probability that a candidate will get an item correct. As the ability estimate increases (to the right), the likelihood of that candidate answering the item correctly increases (up). The line represents the theoretical ICC and each black dot represents a group of candidates with similar abilities. For an item for which the Rasch curve is found to fit, the dots for each group should be on or close to the line of the theoretical curve.

Figure 5.4 Item characteristic curve for an item with good fit

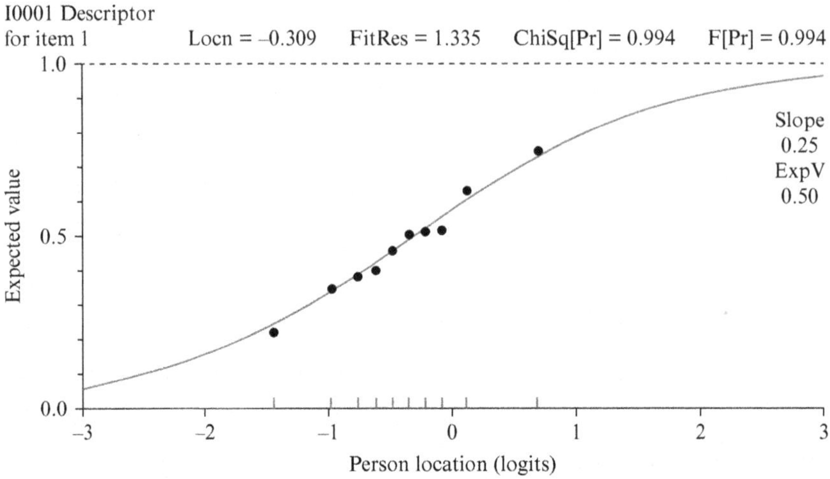

For a BMAT session, ICCs are plotted for a visual inspection of each item's fit. Easier items will have lower difficulty estimates, and the ICC will appear to the left, to indicate that groups of candidates with lower abilities are expected to achieve the correct response. Harder items will have higher difficulty estimates, shifting the curve to the right, indicating that only the higher ability candidates are expected to get the item correct.

The degree of divergence between the dots and the line is reported as a mean square statistic for each item, which has a corresponding chi-square and probability value indicating whether the divergence is significantly different from zero. These form the basis for model fit statistics that are also used to establish each item's degree of misfit, and the nature of any issues that are detected. Different types of misfit can provide diagnostic information for BMAT assessment managers and item writers to review as part of question paper production procedures.

Is there a sufficient level of test reliability?

The concept of reliability in a test relates to the stability of test scores. Theoretically, a test with perfect reliability would result in a candidate achieving an identical score every time they took the test, because the score would represent the true ability of the candidate, free from any sources of error. Of course, this hypothetical ideal is not achievable in practice, rendering the premise untestable because this conceptualisation relies on the candidates' abilities remaining precisely stable across administrations of the test. Therefore, reliability of a test is estimated from the consistency of scores for the same candidate, either between different administrations of a test (test–retest reliability) or within a test (internal consistency).

Test–retest reliability

Test–retest reliability involves the administration of the same form of a test to a sample of candidates on two separate occasions and correlating the scores obtained from the two administrations. This method of estimating reliability has several drawbacks (Ebel and Frisbie 1991:81–82), in particular, the restriction to one form does not reflect variation in items across different forms of the test, and candidates are seeing the same items for a second time, so the responses during the second administration will inevitably be influenced by the first due to memory, meaning that the two administrations are not independent. If the time interval between the two administrations is too great, a process of additional learning or attrition is likely to change the candidates' ability, reducing the validity of the comparison. To date, no test–retest reliability studies have been carried out on BMAT.

Parallel form/equivalent form reliability

Parallel form reliability involves administering two different forms of a test in immediate succession to a sample of candidates and correlating the scores. In order to be considered *parallel forms*, not only must the tests be constructed to the same specifications but the scores on the two tests must have the same mean and standard deviation; otherwise, the two forms are referred to as *equivalent forms*.

To date, no studies on parallel forms or equivalent forms have been carried out on BMAT; this is a possible area for future research, although it can be considered to overlap to a large extent with *internal consistency*, as described in the next section. Data does exist, however, on candidates who have taken BMAT in successive years, which can be considered an example of equivalent form reliability. The usefulness of this data, however, is limited under the administration of BMAT, since candidates only have one opportunity per year to achieve scores. Over the course of a year a number of things might change for each candidate to affect their ability, such as the candidate's level of knowledge or motivation being different across application cycles. As a result, we would not expect a candidate's performance to be the same a year later – the candidate should not be expected to have the same level of ability, meaning that few, if any, meaningful inferences can be drawn from the data.

Internal consistency

The internal consistency of a single administration of a fixed-format multi-item test is usually measured by *Cronbach's alpha* (Cronbach 1951), which focuses on the homogeneity of the responses to items within a test administration. Conceptually, it is the mean of all possible split-half correlations, which are the correlations of candidate scores on two halves of the items in a test – this can be viewed as a version of equivalent form reliability where the two equivalent forms are constructed from the two halves of a single test. Mathematically, Cronbach's alpha represents a conceptualisation of reliability as the proportion of variance in observed scores which is accounted for by variance in true scores, with the remaining variance accounted for by error:

$$\rho_{XX} = \frac{\sigma_T^2}{\sigma_X^2}$$

(Where ρ_{XX} = reliability, σ^2_T = variance of true scores, σ^2_X = variance of observed scores.)

This figure cannot be calculated directly in practice, however, since true scores cannot be known. As an estimate, the proportion of variance of the total scores comprised of the covariance of items, corrected for bias in the estimator for variance (Bol'shev 2001), is used; the standard formula for calculating Cronbach's alpha is:

$$\alpha = \frac{N}{N-1}\left(1 - \frac{\sum_{1=1}^{N} \sigma_i^2}{\sigma_X^2}\right)$$

(Where N = number of items in the test, σ^2_i = variance of scores on item i (for dichotomous items, this is simply $p(1-p)$, where p = item facility), σ^2_X = variance of scores on the whole test.)

Cronbach's alpha statistics tell us about the scores on an administration of a test, but they are sample dependent; in particular, they are affected by the spread of abilities in the candidature, as well as the number of items, and are sensitive to violations of unidimensionality (Andrich 2009b:3). Assuming that the amount of error in the test remains constant, an increase in the range of ability of the candidature will result in an increase in the variance of the observed scores and a higher alpha. As a result, a higher or lower Cronbach's alpha may be a function of the candidature rather than the items in the test, meaning that there are limits on the interpretation of alpha. Nonetheless, it remains a useful measure to compare two administrations of a test with a stable candidature across time. A related CTT statistic which has less sample dependence than Cronbach's alpha is the *Standard Error of Measurement* (SEM), which represents a standard deviation of the error present in the test. As such, the SEM can be used to construct confidence intervals around test scores. The SEM of a set of items can be calculated by the following formula:

$$SEM = \sigma\sqrt{1-r}$$

(Where σ = standard deviation of raw scores, r = Cronbach's alpha.)

Table 5.1 shows the Cronbach's alpha and SEM figures for BMAT for the period 2012–16, based on analyses of the cohort applying to the University of Cambridge, which represents a consistent, relatively stable cohort and thus renders year-on-year comparisons more valid.

Table 5.1 Cronbach's alphas and SEMs for BMAT 2012–16

Year	Cronbach's alpha		SEM	
	Section 1	Section 2	Section 1	Section 2
2012	0.55	0.63	2.57	2.28
2013	0.61	0.57	2.61	2.34
2014	0.71	0.79	2.53	2.12
2015	0.70	0.80	2.58	2.26
2016	0.72	0.79	2.63	2.25

As can be seen in Table 5.1, the majority of internal consistency estimates have been above 0.70 for BMAT Sections 1 and 2, particularly in recent years. This is in the lower range of coefficients considered acceptable; however, the use of internal consistency estimates as evidence of test quality is problematic because a number of factors impact on these values. In fact, Cronbach himself expressed dissatisfaction with over-zealous application of his alpha in scale evaluation (Cronbach and Shavelson 2004). Other researchers have expressed similar concerns that alpha is not always the best indicator of reliability, particularly when multidimensionality is observed in test responses (Sjitsma 2009, Zinbarg, Revelle, Yovel and Li 2005). Given that BMAT Section 1 is designed to assess three specified thinking skills, and Section 2 includes knowledge from four subject disciplines, some degree of multidimensionality in these sections is inevitable. However, the broad domain coverage of these sections is an important feature of the test that contributes to the cognitive validity of BMAT. Although estimates of internal consistency could be improved by making BMAT sections more unidimensional, this would be detrimental to the quality of inferences that could be made based on the test (Zumbo and Rupp 2004).

Another way of improving internal consistency would be to increase the number of responses marked in the test sections by increasing the number of items. This would either increase the testing time, or reduce the time available for each item, which would have knock-on effects for the context validity of BMAT (see Chapter 4 for a discussion of speededness within BMAT), or indeed the practicality of administering BMAT. Due to the limitations of Cronbach's alpha, SEM values should be inspected when considering internal consistency. Because score standard deviation is included in the calculation of SEMs, they are less susceptible to sample dependence; therefore, SEMs can be regarded as more useful reflections of test reliability (Tighe,

McManus, Dewhurst, Chis and Mucklow 2010). The SEM values for BMAT are in line with other MCQ tests of similar length, although the Section 1 values suggest there is some room for these to be improved on the basis of 35 items. The Cronbach's alpha values reported in Table 5.1 dip below 0.60 in two cases and progressively improve for more recent years, whereas the SEM values are relatively consistent throughout, which is encouraging.

One issue to note is that some biomedical schools using BMAT aggregate Section 1 and Section 2 scores to provide a composite score based on all 62 items across these sections. When based on multiple sets of items, rather than a single set, internal consistency can be higher purely as a function of the greater number of items included. For example, composite alphas calculated across all 62 items for the most recent test sessions were 0.83 (2016) and 0.81 (for both 2015 and 2014). This is within the acceptable range for similar tests, indicating that combined aggregates of the sections have good internal consistency. However, the values should be interpreted with caution because Cronbach's alpha is calculated on the basis that individual items contribute to an overall score equally. This is not the case when Rasch scaled scores for the two sections are aggregated together; therefore, these values are merely a rough indicator of the improved internal consistency when scores are calculated using a larger number of items.

In the language testing context, Cambridge English has historically adopted a construct validity approach to developing examinations, unlike other exam boards more heavily influenced by the US psychometric tradition, such as the Educational Testing Service (ETS). Weir (2005:31) describes the focus on internal consistency forms of reliability as 'a fetish with internal consistency among the professional testing fraternity' and points out that very high internal consistency may not be an appropriate aim for tests that seek to evaluate complex and multi-faceted constructs. Over a decade ago, Weir also observed that ETS was acknowledging context validity more readily in the Test of English as a Foreign Language (TOEFL) than they had in the past. Interestingly, a similar change is currently happening in admissions testing contexts, as the SAT has recently been redesigned to have a greater focus on content and learning than has previously been the case (College Board 2015).

Given the narrow ability range of the candidature, the number of test items and, importantly, the broad domain coverage of Sections 1 and 2, the internal consistency of the test sections is acceptable, and respectable when aggregating Sections 1 and 2 together. The reliability of the test sections is routinely monitored in analysis alongside other features, such as item bias, which is evaluated using the procedures described in the following portion of this chapter.

Is there any evidence of item bias?

A test may be considered biased when it produces *systematic* differential performance among test takers of comparable ability on the construct, but who differ on a non-test-related dimension (e.g. in terms of age, gender, race and ethnicity, or physical disability). Bias is a clear threat to test score validity because it prevents the conclusion that ability estimates reflect only the relevant and desired constructs. The BMAT test construction process mitigates bias in test items through the avoidance of culturally bound or sensitive topics and words; however, empirical analysis can still flag individual items that have produced inconsistent performance across different subgroups of test takers. Differential Item Functioning (DIF) analyses (Holland and Thayer 1988, Holland and Wainer (Eds) 1993) can be used to monitor evidence of bias by gender and by school type.

DIF analysis formalises the question of bias by asking whether candidates in a 'focal group', who are indicated to be different on a non-test-related dimension such as gender or school type, have the same probability of getting an item correct in comparison with candidates in a 'reference group' while controlling for ability. The total test score is treated as an indicator of candidate ability for these procedures, which have been employed by Cambridge Assessment researchers with BMAT. An example of this work is presented as a key study below.

Key study – Investigating item bias in BMAT using DIF analysis (Emery and Khalid 2013a)

In the study described here the BMAT performance of different candidate groups (male versus female, independent versus state school) was investigated at the individual item level using the Mantel-Haenszel (MH) procedure (Mantel and Haenszel 1959). The aim was to look for any evidence of DIF in BMAT items by gender and by school sector over multiple years of the test.

Research question

Is there any evidence of DIF by gender or by school sector in BMAT Sections 1 and 2?

Data collection

Candidate-level information (gender and centre number) was matched to BMAT item-level data for test years 2010, 2011 and 2012 (whole cohorts). School type was matched to candidates' centre number (as outlined in Chapter 2). All UK school types other than 'independent' and 'other' were classed as belonging to the state sector. The data of candidates from non-UK schools and those from UK school type 'other' were omitted from school sector analyses. All candidates were included in the gender analyses (see Table 5.2).

Analysis

DIF analyses were carried out using the MH statistical procedure (Holland and Thayer 1988), which uses ability matching by treating the observed total

Table 5.2 Sample sizes for DIF analysis

BMAT year	Gender analysis (N)	School sector analysis (N)
2010	6,225	4,633
2011	6,230	4,681
2012	7,044	4,556

test score as a criterion. In this case, BMAT Section 1 score was used as the criterion for Section 1 items and BMAT Section 2 score was used as the criterion for Section 2 items in each test year. The MH procedure compares the odds of getting the item correct for the reference and focal groups at a given level of ability.

For gender analyses the reference group was defined as male and the focal group as female. For school sector analyses the reference group was defined as independent sector and the focal group as state sector. The following guidelines (Zwick and Ercikan 1989) were used to evaluate the DIF effect size:

- type A items – negligible DIF/functioning properly: items with |delta value| < 1
- type B items – moderate DIF: items with |delta value| between 1 and 1.5
- type C items – large DIF: items with |delta value| > 1.5.

A negative delta value indicates that the item favours the reference group over the focal group and a positive delta value indicates that the item favours the focal group over the reference group. Delta value thresholds of 1.0 and 1.5 (or -1.0 and -1.5) are equivalent to odds ratios greater than 1.53 (or less than 0.65) and greater than 1.89 (or less than 0.53), respectively. Type A items are considered to function properly but type B and C items require necessary revision and action (Holland and Thayer 1988, Zwick and Ercikan 1989).

Results and discussion

Figure 5.5 and Figure 5.6 display example DIF statistics by gender for BMAT Sections 1 and 2 in the 2012 test. The 2012 figures are presented here as these contained the larger delta values found in the study. No delta value in any of these test years was greater than 1 (or less than -1), indicating no instance of DIF by gender. Additionally, there was no gender pattern evident in the delta values by either item position in the paper or item type (e.g. biology, physics). Four items (out of 186) across all three test years had delta values approaching 1 or -1. These were further scrutinised and were found to belong to a mixture of item subtypes.

Figure 5.5 DIF statistics by gender for BMAT 2012 (Section 1) items*

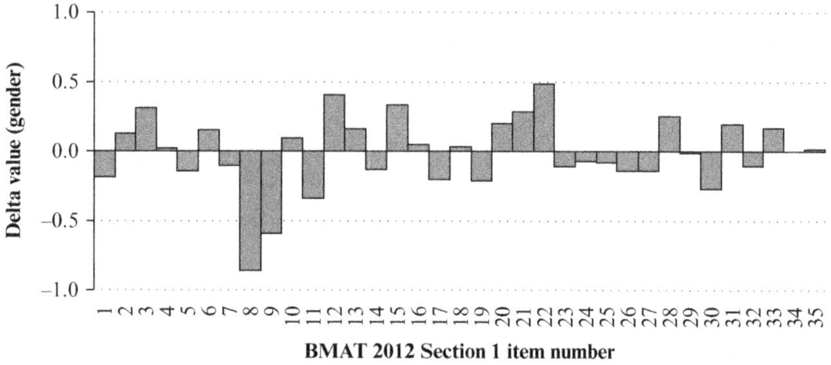

**A positive delta value indicates that the item favours the focal group (females); a negative delta value indicates that the item favours the reference group (males); delta values 1 to 1.5 = moderate DIF; delta values >1.5 = large DIF.*

Figure 5.6 DIF statistics by gender for BMAT 2012 (Section 2) items*

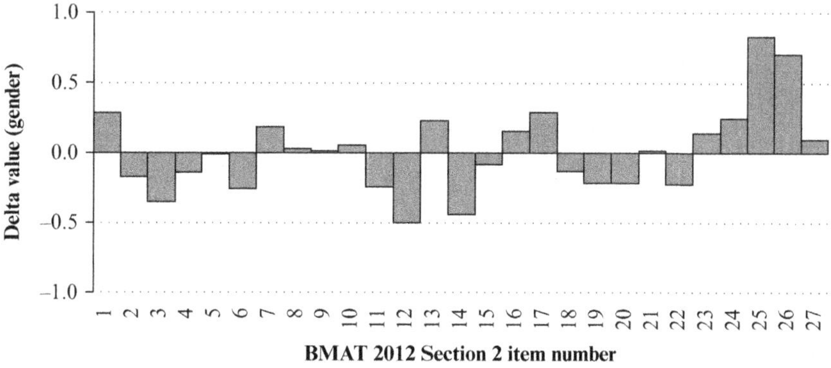

**A positive delta value indicates that the item favours the focal group (females); a negative delta value indicates that the item favours the reference group (males); delta values 1 to 1.5 = moderate DIF; delta values >1.5 = large DIF.*

Figure 5.7 and Figure 5.8 display DIF statistics by school sector for BMAT Sections 1 and 2 in the 2012 test. As for gender, no DIF was evident by school sector in any of these test years (no delta value was greater than 1 or less than -1). Again, no pattern in delta values was evident by either item position or item type and very few items in the school sector analyses yielded delta values in excess of 0.5. A single item across all three test years had a delta value close to 1. This was a mathematics question in BMAT 2012 (item 24 in Figure 5.8), which trended towards favouring state school candidates.

Figure 5.7 DIF statistics by UK school sector for BMAT 2012 (Section 1) items*

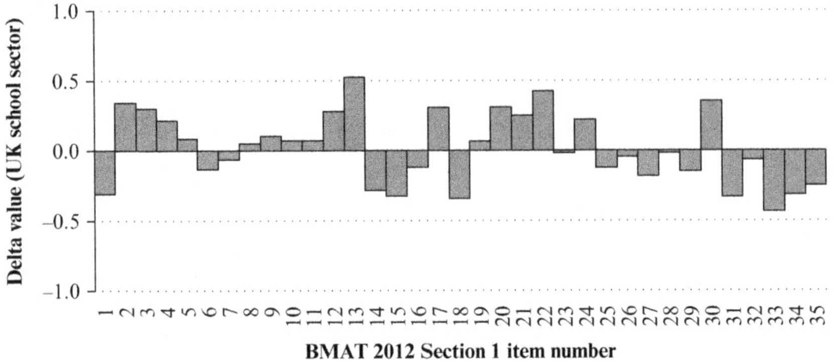

**A positive delta value indicates that the item favours the focal group (state); a negative delta value indicates that the item favours the reference group (independent); delta values 1 to 1.5 = moderate DIF; delta values >1.5 = large DIF.*

Figure 5.8 DIF statistics by UK school sector for BMAT 2012 (Section 2) items*

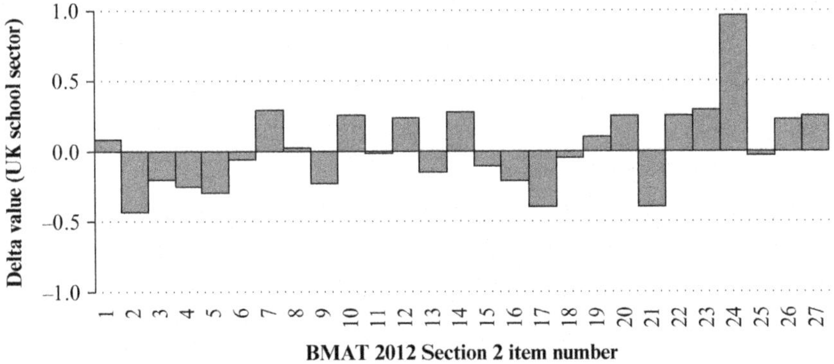

**A positive delta value indicates that the item favours the focal group (state); a negative delta value indicates that the item favours the reference group (independent); delta values 1 to 1.5 = moderate DIF; delta values >1.5 = large DIF.*

In these three years of BMAT data there was no evidence of DIF by gender or by UK school sector using the MH procedure. Emery and Khalid's (2013a) study informed current Cambridge Assessment practices, which include DIF analyses of BMAT as part of routine operational procedures.

However, the contemporary approach uses more advanced Rasch-based procedures, which are outlined briefly in the next section.

Current Cambridge Assessment practice: Item bias

In Rasch terms, DIF analysis tests whether an item has a significantly different difficulty estimate when treated as two separate items, one for each group (Andrich 2009a, Linacre 2016, Thissen, Steinberg and Wainer 1993). That is to say that for any given ability, one group would have a lower proportion of correct responses than the other. This would manifest in ICCs with two separate lines when plotting observed scores for response categories, as illustrated in Figure 5.9. When the ICCs for two groups are plotted parallel to each other side by side, the group represented by the curve on the right found the item more difficult than the group represented by the curve on the left. This indicates that a person of the same overall ability had a different probability of answering the item correctly, associated with their membership of a particular group.

Figure 5.9 Example ICC for an item exhibiting DIF

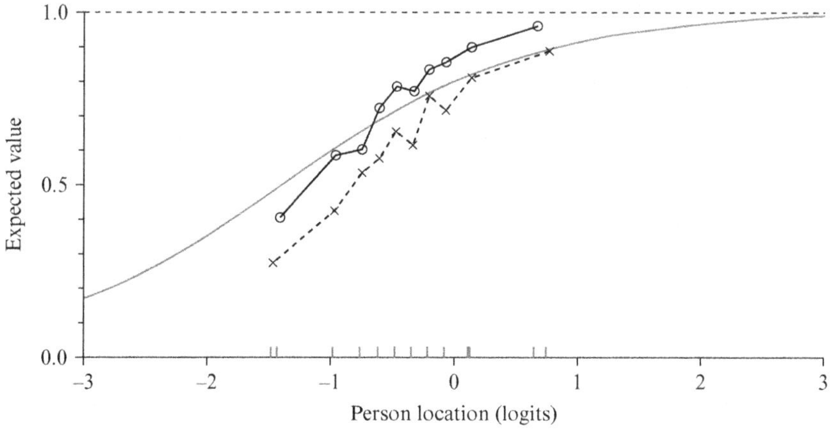

Examining each item in a test sequentially can identify items whose content might be related to the non-test-related dimension, potentially indicating bias in the items identified. Criteria for flagging items displaying different degrees of DIF were developed by Zwick, Thayer and Lewis (1999) based on the MH method, with Rasch-based equivalences outlined by Linacre (2016:422). These criteria are predicated on the detected DIF being both statistically significant and substantive in terms of its magnitude; under Linacre's criteria, an item is deemed to display moderate to large DIF (i.e. potentially be a cause for concern) if the magnitude of the DIF is at least 0.64

logits and a significance test on the magnitude of the DIF being 0.43 logits or greater is significant at p = 0.05. Here, 0.43 and 0.64 logits equate to MH measures of 1 and 2 δ units respectively, based on an equivalence of 1 logit = 2.35 δ units. A significant DIF result does not automatically indicate that an item is unfair, but it does represent grounds for qualitative investigation by subject experts.

The operational DIF analyses of BMAT November sessions covering the period 2013–16 investigating DIF by gender (male versus female) and school type (state versus independent) were reviewed. They produced three items out of a total of 186 displaying moderate DIF. Items with negligible DIF were balanced between those slightly favouring males and those slightly favouring females. Similarly, items were equally balanced between those slightly favouring independent school candidates and those slightly favouring state school candidates (all with negligible DIF). Assessment managers checked the content of all items flagged at these levels to confirm that there were no task features that give an advantage to one group over another. These analyses are conducted immediately following a test session as part of BMAT's quality assurance procedures.

Are the candidates' responses their own?

Measures such as reliability, error and dimensionality are only meaningful if candidates' test scores reflect their ability in the trait under investigation, and are not the result of issues such as pre-exposure to test items or collusion – in other words, that the integrity of the test is preserved. Ensuring that items are not pre-exposed is a question of test material security, and relates mainly to administrative factors. These issues are discussed in Chapter 4 as contextual features of BMAT's administration. Detecting collusion and copying, on the other hand, is a task that statistical analysis contributes to, alongside monitoring of test centres.

Once BMAT MCQs have been scored, a statistical analysis of candidates' response strings is conducted to identify cases with unusually strong patterns of common wrong answers (instances where pairs of candidates have both chosen the same incorrect option for an item) using Angoff's (1974) A index, following standardised procedures (Bell 2015, Geranpayeh 2014). Angoff's A index compares the proportion of common wrong answers between each pair of candidates relative to their overall score, against the pattern observed across the whole candidature; high indices indicate a greater degree of similarity than that observed between other pairs, which may indicate that collusion or copying has occurred. Often, detection of unusual patterns coincides with reports of unusual activity from exam invigilators. The results of statistical analysis are not treated as definitive proof of malpractice, but rather as an indicator; any cases which are flagged from this check are referred to a malpractice panel for scrutiny, which consists of a senior manager from each of three divisions[1] with some responsibility for BMAT. They are joined by one representative from the biomedical or dentistry departments using BMAT and another Cambridge Assessment colleague who is not involved in the development of admissions tests. The panel reviews the results of statistical analysis on a case-by-case basis, alongside other information, such as seating plans and reports from the exams officers at test centres. In some cases, statements are requested from the candidates and further investigations are conducted to gather information, before final decisions on whether to withhold results are made.

5.4 Scoring validity in BMAT Section 3

Are there clearly defined marking criteria that cover the construct?

BMAT Section 3 responses are marked by two markers against the criteria presented in Table 5.3. Scripts are identified only by BMAT number and candidate initials, so markers are blind to demographic information about the candidate. Each marker gives two scores to each response: one for quality of content (on a scale of 0–5) and one for quality of written English (on the scale A, C, E). Candidates have access to the Writing Task marking criteria on the BMAT website.

In arriving at their scores, markers are instructed to consider whether the candidate has:

- Addressed the question in the way demanded?
- Organised their thoughts clearly?
- Used their general knowledge and opinions appropriately?
- Expressed themselves clearly using concise, compelling and correct English?

The marking criteria against which markers judge the essays are presented in Table 5.3.

Prior to 2010, Writing Task responses were given a single, holistic score that reflected the overall quality of the response. The marking criteria incorporated both the content and the quality of written English descriptors above. The mark scheme was altered in 2010, at the request of stakeholder universities, over concerns that some markers may give more weight than others to quality of written English. The new mark scheme was trialled before its first use (Shannon and Scorey 2010) to ensure that examiners were able to apply it as well as the previous scheme, using a re-marking of a sample of scripts from the live 2009 test.

---

1 These are Assessment; Validation and Data Services; and Stakeholder Relations.

Table 5.3 BMAT Section 3 marking criteria

Quality of content

Score	Criteria
5	An excellent answer with no significant weaknesses. ALL aspects of the question are addressed, making excellent use of the material and generating an excellent counter proposition or argument. The argument is cogent. Ideas are expressed in a clear and logical way, considering a breadth of relevant points and leading to a compelling synthesis or conclusion.
4	A good answer with few weaknesses. ALL aspects of the question are addressed, making good use of the material and generating a good counter proposition or argument. The argument is rational. Ideas are expressed and arranged in a coherent way, with a balanced consideration of the proposition and counter proposition.
3	A reasonably well-argued answer that addresses ALL aspects of the question, making reasonable use of the material provided and generating a reasonable counter proposition or argument. The argument is relatively rational. There may be some weakness in the force of the argument or the coherence of the ideas, or some aspect of the argument may have been overlooked.
2	An answer that addresses most of the components of the question and is arranged in a reasonably logical way. There may be significant elements of confusion in the argument. The candidate may misconstrue certain important aspects of the main proposition or its implication or may provide an unconvincing or weak counter proposition.
1	An answer that has some bearing on the question but which does not address the question in the way demanded, is incoherent or unfocused.
0	An answer judged to be irrelevant, trivial, unintelligible or missing will be given a score of 0.

Quality of written English

Band	Criteria
A	Good use of English. Fluent. Good sentence structure. Good use of vocabulary. Sound use of grammar. Good spelling and punctuation. Few slips or errors.
C	Reasonably clear use of English. There may be some weakness in the effectiveness of the English. Reasonably fluent/not difficult to read. Simple/unambiguous sentence structure. Fair range and appropriate use of vocabulary. Acceptable grammar. Reasonable spelling and punctuation. Some slips/errors.
E	Rather weak use of English. Hesitant fluency/not easy to follow at times. Some flawed sentence structure/paragraphing. Limited range of vocabulary. Faulty grammar. Regular spelling/punctuation errors. Regular and frequent slips or errors.
X	A response that is judged to be below the level of an E will receive an X.

The double marks for each response are combined as follows to give the final mark for each candidate. If the two marks for quality of content are the same or no more than one mark apart on the scale, the candidate is awarded the average of the two marks. If the two marks for quality of written English are the same or no more than one mark apart on the scale, the scores are combined like this: AA = A, AC = B, CC = C, CE = D and EE = E. For example, a response given a 4C by one examiner and 4A by the other will get a final score of 4B. A response given 3C by one examiner and 2C by the other will receive a mark of 2.5C.

If there is a larger discrepancy in the marks for either scale then the response is blind-marked for a third time by an experienced marker. The third marker considers only the scale on which the initial discrepancy occurred. If the third mark is the same as, or adjacent to, either of the first two marks then the mean of those two marks is reported. Where the third mark is equally spaced between the first two marks then the mean of all three marks (i.e. the third mark) is reported. All responses awarded a 0 for quality of content or an X for quality of written English are reviewed by an assessment manager to establish whether it deserved such a low mark.

In addition to the Writing Task scores, a scanned image of the response is supplied to the applicant's institution(s). This image provides institutions with a basis for further qualitative assessment of the applicant's writing skills as well as a potential tool for promoting discussion at interview.

Are markers trained, standardised, checked and moderated?

All examiners are recruited based on qualifications (with a minimum of a degree or equivalent), as well as skills and experience set out by recruitment guides appropriate for the level of examiner seniority. More experienced senior examiners are responsible for groups of markers, so the most experienced markers lead those who are less experienced. The more experienced examiners, such as Principal Examiners, are also involved in training more junior ones alongside assessment managers. This approach is informed by studies showing that differences between scores awarded by experienced and inexperienced markers can be reduced through training and standardisation (e.g. Weigle 1999).

New potential markers are required to engage in a ranking exercise. After reading the marking criteria applicants are given eight scripts covering the full range of marks. They are asked to rank these in order of quality of content and to assign a mark on a 3-point scale for quality of English. The aim is to verify that the marker is able to judge the relative quality of responses, although they are not expected to accurately apply the marking criteria at this stage. Assessment managers and Principal Examiners recruit the marking team based on whether potential markers' rankings deviate significantly from what is expected, but also based on interviews.

Marker training and standardisation

Recruited markers attend a compulsory training and standardisation day each year, where markers read through the information available to candidates, the marking criteria and an extract from the official BMAT preparation book, *Preparing for the BMAT* (Shannon (Ed) 2010). Mark schemes have been shown to have a standardising effect on the scores awarded by examiners (Furneaux and Rignall 2000), so the mark scheme for Section 3 is emphasised throughout these sessions, and markers are required to familiarise themselves with it as part of their training. Markers then sit the Writing Task paper under normal test conditions. The markers' own papers are shared out for marking followed by a brief discussion to reflect on the experience of writing their response, and to raise any queries about the application of the marking criteria. These group exercises are used because writing examiners learn mark schemes from their peers and contemporaries (Weigle 1994).

Following the BMAT test session, experienced assessment managers review a large number of scripts to identify examples of candidates' writing that match particular points in the mark scale, both in terms of quality of content and quality of English. The aim is to put together two sets of scripts that contain a representative spread of quality, and for which there is close agreement in terms of the marks that each script should be awarded.

As iterative standardisation has been shown to improve marker reliability (Furneaux and Rignall 2000), two rounds of standardisation exercises are used to prepare markers before marking of live papers begins. First, all markers mark the same four scripts covering a range a quality. Marks are collated and, for each script, a discussion is held of the marks awarded and how these relate to the mark scheme. Where necessary, guidance is given on the interpretation and application of the marking criteria. Another standardisation exercise then requires all markers to mark the same eight scripts. These scripts are chosen to represent a range of quality but include some that may prove difficult to mark (for example, responses where it might be questioned whether the candidate has addressed all of the demands of the question). Again, marks are collated and a discussion held on how they relate to the mark scheme, with any further necessary guidance given.

Marker checking and monitoring

During the live marking period, markers work in teams located together on the same table, led by a Team Leader. These teams are mixed regularly to include experienced markers alongside those who are less experienced. First, second and third marking is all done 'blind' where markers are unaware of the marks given by other markers. Markers take a script, write their marker number on the script, and record marks awarded on a separate sheet. Another marker will take another script and do the same, while yet others might provide second or third marks, and progress the scripts along trays located on the table, indicating the stage of marking. Principal Examiners and Team Leaders submit an evaluation of examiners, indicating the degree of their satisfaction.

Marker behaviour is also monitored statistically, using a 'means model' technique devised by Bell, Bramley, Claessen and Raikes (2007). The mark distribution (mean and standard deviation) of each individual marker is compared to that of the whole group to flag suspected severity, leniency and variability. This method of live marker monitoring assumes that scripts are assigned to markers at random and that, once a minimum number have been marked, we would expect the average mark they award and its standard deviation to be approximately the same as those of all other markers. Markers whose mean score is much lower or higher than others might be exhibiting harshness or leniency, whilst their standard deviation reveals erraticism or, conversely, their failure to use the whole mark range. An assessment manager from Cambridge Assessment oversees this process and answers any queries about the interpretation and application of the mark scheme.

The assessment manager also gives feedback to markers who are flagged, and to markers who are frequently involved in double-marking disagreements. Where there are concerns about a marker's performance, the marker can be dismissed and their scripts re-marked. A feedback session is held at the end of each marking day to address any remaining issues, but markers are not provided information on their marking distributions. There is some evidence that continuous standardisation and feedback can result in a see-saw effect as markers attempt to over adjust (Shaw 2002); therefore, the monitoring for BMAT Section 3 is designed so that assessment managers can control the flow of feedback provided.

From 2017 onwards, Principal Examiners also deal with results enquiries received after results have been released. These were historically marked by the chief examiner for BMAT Section 3, who is always a member of staff from one of the medical or dental schools using BMAT. In the event of an appeal following completion of the results enquiry process, the chief examiner for BMAT Section 3 evaluates all of the previously awarded grades alongside the submission. This arrangement remains unchanged.

Is marking reliable and consistent?

With regard to the consistency of scoring for BMAT Section 3, the *Standards* (2014) make it clear that, since the responses are scored with subjective judgement, evidence should be provided on both *inter-rater consistency* in scoring and (if applicable) *within-examiner consistency* over repeated measurements. In order to unpack that idea we can talk about the need for human markers to be consistent in two different ways: each marker needs to be internally consistent, i.e. given a particular quality of performance, a marker needs to award the same mark whenever this quality appears (*intra-rater reliability*); there also needs to be consistency of marking between markers, i.e. one marker will award the same mark to a constructed response as another marker when confronted with a performance of the same quality (*inter-rater reliability*).

Following the marking period, the level of agreement between the first and second marks is calculated using cross-tabulations, frequencies of mark differences and the percentage of responses that required a third mark. An example cross-tabulation is provided in Table 5.4 and Table 5.5, for BMAT 2015.

Table 5.4 BMAT November 2015 Section 3 marker agreement: Quality of content*

Quality of content		Marker 2						Total
		0	1	2	3	4	5	
Marker 1	0	0	0	0	0	0	0	0
	1	0	64	65	3	0	0	132
	2	0	46	1,087	801	29	1	1,964
	3	0	2	756	3,221	840	9	4,828
	4	0	0	10	858	875	88	1,831
	5	0	0	0	7	95	76	178
Total		0	112	1,918	4,890	1,839	174	8,933

* *59.6% exact agreement (dark shading), 99.3% within one score band (light and dark shading).*

Table 5.5 BMAT November 2015 Section 3 marker agreement: Quality of English*

Quality of English		Marker 2				Total
		X	E	C	A	
Marker 1	X	0	0	0	0	0
	E	0	30	65	4	99
	C	0	46	647	818	1,511
	A	0	7	702	6,613	7,322
Total		0	83	1,414	7,435	8,932

* *81.6% exact agreement (dark shading), 99.9% within one score band (light and dark shading).*

Multi-faceted Rasch analysis (Linacre 2014) is an extension of the Rasch model that can, in addition to person ability and item difficulty, account for additional facets that are seen in scoring that involves judgement. In the case of BMAT Section 3, an analysis was conducted using 2016 data, covering the following facets: 1) candidate ability; 2) marker leniency/severity; and 3) marking criteria (quality of English and quality of content). Among other things, the analysis provides estimates of markers' relative leniency/severity to identify problematic markers, as well as measures of marker consistency.

The multi-faceted Rasch model for BMAT Section 3 exhibited good model fit, explaining over 87% of the variance. Test takers were reliably separated into three strata. As candidates are marked on a 5-point scale in this section of BMAT, one might expect that candidates would be divided into more strata. That they are only separated into just three strata can be explained by the strong BMAT cohort not generally getting scores at the bottom of the scale, as can be seen in Table 5.5.

Quality of markers' marking was generally good. In terms of severity and leniency, markers showed acceptable levels of variation, with the most severe and lenient markers deviating from the mean by less than a quarter of a score point. Only a small number of markers (six of 88) had an infit mean square above 1.5, indicating that the vast majority of markers were marking consistently (Bond and Fox 2001). For the small number of cases where markers are shown to not mark consistently, the findings of these analyses are provided to assessment managers, who provide further training and additional supervision during future marking sessions. If a marker is erratic in their awarding of marks, the assessment manager can decide to dismiss them or exclude them from future marking exercises.

The appeals process allows candidates a re-mark of any section of their BMAT paper. For example, in the November 2015 administration of BMAT, 448 sections were re-marked, with slightly more requests for Section 3 than Sections 1 or 2. After the re-marks for Sections 1 and 2 there were no amendments to the scores from those issued, and nine amendments to Section 3 marks, one of which led to a change greater than one point: the re-mark resulted in a decrease of 1.5 marks in the candidate's quality of content score. The outcomes of the appeals process help to confirm the scoring is valid, but the process also reassures candidates that the mark they receive is the most accurate reflection of their performance that is possible.

5.5 Chapter summary

In this chapter we have answered questions that derive from Weir's (2005) socio-cognitive framework in terms of the scoring validity of BMAT Sections 1, 2 and 3. This was achieved by describing the core analyses that form part of the BMAT yearly cycle, and by presenting results from additional investigations into BMAT's scoring validity. We have also shown how statistics from CTT and Rasch analysis can inform our understanding of test scores, and the importance of understanding the strengths and weaknesses of these models.

Although this chapter emphasises the technical aspects of test validity, it has also presented a critical evaluation of the role that statistical analysis plays in monitoring of a test such as BMAT. Whilst the questions addressed by scoring validity are important, evaluation of the answers in a meaningful way is not possible unless other aspects of validity are considered. Therefore, the methods presented in this chapter and the coefficients they produce should be considered as tools that enable validity to be investigated fully. Many of the statistics outlined favour longer tests with simple items that assess a restricted and simple construct. A test with good fit, discrimination and reliability could be constructed by identifying a simple discriminating item and posing it to test takers repeatedly in slightly different, but many, forms. This approach would certainly be easier and less resource intensive than the production processes outlined in the previous chapter on context validity. However, it would be difficult to favourably judge the construct coverage and theoretical rationale for an admissions test produced in this way. Furthermore, an approach focused on improving psychometric coefficients cannot produce an assessment that satisfactorily evaluates the ability to develop complex arguments.

Cambridge Assessment Admissions Testing's approach, much like that of Cambridge English Language Assessment, is to consider scoring validity alongside other aspects of test validity; this guards against reliably assessing a construct that is not valid or fit for purpose. In particular, test developers have a responsibility to consider scoring validity alongside the rationale for assessing targeted constructs (cognitive validity) and the social impact of bias in assessment (consequential validity), which cannot be achieved without an understanding of the test taker characteristics in a candidature. Weir's (2005) observation that scoring validity is essential, but not sufficient, for presenting an overall validity argument certainly applies to the admissions testing context. In the following chapter, another topic crucial to overall validity of an admissions test is explored – that of criterion-related validity.

Chapter 5 main points

- Coefficients calculated on Sections 1 and 2 of BMAT indicate acceptable levels of psychometric quality.
- Section 3 is assessed by two markers, and Rasch analysis is used to provide evidence of scoring validity for Section 3.
- Statistics can also support detection of malpractice within test cohorts.
- Statistics based on CTT and Rasch analysis can be useful tools for investigating scoring validity of an assessment.
- Commonly reported statistics have specific limitations and weaknesses that should be considered when interpreting them in relation to tests.

6 The relationship between test scores and other measures of performance

Molly Fyfe
Research and Thought Leadership Group, Cambridge Assessment Admissions Testing
Amy Devine
Research and Thought Leadership Group, Cambridge Assessment Admissions Testing
Joanne Emery
Consultant, Cambridge Assessment Admissions Testing

6.1 Introduction

This chapter deals with an aspect of validity that is commonly researched in the admissions testing context: criterion-related validity. Criterion-related validation aims to demonstrate that test scores are systematically related to another indicator or outcome ('criterion') that is relevant to the construct measured by the test. It asks how strongly the criterion of interest is related to scores on the test, and is usually investigated using statistics that indicate the strength of relationships, such as correlation and regression.[1]

Weir's (2005) framework conceptualises two types of criterion-related validity: concurrent and predictive. Concurrent validity seeks to establish a relationship between two or more measures of the same ability that are administered at the same time, where the assessment being evaluated is one of the measures. For example, a medical licensing exam given at the end of medical school would be expected to correlate with other robust measures of clinical performance, and relationships between these variables would be taken as evidence of concurrent validity.

1 Positive correlation coefficients can range from 0 to 1, with higher numbers indicating a stronger relationship between the assessment and the criterion variable. In the context of selection, coefficients above $r = 0$ .35 are considered very useful, while those below $r = 0.3$ are considered moderately useful, and below $r = 0.1$ as weak (Cleland et al 2012).

Box 6.1 Definition of criterion

The criterion variable is a measure of some attribute or outcome that is operationally distinct from the test. Thus, the test is not a measure of the criterion, but rather is a measure hypothesized as a potential predictor of that targeted criterion.

(*Standards* 2014:17)

Predictive validity seeks to establish a relationship between scores from an assessment and a measure of future performance. The criterion variable used to evaluate the assessment typically becomes available after the test has been administered. Criteria used for predictive validity tend to be measures of different, but theoretically related, constructs to the one represented by a test score. They are often outcomes of interest for reasons other than test validation. In the context of admissions tests, criterion variables used in predictive studies tend to be ones that indicate academic success at university. As admissions tests are used to infer an applicant's potential to be successful in their studies, predictive validity is a particularly important aspect of validity in selection contexts.

For selection tests such as BMAT, fitness for purpose is closely bound with the question of whether test scores differentiate between candidates in a way that relates to their future performance. Selection tests and other selection criteria are forms of 'predictive assessment' (James and Hawkins 2004:241) in that they aim to assess *potential* for a future course of study or job role. According to a previous edition of the *Standards* (1985:11), 'predictive studies are frequently, but not always, preferable to concurrent studies of selection tests for education or employment' whereas 'concurrent evidence is usually preferable for achievement tests, tests used for certification, diagnostic clinical tests, or for tests used as measures of a specified construct'. Establishing good predictive validity is often seen as the holy grail of admissions tests and it is generally accepted that predictive studies should be conducted with selection assessments. Indeed, the published research on validity of admissions tests within medical education has largely focused on investigating the relationship between test scores and measures of future course performance (e.g. Emery and Bell 2009, Emery et al 2011, McManus, Dewberry, Nicholson and Dowell 2013, McManus, Dewberry, Nicholson, Dowell, Woolf and Potts 2013).

The emphasis on predictive validity is greater in admissions testing than it is in language testing. Despite this, Weir's (2005) socio-cognitive framework developed in language testing is useful for framing the criterion-related validity of admissions tests such as BMAT. In the opening chapter of this volume, Saville used the framework to pose the following questions in relation to criterion validity:

- Do test scores relate to other tests or measurements? (concurrent validity)
- Do test scores relate to future outcomes? (predictive validity)

When carrying out studies of criterion-related validity, it is important to acknowledge that longitudinal studies of predictive validity can be more practically difficult to conduct than concurrent studies, and are also more susceptible to influence from confounding variables. Weir (2005:209) points out that 'predictive validity is, however, in general beset with problems because of the variables that may interfere with the comparison over time'. In addition to the challenges of tracking test takers over time, the ways that a test is used can impact greatly on the availability of data, resulting in complications when conducting statistical analysis (see Box 6.2 for examples); these issues will be discussed in depth later in the chapter.

In this chapter we present studies on criterion validity of BMAT conducted by Cambridge Assessment researchers, in light of issues highlighted by Weir's (2005) socio-cognitive framework. In addition, we draw on work conducted in other selection contexts, such as occupational psychology, to outline some of the challenges facing admissions testing researchers. The focus is primarily on predictive validity, although a discussion of relevant concurrent validity considerations is included. To provide a clear picture of the issues, the present chapter begins with a non-technical description of the theoretical and methodological issues related to criterion validity. For each of the topics discussed, Cambridge Assessment's approach to them with BMAT is described. Following this discussion, a key study is described in detail and the findings of other studies are summarised briefly.

6.2 Key issues for investigating criterion-related validity of BMAT

There is a clear rationale for establishing criterion-related validity of educational assessments used in selection contexts (Anastasi and Urbina 1997, *Standards* 2014); however, *how* to conduct criterion-related validation in real-world settings is a somewhat murkier issue. The primary challenge in criterion-related validity is that research must be conducted within the real-world practices of selection. Many best practices within the context of medical education, such as multi-faceted selection procedures[2] or extra support and remediation for specific groups of students, pose methodological challenges for criterion-related validation. There are many

2 Cambridge Assessment Admissions Testing advocates that BMAT be used alongside other selection criteria, as this is seen as best practice in medical school admissions (Cleland et al 2012); however, a multi-faceted selection process poses methodological challenges for criterion-related validation.

difficulties with investigating criterion-related validity in the context of medical selection; for example, James and Hawkins (2004) list seven specific challenges for evaluating predictive validity in this context (Box 6.2).

Box 6.2 Difficulties associated with investigating predictive validity of medical selection methods (adapted from James and Hawkins 2004:244)

- Selection assessment could produce qualitative or non-normally distributed data.
- The cohort completing the assessment might be too small.
- Assessment scores may not be recorded after decision making.
- The time from administration of the selection assessment to the availability of outcomes is usually very long.
- Outcome variables are only available for successful applicants, who are a subset of the applicants that completed the selection assessment.
- Measures of validity are sensitive to error variation and are dependent on reliability.
- The outcome may neither be reliable nor valid.

With predictive studies, as with most methodologies, a researcher must fully understand the theoretical issues at play, appreciate the situational constraints in studying a real-world phenomenon, and then make and defend a series of expert judgements about how to conduct the desired research. In this part of the chapter, we describe some of the key theoretical and methodological issues in criterion-related validation, and the approach that Cambridge Assessment Admissions Testing takes to researching these areas with BMAT.

Selecting suitable outcome criteria

When considering criterion-related validity, one of the first issues that must be addressed is what criterion a test should be related to. The answer to this question in the context of admissions testing is not clear-cut (Stemler 2012), and researchers must develop a rationale for what they will measure and at what point in time they will measure it. As predictive validity is a key concern of admissions tests, we focus the discussion on selecting outcome criteria for predictive validity studies.

Some researchers approach predictive validity as a purely empirical issue in which any selection variable can be justified if it relates to a desirable outcome. To illustrate this approach, Hopkins, Stanley and Hopkins (1990:82) use an example of selecting employees for sales positions; they argue that: 'If people who indicate that they prefer strawberry to vanilla ice cream become more successful salespeople, then that would be a relevant item for inclusion in the screening test for sales people.'

This approach rejects the need for theoretical or logical accounts that attempt to explain the relationships being investigated, particularly when tests are used in selection. Applied to admissions tests, the position advocated by Hopkins et al (1990) typically means that the criterion becomes the focus of validation studies rather than the assessment being validated. For admissions testing researchers adopting this approach, the validity of the outcome measure, normally a grade point average (GPA), is considered self-evident; therefore, any variable that predicts the desirable outcome can be validated as a selection variable.

Cambridge Assessment takes a different position on criterion-related validity in admissions tests. Selecting suitable outcome criteria should be based on the theory behind the test construct, and this is a fundamental consideration in undertaking criterion-related validity studies. Although predictive validity is particularly important in selection contexts, it is still treated as one aspect of overall validity. In addition, we do not treat outcome measures uncritically; instead we recognise that many outcome measures are available in the higher education context and that relationships worthy of investigation should be identified on theoretical grounds. In this regard, we agree with Sireci's (1998:98) observation that: 'Because no one criterion is sufficient for the validation of a test, and because criteria must also be validated, criterion-related studies were only a part of the larger process of construct validation.'

As admissions tests are intended to help select students most likely to be successful in a given endeavour, a theoretical approach to selecting outcome criteria should focus on indicators of success in that endeavour. However, indicators of success can vary on a number of dimensions. Firstly, they can be measured at different points in time, ranging from 'proximal' indicators which are measured fairly close to the assessment, to 'distal' indicators, which are measurements taken far into the future. For example, in professional education, such as to become a doctor or a lawyer, admissions tests could predict success in the first year of study (a proximal outcome) or success as a professional five years after graduation (a more distal outcome). In medical education, there is debate about whether the aim of an admissions test is to select students who have the capabilities to succeed academically on the course or those who will eventually make good doctors. These aims may not be easy to marry and require different criterion measures. Cleland et al (2012:6) point out that attempting to predict who will be a good doctor can be problematic because 'this is a somewhat indeterminate and distal criterion, in the sense that performance as a doctor is not a discrete construct and is temporally distant from selection'.

While there is continuity of development between study and professional practice, the skills needed for success in these endeavours likely differ (Shultz and Zedeck 2012). Figure 6.1 depicts some of the criteria that could be used to assess predictive validity in a medical selection context.

Figure 6.1 Examples of criteria for measuring success in the progression of medical education

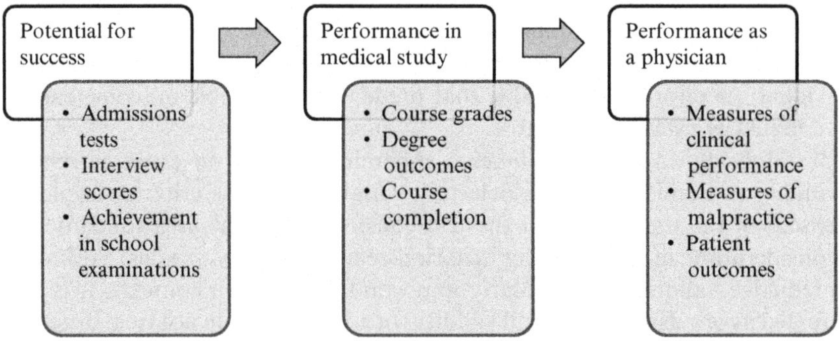

While it might be appealing to determine whether an admissions test can predict professional performance, there is great potential for spurious results from this type of analysis due to confounding factors.[3]

> Naturally, the most interesting outcomes to predict would be those that are more distant in time . . . The tension from a psychometric perspective, however is that the greater amount of time that elapses between instruction [or test administration] and assessment, the more mediating variables can creep in that impact on subsequent performance (for good or ill) making it difficult to link outcomes to predictors (Stemler 2012:10).

In this regard, Woolf, Potts, Stott, McManus, Williams and Scior (2015) argue that selection for training should also deselect those who are unsuitable for clinical practice, because once applicants are accepted onto a training course nearly all of them qualify to practise. On the other hand, it is expected that the learning and experience provided by the university through teaching and apprenticeship ultimately shapes a trainee's development in the medical

3 While attempting to establish predictive validity of an admissions test based on distal performance outcomes may be inadvisable, universities may well want to review their selection process as a whole, in light of the proximal and distal performance of their graduates (Stemler 2012).

or dental profession; therefore, screening out individuals before they have benefited from this training needs a strong justification, particularly because non-academic skills have a stronger theoretical relationship with suitability for clinical practice than academic abilities. In relation to this, Niessen and Meijer (2016) have suggested that optimising training of non-academic skills would be preferable to selecting students on the basis of these skills.

In the case of BMAT, the test construct focuses on potential for the course of study (a proximal outcome), rather than predicting who will make a good doctor, although the former (passing the course) is a necessary condition for the latter. There are a number of different ways to look at proximal outcomes related to performance on a medical course. Many would argue that the purpose of admissions tests is to deselect those applicants who are unlikely to succeed and that test scores should not be expected to differentiate between candidates beyond an 'adequate' or cut-off level. Others believe that the purpose is selection of the very best candidates in terms of course performance. Whether criterion measures should indicate excellent, adequate or poor performance is therefore a decision to be made in establishing a test's predictive validity.

BMAT aims to help schools select from the applicant pool those who have a good chance of completing the course of study successfully whilst rejecting those who are least likely to succeed. It is therefore desirable to show that BMAT scores relate to either future course performance itself or to other, known indicators of this. Of course, scores on any selection test only show us what a candidate *could* achieve in the future rather than what they necessarily *will* achieve, which is shaped by many additional factors.

The wider literature on admissions tests shows that first year grade point average (FYGPA) is one of the most common measurements of course performance used for establishing predictive validity. An acknowledged limitation of this approach is that achievement on a course only reveals part of the spectrum of learning and achievement produced through study in higher education (Stemler 2012). Other criteria that might be used to assess predictive validity include rates of attrition and course completion, but these are only useful in contexts where the outcomes occur regularly and are theoretically related to the constructs assessed by a test, such as when students are not progressing due to academic failure.

Cambridge Assessment researchers use measures of academic performance on biomedical courses, including GPA, as a criterion in predictive studies, in line with conventions established by other researchers in educational assessment. We also identify course performance indicators that align theoretically with the cognitive processes and skills assessed by BMAT outlined in Chapter 3. This is done on a case-by-case basis in collaboration with university tutors, in order to acknowledge the complexity of teaching and learning contexts in schools of medicine and dentistry. Commonly this includes grades for particular course components, grades during early years designated as pre-clinical, and course completion when there are concerns about students' abilities to cope with the science-based study required on a course.

Concurrent validity in the admissions testing context

Concurrent validity is a key component of criterion-related validity; however as the purpose of an admissions test is geared towards selecting for good future performance, concurrent validity is considered less often than predictive validity for admissions tests. Additionally, there are a number of challenging issues that arise when considering concurrent validity for a test used in selection for the healthcare professions.

In the language testing context criterion-related validity has a strong focus on concurrent validity. Relating test scores to other well-established measures of language performance helps to establish the validity of an instrument. Concurrent validity is particularly useful when validating a new tool that acts as a more efficient substitute for an established assessment. In this regard Anastasi and Urbina write:

> Because the criterion for concurrent validity is always available at the time of testing, we might ask what function is served by the [new] test in such situations. Basically, such tests provide a simpler, quicker, or less expensive substitute for the criterion data. For example, if the criterion consists of continuous observation of a patient during a two-week hospitalization period, a test that could sort out normal from disturbed or doubtful cases would appreciably reduce the number of persons requiring such extensive observation (Anastasi and Urbina 1997:119).

One of the immediate challenges to conducting concurrent validity studies on BMAT is that there is not an established measure of the same construct available against which to correlate BMAT test scores, nor is there a common framework of standards that define what a medical student should be able to do at entry into medical school[4]. In language testing, there are established frameworks of language proficiency, such as the Common European Framework of Reference for Languages (CEFR, Council of Europe 2001), which support concurrent validation studies by providing a common rubric against which skills measured on different assessments or qualitative measures can be interpreted. A common framework in language testing also

4 Medical schools frequently use competency frameworks that guide their curriculum and provide detailed statements of what students should be able to do at the end of medical school. However, as these competencies are largely developed through the training provided in medical school, they are not appropriate for establishing a framework of abilities for entering medical students.

supports concurrent validation through 'comparability studies' of different exams that are benchmarked to assess the same levels of the framework.

Medical education currently lacks a common framework that can be used to benchmark potential for medical education. The Association of American Medical Colleges (AAMC, 2014) has recently made a first step in this regard by proposing a series of core competencies for 'entry into medicine' which is being adopted by medical schools in the US and Canada for graduate entry into medical study. The competencies identified by the AAMC link closely to the skills assessed by BMAT sections (see Chapter 3). However, at present, the AAMC's competencies lack structured definitions of levels of ability. In the UK, in which entry into medicine is predominantly at the undergraduate level, there is not yet consensus as to what competencies an entering student should have. Without a common framework, the admissions tests used for medicine and dentistry in the UK (BMAT, United Kingdom Clinical Aptitude Test (UKCAT) and Graduate Medical School Admissions Test (GAMSAT)) conceptualise potential for success at medical school in different ways. From a cognitive validity perspective, the tests are assessing different constructs (although all are described as aspects of potential for biomedical study), and thus comparisons of the scores between these tests would be problematic to interpret.

Of course, potential for success in biomedical study is represented in various ways, not just by admissions test scores. The most commonly used selection criteria are measures of academic achievement at school. Within the broader literature on admissions tests for higher education, secondary school GPA is frequently considered as a criterion for concurrent validity. Admissions test scores and school-based qualifications, such as A Level grades, are typically determined in the late stages of secondary school, so studies examining these variables are often considered as concurrent validity designs (Coates 2008). While one can consider school-leaving qualifications as a concurrent measure for evaluating test validity, a closer look at the timing and constructs in the UK context prompts us to re-examine this position.

Cambridge Assessment Admissions Testing has investigated the relationships between BMAT performance and A Level achievement, which can be conceptualised as a concurrent or predictive criterion. To contextualise Cambridge Assessment's work on BMAT's relationship with A Level grades, we must address the grey area between predictive and concurrent validity.

The *Standards* (2014) pose that 'historically, two designs, often called predictive and concurrent, have been distinguished for evaluation of test-criterion relationships' (2004:17). While researchers tend to agree on distinguishing between these two designs for criterion-related validity, there is debate over where the dividing line is drawn. Traditionally, in occupational psychology settings, the distinction between concurrent and predictive validity designs is based on whether the criterion was measured at the same time as the assessment being validated (Barrett, Phillips and Alexander 1981). In contrast, Anastasi and Urbina state:

> The logical distinction between predictive validity and concurrent validation is based not on time, but on the objectives of testing. Concurrent validation is relevant to tests employed for diagnosis of existing situations, rather than prediction of future outcomes. The difference can be illustrated by asking "Does Smith qualify as a satisfactory pilot" or "Does Smith have the prerequisites to become a satisfactory pilot?" The first question calls for concurrent validation; the second for predictive validation (Anastasi and Urbina 1997:119).

Sometimes it is easy to distinguish between concurrent and predictive validity. When a criterion is measured well into the future from the point of an assessment, and is intended to provide evidence that an assessment can meaningfully predict future outcomes, it is clearly predictive validity. This is the case when admissions tests are correlated with measures of academic performance at university. However, in other cases it can be very difficult, and potentially unimportant, to distinguish between concurrent and predictive validity.

One confusing issue is that the word 'prediction' is used in two ways as explained by Anastasi and Urbina (1997:119): 'criterion-prediction validation procedures indicate the effectiveness of a test in predicting an individual's performance in specified activities . . . the term 'prediction' can be used in the broader sense, to refer to prediction of the test to any criterion situation, or in the more limited sense of prediction over a time interval'. Therefore, a statement that 'assessment X predicts Y' may refer to a statistical correlation that is either concurrent or predictive. In this volume, we use 'predict' in the broader statistical sense, to describe a relationship between two variables.

To illustrate the challenge in distinguishing between concurrent and predictive validity, let us consider research designs that correlate A Level grades (a measure of academic achievement) with BMAT scores (see Figure 6.2).

Figure 6.2 Typical A Level and BMAT arrangements in the UK

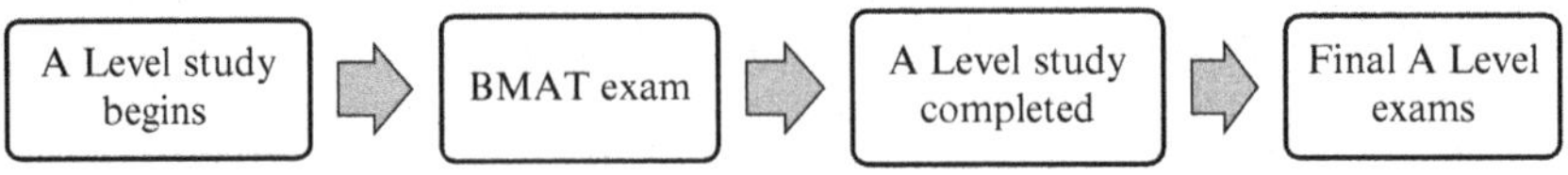

Studying for school examinations tends to begin in advance of sitting a university admissions test, and awarding for some components that contribute to the final grade can occur early in the course of further education study. For qualifications or assessments that are composed of various subcomponents awarded throughout a course of study, the question of when it was administered is not a simple one to address. On the other hand, final grades for school-leaving qualifications might not be available until after the results of the admissions test are released; this makes it reasonable to treat A Level grades as criteria predicted by scores on the admissions test.

Research on A Level performance and BMAT scores can be regarded as examples of concurrent or predictive validity studies, depending on the intended use of BMAT scores in the selection process. Due to the difficulties in timing as explained above, we do not describe research investigating school qualifications and test scores as concurrent or predictive validity. Instead, those using the research can determine whether they would consider the studies as concurrent validity, or predictive validity, or whether to consider the results more generally as evidence of criterion validity, which may be informed by their intended interpretation of the findings.

Exploring these relationships is still important, because it is desirable that BMAT scores should relate to other measures of potential for biomedical study. However, criteria used in student selection should aim to have *incremental* predictive validity over other criteria, contributing some unique information on applicants' potential. For example, we would expect BMAT scores to be related to academic measures such as A Level attainment, which are known predictors of future course performance. On the other hand, a high degree of shared variance might imply redundancy of measures (unless there was doubt about the predictive equity of A Level grades for different groups of applicants). Given that the selection process generally begins before final A Level grades are available for most university applicants, a positive relationship between BMAT scores and A Level attainment (as an outcome criterion) will prove useful to selecting institutions. An example of how BMAT scores have been shown to predict both high and, importantly, insufficient A Level attainment (the failure to achieve minimum conditional offer grades and therefore face a late rejection) is presented later in this chapter (Emery 2007c). In line with Anastasi and Urbina's (1997) focus on distinguishing between concurrent and predictive validity based on the intended use of scores, these findings can be interpreted as either aspect of criterion-related validity.

Box 6.3 BMAT scores' correlation with A Level grades

Tip: BMAT scores have been shown to correlate with A Level grades. This can be useful to schools making admissions decisions before A Level grades are known.

One other aspect of concurrent validity that has not been investigated is the relationship between scores achieved on two different versions of BMAT. Administering two test versions of a test to the same group of students can be used to establish parallel forms of reliability (see Chapter 5 for a description of this), and to investigate the equivalence of writing tasks in BMAT Section 3. Conducting these studies in the future will provide concurrent validity evidence for BMAT.

Methodological challenges

Establishing predictive validity evidence is a priority for tests like BMAT as relevant outcome data becomes available for the test takers. This evidence is important to stakeholder institutions and to test takers themselves, so predictive validity formed the focus of much early research work on BMAT. However, it is difficult to establish predictive validity evidence for university selection tests because methodological issues systematically reduce the strength of correlations that are observed in datasets used for investigating predictive validity. In this part of the chapter, we present three of the main ways that correlations are attenuated in selection contexts, using simulated example datasets. Following an overview of these issues, the approach to presenting predictive validity analysis adopted by Cambridge Assessment researchers is outlined.

Range restriction

Range restriction arises because predictive validity must be calculated from the pool of accepted applicants, whose test scores represent a selected range that is higher and narrower than that of the overall applicant pool. The course performance of applicants who were rejected with low test scores cannot be known and researchers are restricted to looking for differences in course performance between selected applicants, who typically achieved in the range of scores deemed adequate by selectors. Test scores on BMAT can be used in a variety of ways and this can impact substantially on the relationships observed in analyses. The rejection of low scorers, particularly if there is a minimum score that applicants must achieve to be accepted onto the course, gives rise to restricted ranges of test scores and shapes of scatter that limit the strength of relationships. A detailed description of various types of range restriction is available in Bell (2007), but for the purposes of explaining the concept of range restriction, a single hypothetical example will suffice. Low scorers can be rejected by setting a minimum score, which is often referred to as applying a cut-score or hurdle; this method is commonly used in selection settings and results in the forms of range restriction that are easiest to conceptualise.

Consider an idealised situation where the sum of an applicant's scores on BMAT Section 1 and 2 is correlated with FYGPA at $r = 0.492$ (see Figure 6.3). Of course, applicants to the course that are located in the bottom left of the plot are unlikely to be accepted onto the course; therefore, their FYGPA would not actually be observed.

Figure 6.3 Idealised correlation between BMAT scores and FYGPA

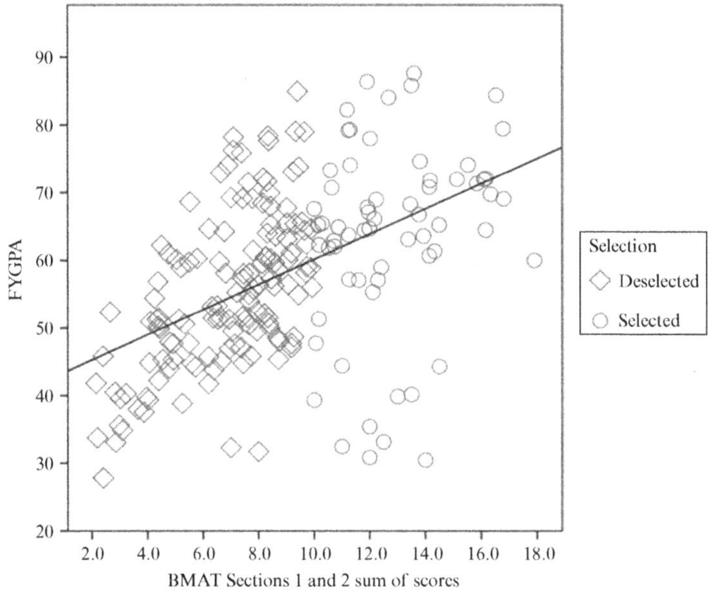

If the admissions process applied a hurdle so that only applicants with a combined BMAT Section 1 and 2 score of 10 or above were accepted onto the course, only those applicants on the right-hand side of Figure 6.3 would have course performance data available for analysis, resulting in Figure 6.4. When the correlation between the two variables is calculated only using the data observed after applying a hurdle, the coefficient indicates a much weaker relationship of $r = 0.218$. As the correlation coefficient is an estimate of the relationship that exists between the two variables, the observation of a weaker relationship is described as an attenuation of the estimate. The observed statistic is much weaker than the relationship that would be observed if the data in the entire population was available.

This simplified example demonstrates one of the major challenges with estimating the relationship between a variable used for selection and an outcome score. While use of a cut-score for accepting applicants onto a course may be appropriate for some selection contexts as an admissions practice, it can exacerbate problems in assessing predictive validity. One method for dealing with this issue is to apply formulae that correct the strength of the coefficient based on the distributions of the variables (e.g. Sackett and

Figure 6.4 Correlation between BMAT score and FYGPA after selection using a cut-score on BMAT

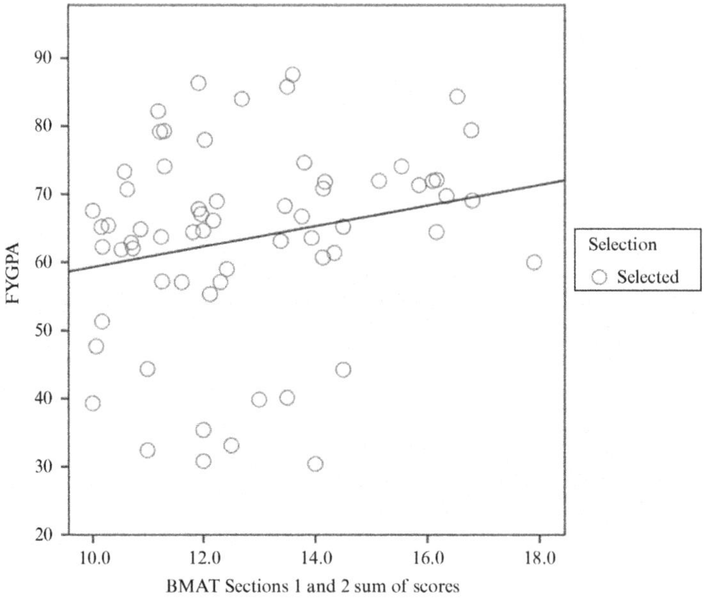

Yang 2000). This has been used in research on admissions tests by McManus, Dewberry, Nicholson, Dowell et al (2013) and represents a suitable solution for the example we have outlined. However, we should recognise that the situation represented in Figure 6.3 and Figure 6.4 is a simplistic one. It is far more common for biomedical courses to use multiple stages in their selection process. This means there might be hurdles applied on various selection criteria that restrict the range of observed scores in different ways, either directly or indirectly. Furthermore, predictive studies often use more than one outcome as criteria, which can complicate things even more. In some instances, collegiate systems used by Oxford and Cambridge can even mean that subgroups within a course cohort had different hurdles applied to the selection criteria that were used, possibly in a different order. Without a detailed understanding of the mechanisms used in selection, it can be very difficult to unpick the ways that a final cohort of students was derived. In general, the greater the reliance on a test score in selection, the more that range restriction becomes an issue when calculating correlations.

Compensatory selection

Within a multi-faceted admissions process, poor performance on one selection criterion (an admissions test) might be compensated for by good

Figure 6.5 Idealised correlation between BMAT scores and FYGPA indicating outlier scores

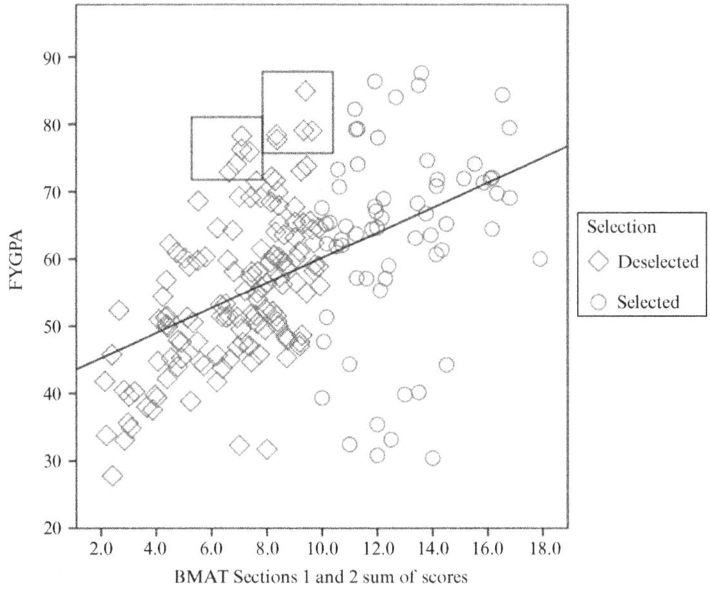

Figure 6.6 Correlation between BMAT score and FYGPA when the candidates with outlier BMAT scores are also selected

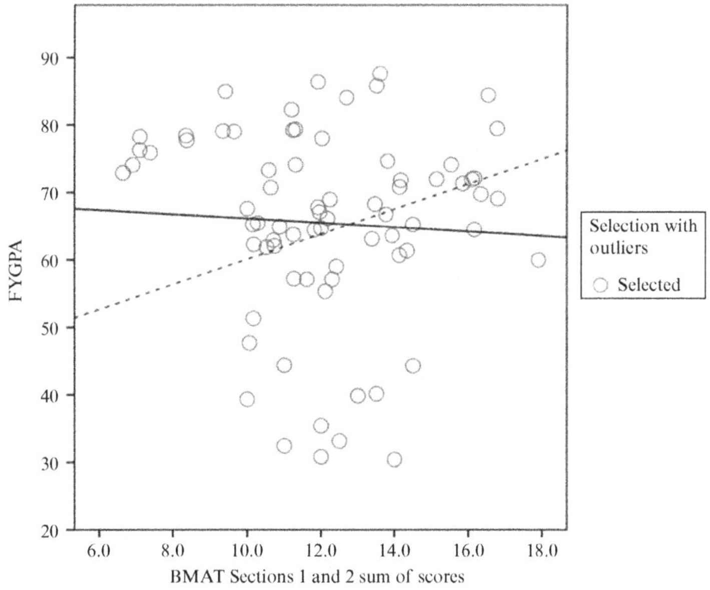

performance on another (e.g. academic achievement, interview). While an appropriate practice for university admissions, this again creates problems for analysing predictive validity. The compensatory use of assessments in multi-method selection procedures means those accepted onto a course with low test scores tend to have performed well on other selection measures. These candidates are therefore atypical of low test scorers in general terms of their potential for succeeding on the course. Compensation in selection processes can make predictive relationships appear, statistically, to be non-existent or even negative. In order to illustrate the effects of compensatory selection on predictive relationships, let us reconsider the hypothetical scenario described previously. Figure 6.5 depicts the idealised correlation between BMAT combined scores and FYGPA as before, but several outlier scores have been highlighted by the boxes, which represent candidates who achieve just under the hurdle of a combined BMAT Section 1 and 2 score of 10. Such candidates may be selected if they have strong performances on other admissions criteria (e.g. school grades or interview scores) that indicate they will be successful on the course. In other words, high performance on some selection criteria can be used to compensate for lower performance in another, allowing the admissions tutor to identify applicants more likely to succeed on the course, when compared with other applicants who achieved the same test score.

Figure 6.6 shows the resultant correlation between BMAT scores and FYGPA when these candidates are selected alongside those above the hurdle. As we can see, the observed correlation, represented by the solid line, is weak and negative (r = -0.058). Inclusion of the outliers has rendered the population correlation, represented by the broken line, undetectable. This is an extreme example because it assumes that the admissions tutor is very accurately identifying those applicants who do not meet the test score threshold but are likely to do well on the course. However, it illustrates how selecting a small number of applicants who are atypical for their test scores can impact on criterion validity.

Again, it should be recognised that the situation represented in Figure 6.5 and Figure 6.6 is more simplistic than actual selection contexts. It is common for biomedical courses to consider multiple selection criteria in their procedures, which may be weighted in various ways. Furthermore, qualitative data and contextual information such as indicators of low socio-economic status are often considered alongside other selection criteria.

Confounds on the outcome variable selected as a criterion

Predictive validity is also affected by potential confounds on the outcome variables. For example, academic outcomes in university can be affected by teaching quality and practice over a course of study. Similarly, outcome measures can be affected by unreliability in course assessments, for example, introduced by subjective marking of assignments. The potential for grades to be confounded as an outcome variable is described by Stemler:

> Grades can be difficult to interpret because they are so frequently influenced in non-uniform ways by other factors. For example, not everyone goes to the same university. Not everyone in the same university takes the same courses. Not everyone in the same courses has the same instructor. Sometimes the interpersonal relationship (either good or bad) that a student has with an instructor colors the instructor's evaluation of the student's content mastery. Each of these outside factors, and many more, can influence final course grades in ways that are not always related to the cognitive abilities and traits that reside within the student (Stemler 2012:8).

The example given by Stemler illustrates the issues that may arise when aggregating grades to serve as outcome data across institutions, courses or years. Collapsing data can produce outcome variables that vary in ways not related to the construct of interest.

In medical education, courses within a university tend to be consistent with all students undertaking a relatively homogenous curriculum of study. Similarity in the course of study undertaken by students reduces the potential for confounds on GPA as an outcome criterion. One caveat to this is that biomedical courses typically include optional components that are selected by the students. Thus, cumulative GPA may be made up of different sets of marks across subgroups of students. This can mean that GPA appears to be comparable across all students, when it is actually composed of differing proportions of assessment types, and actually represents a mixture of sub-constructs. In addition, selection of optional components is unlikely to be random, and may have a systematic relationship with abilities assessed as part of selection. For example, those students confident in their mathematics abilities are more likely to select study options with substantial quantitative components. Further down the line, choices about the medical specialty to pursue might be linked to the communication skills that were assessed during interviews. All of these factors can reduce the reliability of GPA as an outcome measure in predictive validity analysis. However, while we acknowledge the limitations in using GPA in predictive studies, we maintain that within biomedical programmes it is a valid outcome criterion. On this issue, other admissions testing researchers agree, and Stemler writes: 'It is perhaps the case that [first year] GPA is the best that we can hope for as a proxy of domain-specific knowledge at this time' (Stemler 2012:8).

In conducting predictive research, it is important to recognise the limitations of measures that represent academic achievement in university, and to interpret findings whilst considering these issues. We should not assume that everyone's experience when studying will be the same. Indeed, there can be phenomena that change the learning context systematically in line with the constructs being assessed. This would reduce observed relationships between a selection measure and outcome measures. For example, a medical or dental school might identify those candidates with deficits in their scientific knowledge (using the selection test or early indicators of performance on the course). The department can bring this to the attention of the student, increasing the likelihood that the student focuses on this area more than their fellow students. In some instances, the university may offer extra support to students. This is particularly common with written communication skills where students are referred to central support services if their writing is not good enough. If these interventions and influences on behaviour are effective, they can mask the relationships between performance on the selection measure and course outcomes.

Finally, it should be noted that motivation has a large part to play in students' learning and study behaviour, and has been linked to course performance outcomes (Kusurkar, Ten Cate, van Asperen and Croiset 2011). Although biomedical students are typically assumed to be highly motivated, motivation is not considered a stable characteristic and is dependent on contextual factors (Pelaccia and Viau 2017). For example, Wouters, Croiset, Galindo-Garre and Kusurkar (2016) showed that the motivation of applicants to study medicine was high immediately after selection, but decreased rapidly after entering medical school. Thus, changes in motivation over a course of study or even during the transition from secondary to higher education may weaken the relationship between performance on a selection test and outcome measures.

In summary, course performance is affected by a great many variables beyond what the test aims to measure. Course performance will be influenced by a multitude of factors, including the educational environment and the personal circumstances of a student, in addition to academic potential as measured through an admissions test. Even variables traditionally considered as stable, such as personality traits, are now acknowledged to include some plasticity and adaptability (Ferguson and Lievens 2017). Therefore, it is important to recognise that situational context will account for some variances in learning behaviours, which will also impact on course outcomes. The moderating effects of factors such as conscientiousness, motivation and non-academic issues on the relationship between academic ability and course performance should not be underestimated given the amount of variance that remains unexplained by academic ability measures. A single outlying data point from a candidate who has a good test score but fails the course for unrelated reasons can have a large impact on the size of a correlation coefficient. For these reasons, the magnitude of correlation coefficients regarded as beneficial between selection tests and future performance are lower than would normally be expected. In addition, the potential for confounds to reduce the reliability of the criterion increases with the length of time between the test administration and the measuring of the outcome being predicted.

The Cambridge Assessment approach to reporting predictive validity

When describing the methodological issues that result in weaker observed correlation coefficients, we have stressed that the examples used are simplified versions of how selection functions in practice. The ways that actual procedures influence the findings of predictive research are complex and easily overlooked. In fact, the example used to illustrate range restriction actually included a compensatory selection method, even if the hurdle were applied strictly without considering other selection variables. This is simply because two separate BMAT sections were combined to form an aggregate score. Applying a hurdle in this case means that scores on the two sections effectively compensate for each other, so that the hurdle can be reached by a low score on one section with a higher score on the other. Whilst this might be suitable for an admissions policy, it means that relationships between the two section scores would be weaker in the selected group than they are in the wider pool of test takers. As the section scores are expected to predict specific course components differently, the interactions can have further impact on the relationships observed in predictive validity studies.

For selection tests, valuable criterion validity evidence can be obtained from a pilot year of the test where selectors are blind to applicants' scores. The use of such a pilot year can help overcome issues of range restriction and compensatory selection. If it can be shown that candidates scoring low on the test have a very low chance of being offered a place of study following interview when scores were unseen by selectors (the criterion being the admissions decision) then this provides justification for setting a cut-score on the test in future years. Concurrent validity would be evidenced by high agreement between the (hypothetical) admissions decisions made by test scores and the admissions decisions made by selectors blind to those test scores, perhaps on the basis of interviews. Such evidence would allow an institution to apply a future cut-score on the test as a hurdle to the interview stage so as to focus their interview resources on applicants with a reasonable chance of gaining a place of study.

It is not always practical to pilot an admissions test and ignore test scores when making selection decisions. Admissions tests are often introduced in response to specific logistical issues, such as heavy oversubscription or ceilings in applicants' school-leaving qualifications. In these contexts, it might be necessary to use test scores immediately in some way. Even if a hurdle is not applied, it can be difficult to justify the logistical demands of administering a test if admissions tutors do not have access to test scores. Additionally, there are ethical implications of requiring applicants to sit an exam where the scores will not be considered. This means that studies of criterion-related validity are often conducted in the context of real-world selection, requiring researchers to consider how the pool of accepted students has been shaped by admissions decisions.

Given the complexity of the selection contexts we have outlined, Cambridge Assessment recommends that uncorrected correlation coefficients are reported for predictive validity studies, alongside an account of the decisions that resulted in the student cohort that was selected. In order to acknowledge the tendency for coefficients to be attenuated by various issues, guidelines for interpreting uncorrected coefficients can also be included with results, such as those in Table 6.1, which were published by the US Department of Labor, Employment and Training Administration (1999). Alternatively, Cleland et al (2012) provide similar principles for interpreting correlations in the medical admissions context.

Table 6.1 Guidelines for interpreting correlation coefficients in predictive validity studies

Validity coefficient	Interpretation
Above 0.35	Very beneficial
0.21 to 0.35	Likely to be useful
0.11 to 0.20	Depends on circumstances
Below 0.11	Unlikely to be useful

Source: US Department of Labor, Employment and Training Administration (1999)

As with all rules of thumb used to interpret statistical analyses, these values should not be interpreted blindly. It is important to try and obtain as many details relating to the selection procedure used as possible.

One final point that can help deal with the methodological challenges described here is not actually part of our approach, but more of a lesson learned from conducting predictive studies. Most, if not all, of the predictive validity work conducted by Cambridge Assessment has been retrospective. In other words, the studies have been designed and conducted once course outcomes became available, by accessing historical records. From our experience, retroactively describing all of the selection decisions made in application cycles can be difficult to complete with precision. Therefore, it can be advantageous to plan predictive studies prospectively, as this enables the selection decisions used at various stages to be documented in their entirety. In future, we intend to plan predictive research prospectively, as this could allow statistical corrections to be used on observed correlations with confidence.

Box 6.4 Key recommendations from the Cambridge Assessment approach to predictive validity

- Select outcome criteria that are theoretically relevant to the test construct.
- Criterion validity is best established during a 'pilot' year in which the test is administered but admissions decisions are made 'blind' to test results.
- Uncorrected correlation coefficients can be reported alongside descriptions of the selection context and guidelines for interpreting attenuated coefficients.
- It can be useful to plan predictive studies prospectively.

Collecting and collating data

Conducting research on criterion-related validity is dependent on collecting data that is external to the test scores themselves. However, there are difficulties with collating datasets with sufficient sample sizes, as selected cohorts for biomedical courses tend to be small.

Some researchers advocate conducting multiple site or multiple cohort studies to increase statistical power (e.g. McManus, Dewberry, Nicholson and Dowell 2013). A recent big data initiative will enable large-scale predictive validity studies to be conducted more easily in the UK, by collating data from test providers, medical schools and the royal medical colleges into a UK Medical Education Database (UKMED). Big data can offer opportunities to better understand the factors that contribute to success in medical study, and UKMED seeks to support large-scale medical education research by allowing researchers to combine and analyse anonymised datasets. This will encourage studies with large sample sizes and greater statistical power.

The UKMED project is managed by the medical regulator in the UK, the General Medical Council (GMC), and Cambridge Assessment is in the final stages of contributing BMAT data to the database, whilst considering some of the data privacy concerns raised by commentators (e.g. Best, Walsh, Harris and Wilson 2016). The larger scale studies enabled by big data approaches are useful for investigating how the predictive validity of an assessment might generalise across different contexts; however, there are several issues with research using data from different institutions across multiple years. Firstly, adopting Hopkins et al's (1990) approach of treating any variable that correlates with performance as a valid selection criterion could lead to selection methods with no theoretical basis being used, which would also result in unintended side effects for the professional workforce.

To safeguard against identifying spurious relationships, we advocate cautious use of large databases by relying on theory to develop hypotheses about expected relationships. Formulation of relevant hypotheses should include consideration of consequential validity and test taker characteristics. For the UKMED project, research proposals are scrutinised by a group of researchers, which includes a member of the Cambridge Assessment research team that focuses on admissions testing research. Furthermore, Cambridge Assessment also participates in UKMED's Advisory Board, which is the governance structure for the project.

Other methodological issues result from difficulties in obtaining the relevant information about how procedures were applied. If precise details about different selection practices (e.g. hurdles and compensatory selection methods) are not known, it can be difficult to validly adjust for them. As mentioned earlier, this presents complicated issues when considering a single course of study, so documenting the impact of these issues across multiple courses can be even more complex. Furthermore, biomedical courses differ in their composition, affecting the comparability of outcomes across courses, or even within courses that have optional components. The impact of this variability can be reduced by standardising indicators of course performance within cohorts before including them in statistical models, but this does not entirely mitigate the issues faced when combining data across consecutive years of study.

Moreover, different courses, or even course components, can have varying relationships with test sections or selection methods, due to differing candidatures or content focus. For example, one course might have more components that focus on natural sciences than another course that has more assessments that rely on written communication. Performance in these courses would theoretically have different relationships with BMAT Sections 2 and 3. Treating both courses as the same by including them in one analysis can mask nuanced relationships between course outcomes and selection criteria with different emphases, which might be more easily detected using separate analyses.

Therefore, smaller scale studies can contribute effectively to establishing the predictive validity of admissions tests and should not be automatically overlooked in favour of studies with greater statistical power. The approach adopted by Cambridge Assessment researchers in this regard is to collaborate with admissions tutors at universities using BMAT, in order to support them with their own evaluations of predictive validity, which tend to be smaller scale than multi-site studies. This acknowledges that the test users are experts with substantial knowledge of the selection context, whereas Cambridge Assessment researchers tend to be more familiar with issues in educational assessment, such as the impact that various methodological challenges can have on statistical analyses. Most, if not all, BMAT users have conducted their own evaluations of the test, which typically include analysis of predictive validity. This allows individual departments to interpret results in the context of their own courses, in order to satisfactorily show that selection procedures are suitable to institutional committees.

There is often mutual sharing of BMAT data, admissions information, admissions decisions and course performance data between Cambridge Assessment and the institutions using BMAT, which allows both organisations to monitor the predictive validity of BMAT for admitted applicants. These studies provide valuable insights into BMAT's validity; however, Cambridge Assessment researchers arrange to analyse data on a case-by-case basis for each study. As personal data is often required to match course data to BMAT scores, we review data protection issues separately. The on-course performance of students who have taken BMAT is not routinely collected from universities in the same way as some other test providers; this reflects a cautious approach to data protection throughout the Cambridge Assessment Group, which is informed by recent discussions on the opportunities and risks presented by use of student data (e.g. Trainor 2015).

Box 6.5 Key points on data collection

- Small-scale studies can provide important findings that complement large-scale studies.
- Each course or institution's selection procedure is unique and test developers can collaborate with test users to investigate predictive validity.
- BMAT data is being included in a database managed by the GMC, which will support large-scale research into the validity of selection criteria.
- Cambridge Assessment collaborates with universities on a case-by-case basis, and does not routinely collect large amounts of data on candidates from biomedical departments.

Data on selection criteria (e.g. A Level results) is available via the Universities and Colleges Admissions Service (UCAS) to biomedical and dentistry schools for all university applicants rather than just those admitted, as is candidate-level demographic information. This can permit research into institutions' selection processes in general, such as the fairness of admissions offers for different candidate groups, the relationship between demographic variables and selection criteria, and the factors that best predict admissions offers. Predictive validity studies on BMAT are typically single-institution studies using one or more cohorts, which helps reduce confounds on the outcome variable (as described by Stemler 2012). While cohorts tend to be analysed separately, it is sometimes necessary to combine them across years for courses which have particularly small numbers, such as graduate-entry courses (Devine and Gallacher 2017). Findings from separate analyses often illustrate the variability in the strength of correlations that can be found even within the same course, resulting from different admissions decisions, applicant cohorts or course assessments. Outcome data usually consists of early course examination results (e.g. end of Year 1 or Year 2 examination average).

Predictive equity and its role in test fairness

An aspect of predictive validity research that is crucial to investigating test fairness is that of *predictive equity*. This is discussed in detail in Chapter 2, and is illustrated by research into test fairness and bias issues (Emery et al 2011). To recap here, if a test is biased *against* a particular candidate group then we would expect test scores to systematically *under*-predict future course performance for that group (i.e. they go on to perform better than predicted on the course), and vice versa. If BMAT scores fairly reflect ability on the construct of interest regardless of candidate group then scores should predict future course performance equitably for different groups, assuming that other factors are equal between them.

Candidate school sector information and candidate gender are therefore included as additional predictor variables in Cambridge Assessment Admissions Testing regression analyses of course performance on BMAT scores and it is possible to investigate any other candidate-level variables that may be a fairness concern. If a given BMAT score predicts equal course performance, on average, between different candidate groups then this provides strong evidence that the test is fair and unbiased even when test score differences are evident between groups. Analyses to date have consistently shown BMAT to predict course performance equitably regardless of candidate background variables such as gender, school type, school sector and social deprivation indicators.

6.3 Research

In the previous parts of this chapter, we have described the theoretical and methodological issues involved in conducting criterion-related validity, and the approaches to addressing these that are used in BMAT research. Research into the predictive validity of BMAT is regularly conducted by Cambridge Assessment Admissions Testing in collaboration with the universities who use the test. In this section, we present a longitudinal study – conducted when BMAT was first introduced at Cambridge Medical School – which provided foundational evidence of BMAT's predictive validity to support its use as an admissions test for medical study (Emery and Bell 2009). We then summarise some of the other predictive validity studies which have been conducted, with a focus on the diverse contexts that BMAT is used in.

Key research study – The predictive validity of BMAT for pre-clinical examination performance (Emery and Bell 2009)

Main findings

- BMAT makes a significant contribution to predicting performance in medical study.
- BMAT makes a unique contribution to predicting performance when considered alongside other selection criteria.
- Section 2 correlated most strongly with performance in pre-clinical courses.

Introduction and context

The following study was one of the earliest pieces of predictive validity research carried out with BMAT, and provided foundational evidence for use of BMAT in medical student selection (Emery and Bell 2009). This investigated the predictive validity of BMAT (and its predecessor, Medical and Veterinary Admissions Test (MVAT)) in the first four years of use as a selection tool at the medical school of the University of Cambridge. Outcome variables investigated were first and second year medical school performance (both examination marks and examination classification) in four individual cohorts of students.

BMAT was introduced in order to address several problems that University of Cambridge's medical school was facing. Firstly, the applicant pool comprised students with very high, but similar levels of prior academic achievement (A Level grades or equivalent), making it difficult to distinguish between applicants. In addition, there were other problems with reliance on prior school achievement as a selection criterion, such as the need to consider non-UK applicants, the attainment advantage of those attending private schools, the poorer performance of various social groups and the fact that only predicted A Level grades are available at the time of application. BMAT was used as an *additional* source of information to help selectors differentiate between those with the high prior attainment and to compare students from different educational backgrounds and countries.

With such strong competition for places, it is important to establish that a selection measure has predictive validity if test takers and institutions are to have faith in its fitness for purpose. The aim of this study was therefore to determine whether BMAT scores were a significant predictor of early medicine course performance (science-based examinations) in four cohorts of students who were all admitted with the highest A Level grades possible at the time. If selection test scores can significantly predict course performance in students admitted with uniformly high A Level grades (or significantly predict course performance after controlling for A Level grades) then they are a useful addition to the selection process and will be beneficial in increasing student success rates (Kuncel, Hezlett and Ones 2001). The magnitude of the predictive relationships and their variability over course components and cohorts was investigated, given that this appeared to be a typical finding elsewhere (Julian 2005). Whether BMAT Section 1 or Section 2 showed the stronger predictive relationship with course examinations was also of interest.

Research questions

1. Does BMAT significantly predict end of Year 1 and Year 2 examination performance in four cohorts of students entering the medicine course at the University of Cambridge[5]?
2. What is the relative magnitude of the predictive relationship for Sections 1 and 2 of the test?

Data collection and analysis

The medicine course at the University of Cambridge is a 'traditional' (rather than 'integrated') course in that it consists of three years of pre-clinical study followed by three years of clinical training. The first two years are heavily science based. For the cohorts in this research, students completed three core first year courses and four core second year courses, each assessed in examinations at the end of the academic year. The examinations each consisted of a mixture of short-answer, essay and multiple-choice questions based on lecture and practical material. Third year outcome data was pass/fail in nature (and composed of a large number of course options not necessarily related to medicine) and so was not included in the study. Pre-clinical course examinations were the focus of this study as BMAT focuses on academic readiness for demanding science-based study and not clinical skills/fitness to practice.

Scores for Sections 1 and 2 of the test correlated at around 0.4 in these cohorts (as they do in general). It should be noted that Cambridge Assessment did not mark Section 3 prior to 2004 and the University of Cambridge did not use BMAT Section 3 (Writing Task) scores in selection in these test years (2000–03), instead considering candidates' responses as a qualitative piece of evidence and to promote discussion during the interview. Thus, Section 3 scores were not analysed in this study. No BMAT cut-score was applied as a hurdle to the interview stage for these cohorts of applicants, meaning that a full range of BMAT scores was technically possible.

5 BMAT was known as MVAT prior to 2003 so the first three cohorts in this study sat MVAT rather than BMAT.

Examination data for the first and second years of the medicine course was supplied by the University of Cambridge and matched to students' MVAT/BMAT results. Examination data consisted of a total (percentage) mark for each course component plus an overall (percentage) mark and examination classification for each year. First year examination classes were, in descending order of merit: 1st, 2nd, 3rd, Fail. Second year examination classes further subdivided the 2nd class into higher and lower categories. Attrition rates are very low at this institution and numbers were too small to permit its analysis for these cohorts. Around one fifth of each first year cohort and one sixth of each second year cohort was awarded a 1st class.

Numbers of students with complete data in each cohort were 255, 250, 247 and 250, respectively. A small number of students in each cohort could not be matched to MVAT/BMAT results. Fewer than 10 students in each cohort were aged over 21 at the time of course entry. Students gave permission for their examination and test scores to be used for research purposes when registering for the test and data was anonymised after matching. The four cohorts were analysed separately.

Pearson correlations were employed with the examination marks data, which were continuous and normally distributed. Upward adjustments of the correlation coefficients for range restriction were not applied because the complexity of the selection process, a compensatory mixture of qualitative and quantitative information, made them inappropriate (Sackett and Yang 2000). Raw, uncorrected correlation coefficients were therefore presented throughout the results. Logistic regression analyses were employed with the examination classifications in each year, modelling the probability of achieving a 1st class result as a function of BMAT Section 1 and BMAT Section 2 scores.

A Level grades could not be included as an additional predictor variable in this study as there was a ceiling in grades for the cohorts included. A Level grades AAA were required for course entry for these cohorts, which was the maximum attainable outcome at the time (prior to the introduction of the A* grade in 2010).

Results

The score distributions of those offered a place versus those rejected in each cohort shows that those who received an offer had a higher mean and narrower range of test scores than those who were rejected but there was considerable overlap in their distributions. A number of applicants with relatively low test scores were offered a place each year and a number of high scorers rejected due to the compensatory nature of the selection process.

1. Correlations with course examination marks

Table 6.2 displays the Pearson correlation coefficients between MVAT/BMAT scores and the Year 1 and 2 examination marks. It can be seen that the strength of the relationships varied across the cohorts and course components but they were consistently stronger for Section 2 of the test (Scientific Knowledge and Applications) than for Section 1 (Aptitude and Skills) in these students. The majority of coefficients for Section 2 fell within the 'very beneficial' range (above 0.35) or the 'likely to be useful' range (above 0.21). Correlation coefficients were slightly weaker for the second year examinations, an outcome expected given that predictive relationships typically weaken with increasing time intervals (Julian 2005). The exception was Section 1 for the BMAT 2003 cohort, which correlated more strongly with their second year examination performance.

Table. 6.2 Pearson correlation coefficients between BMAT scores and examination performance

Section 1 – Aptitude and Skills

	Year 1 examination components			
Cohort	**Homeostasis**	**Molecules in medical science**	**Functional architecture of the body**	**Total mark**
MVAT 2000	0.22***	0.27***	0.19***	0.24***
MVAT 2001	0.19**	0.17**	0.12**	0.18**
MVAT 2002	0.18**	0.22***	0.14*	0.19***
BMAT 2003	0.1	0.12*	0.11*	0.13*

	Year 2 examination components				
	Biology of disease	**Human reproduction**	**Neurobiology and human behaviour**	**Mechanisms of drug action**	**Total mark**
MVAT 2000	0.15**	0.13*	0.18**	0.24***	0.17**
MVAT 2001	0.12*	0.09	0.11	0.19***	0.11
MVAT 2002	0.20***	0.12*	0.04	0.22***	0.11
BMAT 2003	0.17**	0.20***	0.24***	0.16**	0.22***

Table. 6.2 (continued)

Section 2 – Scientific Knowledge

	Year 1 examination components			
Cohort	**Homeostasis**	**Molecules in medical science**	**Functional architecture of the body**	**Total mark**
MVAT 2000	0.45***	0.41***	0.40***	0.44***
MVAT 2001	0.28***	0.35***	0.26***	0.26***
MVAT 2002	0.46***	0.41***	0.41***	0.45***
BMAT 2003	0.28***	0.27***	0.16**	0.26***

	Year 2 examination components				
	Biology of disease	**Human reproduction**	**Neurobiology and human behaviour**	**Mechanisms of drug action**	**Total mark**
MVAT 2000	0.38***	0.34***	0.35***	0.36***	0.26***
MVAT 2001	0.29***	0.24***	0.24***	0.31***	0.18**
MVAT 2002	0.40***	0.17**	0.24***	0.42***	0.23***
BMAT 2003	0.23***	0.22***	0.27***	0.23***	0.25***

Note: * $p < 0.05$, ** $p < 0.01$, *** $p < 0.001$

MVAT 2000 N = 255, MVAT 2001 N = 250, MVAT 2002 N = 247, BMAT 2003 N = 250

2. Prediction of high examination attainment (1st class)

The logistic regression plots in Figure 6.7 show the probability of achieving a 1st class examination outcome in Years 1 and 2 as a function of students' MVAT and BMAT scores. The x axes cover the actual range of scores achieved by each cohort. The steeper the curve, the stronger the predictive relationship (a horizontal function indicates no predictive relationship). Figure 6.7 shows that students' Section 2 (Scientific Knowledge and Applications) scores strongly predicted their probability of achieving a 1st class outcome in Year 1 and continued to significantly predict this in Year 2. Again, the plots suggest that relationship was stronger for Section 2 of the test in these cohorts (functions are consistently steeper than for Section 1). That is, an increase in Section 2 scores had the greater impact on the probability of achieving this outcome than did an increase in Section 1 scores. Note that the lowest Section 2 scores were associated with a very low probability of achieving a 1st class outcome in both years of the course. Odds ratios show the change in odds for every one point increase in scores on the x axes.

Figure 6.7 Logistic regression functions showing the probability of achieving a 1st class examination outcome in Years 1 and 2 as a function of MVAT/ BMAT Section 1 and 2 scores

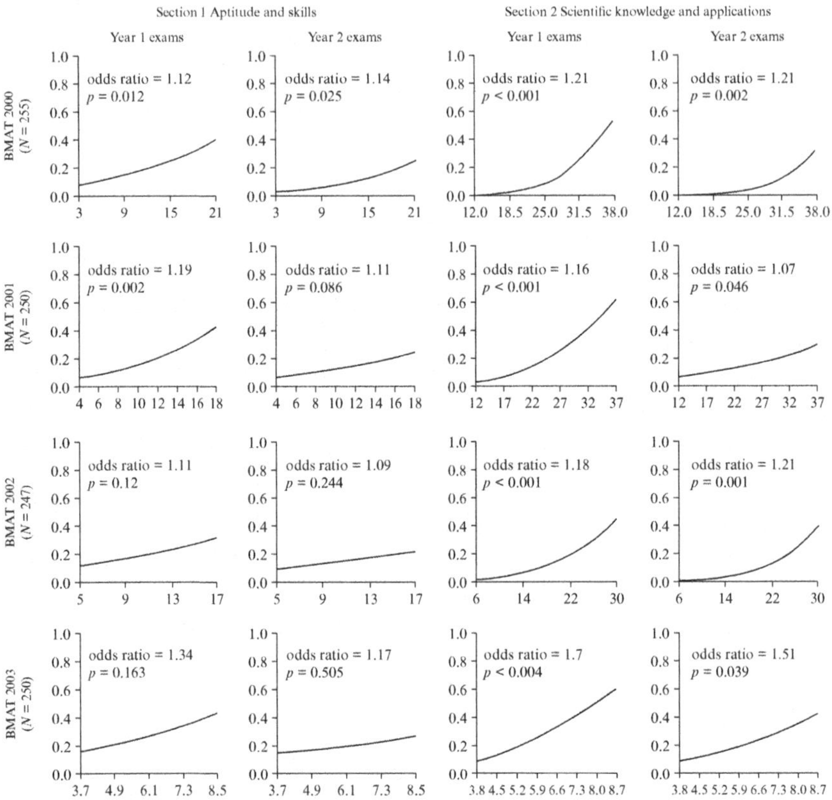

Discussion

The results of this early study into the predictive validity of BMAT support the utility of the test for medical student selection. Correlations with examination marks compare favourably with those reported for the US Medical College Admission Test (MCAT), e.g. Julian (2005), particularly given that there is very little variability in prior attainment in this case because A Level grades were at a maximum in these four cohorts. This indicates that the test has incremental validity on top of prior academic achievement. Students who were accepted onto the course with low test scores, particularly on Section 2 (Scientific Knowledge and Applications), were unlikely to achieve the highest examination class. BMAT therefore appears to fulfil its purpose in identifying valid differences in the thinking skills and scientific reasoning of those with the highest possible A Level grades: differences that relate to future course performance (i.e. potential for biomedical study).

The correlations presented here are likely to be underestimates of the true predictive validity of BMAT. This is because correlations are attenuated for any criterion that counts towards selection due to the narrowing of score ranges (we cannot know how applicants rejected with low scores would have gone on to perform). Despite the lack of a cut-score at this institution and cautious use of the test in its earliest years, the scores of the accepted applicants showed a restricted range. The effects of compensatory selection on hampering the predictive relationship (i.e. the notion that accepted low scorers are likely to be atypically able) must also be kept in mind. The variation in the strength of correlations between cohorts even at the same institution is a typical finding (Julian 2005). For this reason, caution should always be exercised in citing a single number as a test's predictive validity coefficient.

Most of the correlations for Section 1 (Aptitude and Skills) were statistically significant but correlations were consistently stronger and logistic regression functions steeper for Section 2 (Scientific Knowledge and Applications) of the test in these cohorts. The findings from this early study are in line with many subsequent studies on the predictive validity of BMAT, which have also shown that Section 2 has stronger predictive validity. This finding also agrees with reported findings regarding the predictive validity of A Level chemistry and biology for early medicine course performance (e.g. McManus et al 2005). Stemler (2012) proposes predictive validity be tied to both domain-specific ability and domain-general ability. While Sections 1 and 3 in BMAT test domain-general ability (critical thinking skills and writing ability) and Section 2 assesses domain-specific ability (scientific reasoning), the criterion used for establishing predictive validity (course marks) is based on performance in pre-clinical courses, which is generally a measurement of domain-specific achievement. While the development of critical reasoning and problem solving skills is a common aim of medical education, a ubiquitous problem in establishing the predictive validity of critical thinking skills tests is that it is a domain-general ability that is rarely assessed within higher education (Stemler 2012).

Scientific reasoning with subject-specific knowledge (as assessed in BMAT Section 2) may predict course performance well because it additionally assesses motivation and interest in the area (Kuncel et al 2001, McManus et al 2005). A high BMAT Section 2 score suggests that a candidate thoroughly understands the scientific basics that underpin medical study and it is perhaps unsurprising that a poor score here is associated with a very low chance of obtaining the highest examination class.

It is widely accepted that there is much more to being a good doctor than academic success. However, success in science-based examinations is a necessary factor for progression to clinical training and a medical career regardless of whether it is sufficient for becoming a good doctor. It is the former and not the latter that BMAT aims to predict.

Summary of other relevant research

Cambridge Assessment has continued to investigate the predictive validity of BMAT for performance on medicine and veterinary medicine courses at the institutions using the test. This is particularly important to new institutions and courses adopting the test. In summary, the *strength* of the predictive relationship between BMAT scores and course performance varies between institutions, courses and cohorts. This variation may be explained by differences in how BMAT is used at different institutions, and aspects of the educational context that vary between and within courses. However, correlations are typically positive, with both Sections 1 and 2 of the test significantly predicting early course examination performance.

Results for Section 3 (Writing Task) are more mixed with regard to early course performance. In some cases, a relationship between BMAT Section 3 scores and indicators of course performance have not been observed, whereas in others Section 3 scores have been the strongest predictors of performance. Unsurprisingly, our findings indicate that Section 3 scores are more likely to correlate with modules assessed using written components, even where they do not correlate with overall course performance. This suggests it is useful to consider the content of course modules and how they are assessed, when interpreting observed relationships. Studies investigating criterion-related validity of BMAT in undergraduate courses, graduate-entry courses, and using A Level performance as a criterion are presented in the next sections.

Undergraduate course performance

Whilst BMAT Section 2 tends to be the most consistently strong predictor of undergraduate course performance, this is not the case at all institutions and courses, or for all cohorts. For instance, Emery (2007a) showed an equally strong predictive relationship for both Sections 1 and 2 of BMAT for the University of Cambridge's 2004 veterinary medicine course but, in the following cohort (Emery 2007b), Section 2 was the stronger predictor of Year 1 course performance. As described in more detail below, Section 2 was not found to predict course performance in a graduate-entry medicine course (Devine and Gallacher 2017). In one institution, the Writing Task (Section 3) emerged as the strongest predictor of performance in two BMAT cohorts, with significant correlations in the range of 0.171 to 0.343 (e.g. Scorey 2009a).

Scorey (2009b) conducted predictive validity analysis of BMAT for undergraduate medicine performance at University College London (UCL), using successful applicants from the BMAT 2003–07 cohorts. BMAT had been used for selection purposes during these years, so direct range restriction was likely to have weakened the observed correlations. These analyses found that Section 3 scores significantly predicted early course performance (individual exam components as well as aggregate marks) in the 2004 and 2007 BMAT cohorts (correlations between 0.114 and 0.173). Moreover, Section 3 significantly predicted the probability of failing the second year of the course in the 2004 cohort; that is, as Section 3 scores increased, the probability of failing the course decreased. It should be noted that this study also revealed that Sections 1 and 2 predicted course performance in several BMAT cohorts and correlations tended to be stronger than the Section 3 correlations (correlations up to 0.254); however, there was some variation in correlation strength across all cohort and course year combinations.

Although such variation is a typical finding in predictive validity research, the reasons for these differences are difficult to establish. Differences in course content, teaching and examinations, and the ways scores are used in selection, will affect the nature of the predictive relationship but, for different cohorts on the same course, characteristics of the cohorts themselves or the way in which they were selected may be responsible for the observed differences.

Of particular note are the plots in Figure 6.8 (from Emery 2007b). In this cohort, unusually, there were sufficient numbers to permit analyses predicting a *poor* Year 1 medicine course examination outcome. In these analyses, students attaining a 3rd class result, failing the examinations or having left the course were categorised together (N = 20). It can be seen that, whilst BMAT Section 1 scores had little impact on the probability of this outcome (the x axes cover the score ranges of those who entered the course), students who were admitted onto the course with a low BMAT Section 2 score had a

Figure 6.8 Logistic regression functions showing the probability of achieving a poor examination outcome in Year 1 as a function of BMAT Section 1 and 2 scores (Emery 2007b)

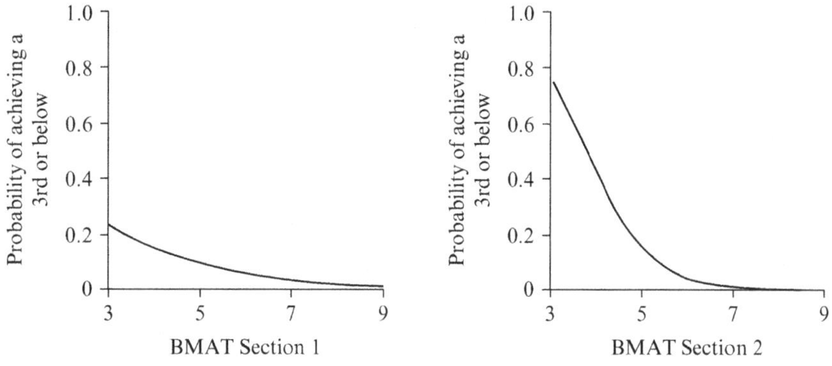

high probability of a poor examination outcome. Those who were admitted with a BMAT Section 2 score of 5.0 or more had a very low probability of this poor outcome. This is an important finding given that all those admitted had achieved the maximum possible A Level grades in sciences prior to course entry.

Graduate-entry medicine

Cambridge Assessment Admissions Testing also investigates the predictive validity of BMAT for accelerated (graduate-entry) medicine course performance. More than a dozen UK universities offer accelerated (4- or 5-year) medicine courses for graduates with a degree in a scientific discipline; BMAT is currently used by three medical schools for graduate-entry selection. Graduate-entry courses also receive a large number of applications and the selection process is highly competitive. BMAT is a useful selection tool in the graduate-entry context because applicants have widely varying educational backgrounds and thus, are likely to have varying levels of foundational knowledge across the physical and biological sciences. An admissions test such as BMAT also allows broader access to graduate-entry medicine courses. For example, the additional information provided by BMAT enables admissions tutors to consider applicants from 'non-traditional' backgrounds, graduates from disciplines other than biosciences, and applicants who may be 'late developers' (i.e. with poorer A Level results but with a good degree classification). BMAT provides a common point of comparison between applicants from diverse backgrounds.

Recent analysis investigated the predictive validity of BMAT for graduate-entry medicine performance at the University of Oxford (Devine and Gallacher 2017), where shortlisting was done through grading of the applications by college and faculty tutors, with BMAT scores used only to differentiate candidates on the borderline of the shortlist; however, the score distributions indicated indirect range restriction of BMAT scores in the pool of shortlisted applicants. At Oxford, the preliminary examinations in medicine for graduates are made up of core and clinical examinations (awarded with a pass or fail), and five extension modules (awarded with percentage marks). In Devine and Gallacher's analysis, the five extension modules were included as outcome variables. Section 1 scores predicted average performance on the extension modules and correlated with performance on two course modules (correlations between 0.184 and 0.344). Section 3 (quality of content) scores were also found to correlate significantly positively with performance on the extension modules (correlations between 0.289 and 0.331). However, no significant correlations emerged between Section 2 scores and performance on the extension modules.

It is unclear why Section 2 scores did not correlate with performance on the extension modules in this cohort but it may be that knowledge of the secondary education level science curriculum has been replaced with more relevant biomedical knowledge from candidates' undergraduate degrees. That is, some graduate-entry applicants may not perform well on Section 2 if they can no longer recall the foundational knowledge, but may be able to learn medical knowledge more easily than expected due to knowledge gained during their undergraduate degree programme. This would reduce the strength of the relationship between Section 2 and course performance. Further work is needed to investigate this null finding, including analysis of performance on the core examination, which, due to its focus on basic facts and principles may have a stronger relationship with Section 2.

Nonetheless, the significant positive relationships between the other two BMAT sections and course performance suggest BMAT scores are likely to be useful for selection to graduate-entry medicine. In particular, the significant relationships identified between Section 3 scores and performances on the extension modules were encouraging, because scores from written essay tests have typically varied in their relationships with performance in medical study. For example, research looking at the essay component of the old (1992–2012) MCAT showed that writing section scores correlated only with some outcome variables, leading Hojat, Erdmann, Veloski, Nasca, Callahan, Julian and Peck (2000) to conclude that written communication skills are more closely associated with clinical practice than with achievement in the basic sciences.

A Level performance as a criterion

The criterion validity of BMAT with A Level outcomes has been investigated by Cambridge Assessment researchers (Emery 2007c). Given that only predicted A Level grades are available at the time of university application for most, selectors generally rely upon teachers' predictions for the majority of candidates. It is therefore of interest to stakeholder institutions if BMAT scores are correlated with outcomes at A Level, particularly to prevent places being offered to candidates who are unlikely to make the minimum grades required for entry. Whether BMAT scores correlate with two different A Level outcomes in a cohort of applicants (N = 460) was explored. These two outcomes were: the highest possible A Level outcome at the time of the study (grades AAA), and a poor outcome (failure to achieve the minimum offer grades of BBB). Correlations between BMAT scores and A Level points (a continuous variable) were also carried out.

Correlations between BMAT scores and A Level points in the applicant group were 0.36 for Section 1, 0.36 for Section 2 and 0.26 for Section 3. All three BMAT sections also showed a strong positive relationship with the probability of achieving grades AAA in the applicant group (the probability being under 0.2 in applicants with Section 1 and 2 scores of around 3.0, compared to around 0.7–0.8, respectively, in those with Section 1 and 2 scores of approximately 6;

the probability was around 0.3 for a Section 3 score[6] of 4.5, compared to 0.6 for a score of 10.5). Importantly, BMAT Section 2 scores were a particularly strong predictor of failing to achieve at least grades BBB at A Level in the applicants who had been made an offer of a place conditional upon achieving these grades. It is particularly encouraging that all three sections were predictors of this outcome; Section 2's is perhaps unsurprising, given that applicants to biomedical school typically study two or more sciences at A Level.

Of the 178 candidates who had been made a conditional offer, 32 were rejected due to not achieving the BBB A level grade requirement. Those scoring around 3.0 on BMAT Section 2 had over a 0.5 probability of rejection at this late stage whereas those scoring around 5.0 had only a tenth of that probability (see Figure 6.9).

The use of BMAT scores as a potential early indicator of A Level performance is likely to become increasingly important given the proposed discontinuation of A Levels in their current form, which will increase universities' reliance on predicted A Level grades.

Figure 6.9 Logistic regression function showing the probability of a late rejection (failure to achieve A Level grades BBB) as a function of BMAT Section 2 scores (from Emery 2007c)

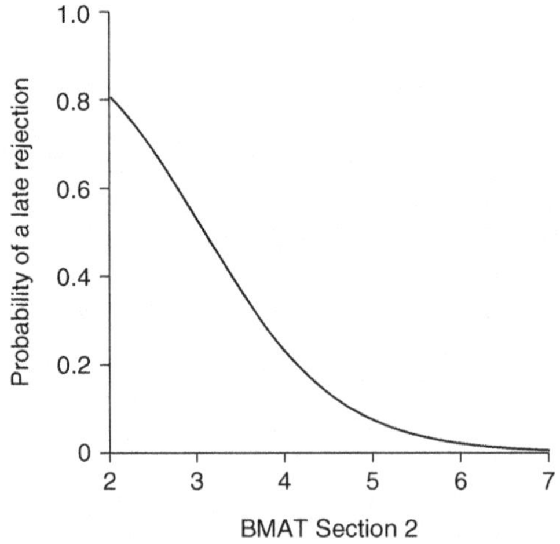

6.4 Chapter summary

In this chapter we outlined the importance of showing a relationship between test scores and other variables (criterion-related validity). We have detailed

6 Emery (2007c) was conducted when Section 3 scores were awarded on a scale from 1 to 15.

the difficulties and limitations that are inherent to this field and outlined the approach adopted by Cambridge Assessment Admissions Testing with regard to measuring and reporting criterion-related validity.

For assessments used in selection such as BMAT, the relationship we are interested in primarily is with the future outcome that the test score is designed to predict (*predictive validity*). However, the relationship of BMAT with an outcome variable such as A Level performance may be considered predictive or concurrent depending on the intended use of BMAT scores in the selection process. We advocate a theoretical approach to the selection of outcome criteria and typically use measures of academic performance on biomedical courses (such as GPA) as criterion variables in our predictive validity studies. As predictive relationships are likely to be attenuated by range restriction, confounds on the outcome variables and the compensatory nature of the selection process, predictive validity is ideally measured during a pilot year for which BMAT scores are not considered in the selection process. However, where this is not possible we interpret uncorrected raw correlation coefficients according to recommended guidelines and take into account the selection criteria used by medical schools. This chapter also considered issues around the collection and collation of data, in particular the merits and limitations of multi-cohort and single-school studies. Predictive equity was discussed as an element of criterion-related validity that linked to consequential validity and test taker characteristics, which are covered in other chapters of this volume.

Finally, we described predictive validity work carried out on BMAT by Cambridge Assessment Admissions Testing. The studies presented in this chapter were conducted in collaboration with medical schools using BMAT as part of their admissions procedures. The results present good evidence of BMAT's predictive validity, demonstrating that scores on the test add value to biomedical admissions processes. Further work on the magnitude of some relationships between course components and specific test sections would add to this evidence, particularly for Section 3. The positive relationships identified so far are observable in single-site studies, despite the theoretical and methodological difficulties that attenuate observed correlations. Therefore test users can expect a degree of correlation between performance on BMAT and subsequent on-course performance.

Chapter 6 main points

- Tests used for selection are conceptualised as predictors, so predictive validity is more commonly investigated than concurrent validity in admissions testing.
- A range of issues weaken the relationships observed in predictive studies; so understanding the selection processes that were used can aid interpretation of results.
- The strength of predictive relationships between BMAT scores and course performance varies between institutions, courses and cohorts.
    - BMAT shows predictive validity across a range of courses and contexts, although the strength of correlations varies.
    - BMAT Sections 1 and 3 predict course outcomes in graduate entry into medicine.
    - BMAT predicts the likelihood of a student achieving their predicted A Level grades.
- Test users can expect positive correlations between BMAT scores and subsequent on-course performance, and also with likelihood to meet A Level offers.
- Future research may investigate concurrent validity in admissions tests, if suitable competency frameworks are developed.

7 The consequences of biomedical admissions testing on individuals, institutions and society

Sarah McElwee
Research and Thought Leadership Group, Cambridge Assessment Admissions Testing
Molly Fyfe
Research and Thought Leadership Group, Cambridge Assessment Admissions Testing
Karen Grant
Lancaster Medical School

7.1 Introduction

This chapter explores consequential validity, which refers to the impact that a high-stakes test, such as BMAT, has on all its varied stakeholders (including candidates, teachers and universities), on teaching and learning, and on society more broadly. Weir's (2005) socio-cognitive framework considers the social consequences of test use as part of overall validity and Cambridge Assessment Admissions Testing also adopts this position, treating the consequences of using an admissions test as part of overall validity (Messick 1995).

Box 7.1 Definition of consequence in educational assessment

Consequences: The outcomes, intended and unintended, of using tests in particular ways in certain contexts and with certain populations.

(*Standards* 2014:217)

In this chapter we describe the way that Cambridge Assessment Admissions Testing investigates the social consequences of BMAT and supports positive impact (*impact by design*). The features of BMAT that support student revision and promote valuable thinking skills ('positive washback') are discussed. This includes a description of how stakeholder needs are addressed through collaboration with institutions using BMAT. At a time of heightened media scrutiny of fair access to higher education, the role of BMAT in supporting transparent admissions processes to heavily over-subscribed courses is outlined by Professor David Vaux, an Admissions Tutor at the University of Oxford. Two key studies are presented in this chapter. The first study details findings from a survey of BMAT candidates on their test preparation activities, which was conducted to understand how preparing for tests like BMAT can impact upon student learning and test performance. The second study explores candidates' attitudes towards admissions tests and the wider process of applying to study medicine, again using survey methods.

7.2 Consequential validity in medical selection

Within the field of medical education, consequential validity tends to be viewed as issues relating to the interpretation and use of test scores (Downing 2003). As will be fully described in the following section, we adopt a broader view on consequential validity that not only includes score use and interpretation, but extends to important issues such as test preparation behaviours, equity and stakeholder perceptions. We feel that this approach is particularly important when considering consequential validity within the context of admissions to medical study.

High-stakes testing for university admission directly affects the choices, careers and experiences of thousands of young people aiming to follow a particular educational path. The institutions that use these tests are also affected; at a micro level (in the effect it has on their admissions decisions and the performance of the cohort they select) and in a wider sense (in linking their reputation to the assessment). More broadly still, at the societal level, issues of social justice, fair access and public confidence in assessment are all relevant to high-stakes testing, and in particular to admission to medical school.

The social impact of BMAT extends to issues such as the diversity of the physician workforce and public health. The British Medical Association (BMA) argued in 2009 that 'doctors should be as representative as possible of the society they serve in order to provide the best possible care to the UK population' (British Medical Association 2009). The General Medical Council (GMC) reported in 2011 that the medical profession has made significant strides in terms of diversity and change in recent years, with large increases in the number of doctors who are female and from ethnic minorities. However, in 2012, Higher Education Statistics Agency (HESA) data demonstrated that the proportion of applicants from lower socio-economic groups gaining access to medical study was still lower than desired (Milburn 2012). Under-representation of physicians from lower socio-economic

Figure 7.1 The context of BMAT scores

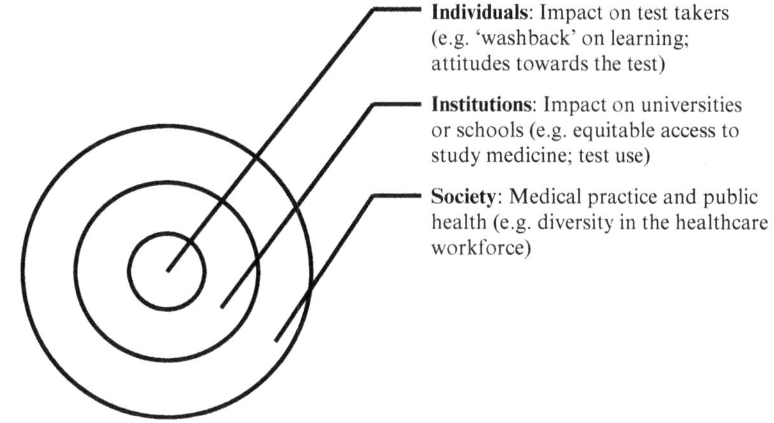
Individuals: Impact on test takers (e.g. 'washback' on learning; attitudes towards the test)
Institutions: Impact on universities or schools (e.g. equitable access to study medicine; test use)
Society: Medical practice and public health (e.g. diversity in the healthcare workforce)

backgrounds in the workforce has a profound impact on society as these doctors are those most likely to work with underserved patient populations (Dowell, Norbury, Steven and Guthrie 2015).

The processes of selection to medicine are complex, with many medical schools using a wide range of evidence, including school academic performance, work experience, 'traditional' (panel) interviews, multiple mini-interviews (MMIs) and teacher recommendations. As a key part of this process, it is important that admissions tests such as BMAT do not act as a deterrent to application, particularly in regard to the entry into medicine of students from lower socio-economic backgrounds.

Defining consequential validity

Consequential validity is conceptually distinct, though related to, the other types of validity discussed in this book. Issues such as cognitive validity, scoring validity and context validity relate primarily to the quality of a test as a measurement instrument ('technical quality') and are the responsibility of the test developers to address (Newton and Shaw 2014). In contrast, consequential validity is concerned with the impact that a test has on an individual, institutions or society ('social value'). Consequential validity must attend to socio-cultural contexts and policies relating to test use. Stakeholders, such as university departments, largely determine how the tests will be used in practice, and so influence the consequential validity of BMAT. Consequential validity is also influenced by the test design, schedule and preparation practices. For BMAT, the approach adopted by Cambridge Assessment Admissions Testing influences the consequential validity of the test, because decisions made by the test developer can impact how the test is used.

Approaches to validation frequently draw on frameworks or models to operationalise validation processes. Weir's (2005) socio-cognitive model, used throughout this volume to frame the validation evidence for BMAT, includes consequential validity as a crucial piece of evidence for scrutinising the fitness for purpose of a test. This aspect of Weir's model is influenced by Messick's (1989) concern with the 'consequences of test use'. Messick argued that any model that did not account for consequential validity was inadequate, as it failed to account for 'both evidence of the value implications of score meaning as a basis for action and the social consequences of score use' (Messick 1995:741).

Box 7.2 Messick's definition of validation

Validation is empirical evaluation of the *meaning* and *consequences* of measurement.

(Messick 1995:742, emphasis added)

While there is consensus that the social consequences of test use are crucial to consider, there is debate over whether these should be included in a 'unified' validity framework (as Weir proposes) or whether 'technical quality' and 'social value' should be conceptualised as separate issues. In the *International Handbook of Research in Medical Education*, Shea and Fortna (2002:110) summarise this issue by stating that 'no-one disagrees that the social consequences of test uses (and misuses) are important. The dispute is whether to call it "validity" or not'. In the wider educational assessment community, Cizek (2012) has argued that ethical and social considerations, such as those discussed in the present chapter, do not fall in the realm of validity. Others have narrowly defined validity to specifically exclude ethical and social evaluations regarding how test scores are used (Borsboom, Mellenbergh and van Heerden 2004). However, even these critics of consequential validity concede that the suitability of a testing procedure depends on more than the properties of the test itself. The *Standards* also recognised that the consequences of introducing an assessment are important to consider when evaluating a test (see Box 7.1).

For a more in-depth discussion of validity theory and the cases made for and against consequential validity, the reader is referred to Newton and Shaw (2014), who treat this topic in some detail. In the present chapter, we adopt the approach advocated in the socio-cognitive framework, by classing these issues as part of validity that need to be evaluated. Like Weir (2005), we advocate treating consequential validity as equal in status to other aspects of validity that are systematically and regularly considered. Consequential validity must be considered alongside other measures of test quality to ensure 'fitness for purpose' as it is possible to have a test that is an accurate measurement instrument, but that has negative impacts due to how it is used (Cronbach 1988). Included within this conceptualisation of consequential validity is an admissions test's impact on the behaviours of potential applicants and on universities using the test.

Consequential validity encompasses three elements: *washback*, *impact* and *differential validity* (Figure 7.2). Washback is effects that the test has on potential test takers or institutions before it is administered, for example, through preparation behaviours. Impact of the test occurs after it has been administered, for example through how test scores are used in the admissions process. In the admissions testing context, because consequences arising from use of a test often impact on future admissions cycles and test administrations, washback and impact can interrelate. For example the perceptions of people who take the test about its fairness may go on to influence how future generations of test takers will view the exam. In particular, views towards an admissions test, and whether these may influence a prospective student's decision to apply to a course, are important aspects of consequential validity.

Figure 7.2 The directionality of impact and washback

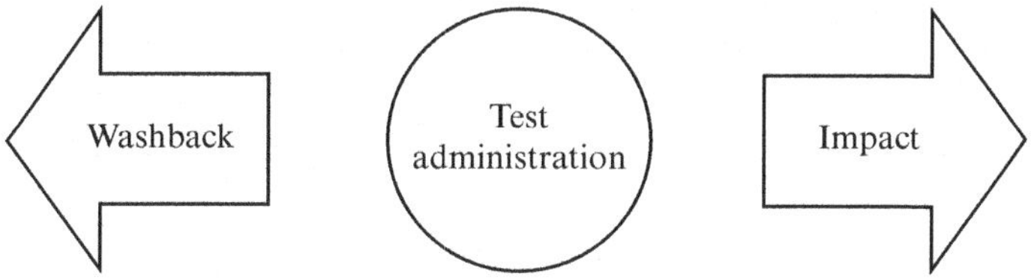

Washback

Washback refers to the influence that an examination has on educational practices. The adage that 'assessment drives learning' is well established in medical education (Newble 2016); 'washback' is a term used widely in the literature on language testing to describe this phenomenon. There is evidence that tests shape learners' preparation behaviours, educational materials, the teaching they receive and the curriculum they follow (Green 2007, Luxia 2007, Newble and Jaeger 1983, Saville and Hawkey 2004). Washback can be positive when test preparation encourages the acquisition of knowledge and skills which are beneficial beyond the context of the test. Conversely, negative washback refers to study behaviour that focuses only on 'learning the test'. Examples of negative washback occur when a test directs students to concentrate on narrow aspects of the curriculum, rewards attempting to 'question spot', or encourages focus on test-taking strategies at the expense of learning. Indeed, recent A Level reforms in

England were introduced to combat such negative washback effects that were perceived to be adversely impacting on learning and understanding: in April 2013, David Laws, the Schools Minister, stated: 'They [school students] and their teachers have spent too much time thinking about exams and re-sitting them, encouraging in some cases a "learn and forget" approach' (Long 2017). To maximise positive washback for candidates it is important to emphasise the relevance, importance and attainability of items in the test and to ensure they are appropriate for the test takers (Green 2003, 2006, Hughes 2003).

Hughes (2003) suggests that positive washback in high-stakes tests can be achieved by testing the abilities whose development you want to encourage, by sampling widely from the curriculum and by ensuring that the test is known and understood by students and their teachers. Green (2003) adds some further details that contribute to positive washback: that success on the test should be perceived to be both important and difficult (but attainable), and that these perceptions are shared by other test takers.

It is worth noting that washback from BMAT will occur in different ways than would be expected in a language testing context, or the context of other high-stakes exams, such as General Certificates of Secondary Education (GCSEs). With BMAT, there is no expectation that schools provide specific preparation for the test, and in fact a key concern of the universities using BMAT is that preparation should not entail significant new learning. However, one could argue that preparing for Section 2 of BMAT would encourage candidates to revise GCSE maths and science, and learn how to apply this knowledge in unfamiliar contexts, enhancing their pre-existing knowledge and developing skills that will be useful for their further study (A Levels and beyond). Furthermore, only a relatively small percentage of students will sit BMAT. Thus, it is unlikely that BMAT will influence the wider system of secondary education, and washback will be observed in terms of impacts on students' out-of-school activities (such as self-directed test preparation) and learning.

Impact

Impact, as described earlier, is the effect that the test has on the full range of stakeholders, and on society more generally. Test takers and selecting institutions are those affected most directly, as the results influence decisions about their future study paths and careers, and their academic cohorts, respectively. Additionally, schools, parents, and national medical and veterinary associations represent just some of the other groups impacted by tests such as BMAT in the wider social sphere.

Perhaps one of the most important impacts of admissions tests for medical study is the observed effect that selection might have on student learning and achievement. Kreiter and Axelson (2013) note that:

> Although effective educational interventions typically produce only small gains in learning, usually with effect sizes of .20 or less, evidence-based selection is comparatively far more powerful. In fact, when well designed, selection procedures in medical education can achieve performance gains easily exceeding 1 standard deviation (Kreiter and Axelson 2013:S51).

Entry to medical school is highly competitive: for 2017 entry, Universities and Colleges Admissions Service (UCAS) received 19,210 applications for approximately 6,000 medical school places (Universities and Colleges Admissions Service 2016). Consequently, medical schools aim to select those who are best suited to studying medicine, and have the best chance of successfully completing the medical degree programme. The role that an admissions test can play in selecting medical students and the positive impact that it can have on student learning and achievement is illustrated in the study by Reibnegger, Caluba, Ithaler, Manhal, Neges and Smolle (2010). Comparison of cohorts of medical students before and after the introduction of an admissions test into the selection process found that the probability of success at medical school was dramatically increased when students were selected using an admissions test compared to those admitted under an 'open' system. The reasons for this increased success rate were not explored but could include: students who performed better on the admissions test were better suited to the intellectual challenge of studying medicine; students who performed better in the test were more motivated to become doctors, and had invested more time and effort in preparing for the admissions test (see Wouters et al 2016). Whatever the underlying reason for the effect, it is evident that selecting a student body with a higher probability of educational success will have a positive impact on the medical school, as well as on individual students.

The impact of an admissions test is only partly explained by the test itself; it will also be determined by the policies surrounding its implementation and the way in which the test scores are used to select candidates. The study by Reibnegger et al (2010) illustrates how a change in government policy can have an impact on both the medical school and its students. Any impact on educational success and dropout rates will also be influenced by the way in which institutions use admissions test scores in their selection processes, and this varies between institutions (see the next section). Therefore stakeholders, including universities and regulatory bodies, play a key role in shaping test impact through the decisions they enact around test use.

Differential validity

Weir (2005) also includes *differential validity* as an aspect of consequential validity, relating to factors that differentially affect the performance of different groups of candidates. Issues of differential validity may pertain to difference in test-related behaviours, attitudes or outcomes by gender, ethnic, socio-economic or other demographic groupings. Although there is diversity in the selection methods employed at different UK medical schools, they universally include academic achievement, in terms of GCSE and A Level grades. This may not be surprising as there is evidence that past academic achievement is a useful predictor of success at medical school (Patterson et al 2016). However, school academic achievement is influenced by factors unrelated to potential: those from lower socio-economic groups tend to underperform relative to their more affluent peers (Blandon and Gregg 2004) even though this difference disappears once they enter higher education (Hoare and Johnston 2011).

One of the rationales for using an admissions test is to provide a standardised measure that levels the socio-economic and educational inequalities inherent in a pool of applicants. It is therefore crucial to evaluate admissions tests for differential validity to ensure that the tests do not reinforce inequity.

Bias is a key issue to consider in differential validity and is defined as score differences between groups that are not related to the construct being assessed. There are different ways of investigating bias, such as Differential Item Functioning (DIF) (Chapter 5) and predictive equity (Chapter 2). In the case of BMAT, there are persistent differences in mean scores, with males performing slightly better than females in Sections 1 and 2, and those from independent schools performing slightly better than those from comprehensive schools overall (see the key study in Chapter 2). However, there is no evidence of these issues being due to test bias, and the conclusion is rather that they are due to construct-relevant variance between the groups, which likely arises from a larger spectrum of socio-cultural influences which impact on students throughout their lives.

While the observed differences in BMAT scores are not attributable to test bias, Cambridge Assessment Admissions Testing is conducting further research to investigate these issues. In the two key studies presented in this chapter, we investigate issues of perceived fairness and test preparation, looking beyond statistical understandings of bias to other issues, which may affect the differential validity of an assessment. Findings from this research have helped shape our approach to supporting test preparation that is equitable, as will be described next.

Cambridge Assessment approaches to consequential validity

Impact by design

Consequential validity is considered in the design of BMAT test materials using the principle of *impact by design* (Saville 2012). This aligns the practice of Cambridge Assessment Admissions Testing with the Cambridge English approach to designing language tests. According to this position, test design and production processes should consider right from the outset the potential uses of the test, in order to maximise positive test impact for candidates. Test developers should also anticipate and mitigate negative impact as far as possible. By following four maxims (see Table 7.1) the positive impact of the test is enhanced as far as possible.

Table 7.1 Impact by design

Maxim 1	**PLAN** Adopt a rational and explicit approach to test development
Maxim 2	**SUPPORT** Support stakeholders in the testing process
Maxim 3	**COMMUNICATE** Provide comprehensive, useful and transparent information
Maxim 4	**MONITOR and EVALUATE** Collect all relevant data and analyse as required

By definition, impact by design principles are integrated throughout the test development and validation cycle (see Chapter 1 for the phases of the cycle), and how the test will be used by stakeholders is considered early in the planning phase. The substantial role that early users of BMAT had in defining the test meant that the intended uses were explicitly included in initial plans and subsequent reviews of BMAT. Cambridge Assessment adopts Saville's (2012) maxims by aiming to support and communicate with stakeholders continuously. The processes for this are outlined in the following portion of the chapter, alongside research that monitors and evaluates the impact of the test.

The socio-cognitive framework

Cambridge Assessment Admissions Testing conducts studies that evaluate the consequential validity of admissions tests. Research in this area tends to be naturalistic, that is, it is focused on exploring existing practices and perceptions. Research and practice on BMAT's consequential validity is framed according to the socio-cognitive validation framework proposed by Weir (2005), which can be used to pose five guiding questions as presented in Box 7.3.

Box 7.3 Questions on consequential validity (Weir 2005)

1. Are actions based on test scores appropriate?
2. Is there a washback effect in the classroom (positive or negative)?
3. Is there any evidence of differential validity?
4. How are candidates preparing for the test?
5. How is the test perceived by stakeholders?

The rest of this chapter considers issues relating to consequential validity, using the criteria proposed by Weir (Box 7.3) as a framework. Thus, we describe the use of BMAT scores by universities, consider washback in the context of BMAT, and present research investigating applicants' preparation behaviours, and their perceptions of the test.

Evidence of differential validity was addressed in Chapter 5, in which work on investigating and preventing bias in BMAT was presented. As part of the work presented here, we discuss research studies that investigated how differential access to test preparation material impacts on test performance, and also how students from different backgrounds perceive BMAT.

7.3 Are actions based on test scores appropriate?

Appropriate score use centres on two issues: the reliability of the test as a decision-making instrument, and how scores are used in practice to make selection decisions.

Based on research presented in earlier chapters of this volume, we know that BMAT scores can effectively be used to support admissions decisions. There is a close relationship between the score interpretation aspect of consequential validity and the criterion-related aspect of validity, which is discussed in more detail in Chapter 6. Ensuring that test scores mean the same thing for all test taker groups (as discussed in Chapter 2, on test taker characteristics, and in Chapter 5, on scoring validity) is another facet of consequential validity. Chapter 2 discusses predictive equity and Chapter 5 describes DIF analyses for BMAT in detail, so they will not be revisited here.

Cambridge Assessment Admissions Testing recommends that BMAT results are used alongside other selection criteria in making admissions decisions. BMAT provides a measure of a student's ability to perform academically in pre-clinical course work; however other attributes, such as interpersonal skills or motivation to study medicine are also important, and frequently assessed in the admissions process. It is also acknowledged that medical schools need autonomy in determining the specific ways in which they use test scores in their admissions process. The way in which BMAT is used within the admissions process is largely determined by the policies and practices of the individual university departments that use it. Thus there are a number of ways in which BMAT is used. For example, some medical schools use 'cut-off' scores and will only consider applications above a minimum score. Others use BMAT scores to conduct an initial ranking to determine which application they will fully review first. Some medical schools use BMAT scores to determine who will be invited for interviews while others consider scores after interviews. Furthermore, some give equal consideration to all three sections, while others may give more importance to scores on a certain section (for example, BMAT Section 2).

The practices around test use are shaped by the particular needs and values of each university.

Due to the range of ways that universities use BMAT in their admissions process, Cambridge Assessment Admissions Testing supports a 'BMAT Liaison Group' in which universities share their admissions practices and discuss the issues they are facing. Cambridge Assessment hosts these twice-yearly meetings, to which representatives of all the faculties that use BMAT are invited. The meeting is an opportunity to update on recently completed research, to recap the key issues from the previous live session, and to explore questions around the nature of admissions test use. This forum also provides support for new institutions using BMAT for the first time. Admissions tutors from universities where BMAT has been used for a number of years are able to outline how the test fits into their own processes of selecting candidates for interview, or for an offer of a place, and can discuss the impact that the test has had on their own admissions rounds for the benefit of new users.

Understanding the ways in which test scores are used (and establishing that the use of scores from high-stakes tests in decision-making processes is justified) is an important aspect of consequential validity for stakeholder institutions. In Box 7.4, Professor David Vaux describes how the University of Oxford uses BMAT in conjunction with other indicators to shortlist candidates for interview, plus the way in which they assess the validity of the test for its intended purpose and its perceived value in their admissions process. This case study describes how Oxford's own monitoring of test use and candidate performance ensures that the actions arising from their use of BMAT scores are appropriate.

Box 7.4 Professor David Vaux[1] on the use of BMAT at the University of Oxford

BMAT was introduced for our undergraduate Medicine admissions in 2003. The primary use of the BMAT test when it was first introduced was as a shortlisting tool. There are far more applicants for Medicine than can be interviewed, so some method was needed for deciding whom to call for interview. In addition, very many Medicine applications are not from the UK, so comparisons have to be made across candidates in different school systems taking different school exams. For instance, in 2013 only 68% of candidates had GCSEs. BMAT is extremely useful in this context as a piece of data that is available for all candidates.

1 Professor David Vaux is Nuffield Research Fellow in Pathology and Tutor in Medicine at the University of Oxford.

How do we use BMAT?
BMAT is one component of the information used to generate a combined score for our initial algorithmic shortlisting process; the other component is a contextualised GCSE score where available. Approximately 90% of our shortlist is drawn from the top-ranked applicants using this combined score; all remaining applications are then inspected individually to ensure that all mitigating circumstances are appropriately taken into consideration, resulting in the addition of the final approximately 10% of our shortlist. The interviewers in each panel at both colleges do not know the BMAT score (or the college choice) during the interview process. College tutors receive BMAT scores and second college interview rankings only after they have submitted their own interview ranking. Tutors then make their final decisions based upon all of the separate items of information available to them.

Assessing the validity of BMAT as a selection tool
We carry out an annual analysis of the relationships between performance on indicators available during the selection process and performance during the course (separated into performance in the first and second year course, the Bachelor of Medicine (BM) examination, and overall performance in the third year Final Honour School (FHS) degree examinations.

Based upon recent comparisons across results for three years (2010, 2011, 2012), the statistically significant factors affecting BM examination performance are the total BMAT score, the mean interview score and gender. Only the total BMAT score and the mean interview score are effects that are stable over time.

There are two statistically significant factors that affect the FHS performance (the average score and the classified outcome) – the total BMAT score and the BM1 result. Both factors explain around 23% of the total variability of the FHS result suggesting they can be useful in predicting the FHS performance. Although the BM1 result is more useful and important in predicting FHS performance, this score is not available during the selection process. Of the information available during the admissions process, only the total BMAT score was shown to be a statistically significant predictor of academic performance.

An ongoing analysis of outcomes at the end of the 6-year standard medical course for the five cohorts for which data is now available suggests that there remain some statistically significant correlations between BMAT performance and performance in clinical finals (second BM examination) six years later, although this is a preliminary analysis and the effects are not seen for all sections of BMAT for all years. This is perhaps unsurprising, as BMAT is designed to assess academic skills that are, perhaps, more important in the pre-clinical years and less relevant in the clinical years, in which assessment of professional practice plays a greater role.

Stakeholder involvement
An important aspect of any test is the extent to which it retains the confidence of its users. Cambridge Assessment Admissions Testing has worked to ensure the engagement of stakeholders in a process of continuous scrutiny of the utility and performance of BMAT. In addition, Cambridge Assessment Admissions Testing has been pro-active in driving future development of BMAT, and ensuring that this evolution is directed by the needs of the stakeholders.

7.4 Is the washback effect positive?

BMAT is designed to both decrease negative washback (time spent on solely test-related knowledge or skills) and promote positive washback, by encouraging the development of academic skills relevant to success at medical school. BMAT is intended to require minimal preparation by students, and focuses on developing skills, such as problem solving, which will benefit them beyond the context of the test. The approaches taken to design positive washback and equitable access to test preparation materials are described in the following part of the chapter.

BMAT's explicit purpose is to help admissions tutors select the candidates with the potential to succeed in fast-paced, demanding, science-based courses (such as the non-clinical parts of medicine courses). This alignment of test content to medical course study is important for positive washback effects. BMAT does not aim to be a context-free measure of intelligence; rather, preparing for BMAT is directly related to school studies and future learning at university.

As discussed in Chapters 3 and 4, the content of BMAT Section 1 is not tied to any particular topics in school curricula and does not require specialised knowledge beyond basic computations for the problem solving items. BMAT Section 3 (Writing Task) also assumes no content knowledge. Nonetheless, the skills elicited by these sections are learnable skills, the practice of which is likely to have a positive effect on future learning.

BMAT Section 2 requires the application of scientific content knowledge. The content knowledge assumed by Section 2 is based on the National Curriculum for England and Wales and the GCSE science and maths specifications for the major UK examination boards. The syllabuses for international qualifications are also reviewed by Cambridge Assessment. As most candidates who are applying to study medicine or veterinary medicine will hold at least an A grade at GCSE (or equivalent) in two or three science subjects, and will be studying a combination of sciences for their A Levels, BMAT candidates should find that their preparation focuses on revising and refreshing knowledge rather than learning large amounts of new material.

For mature students, preparing for BMAT Section 2 may require greater effort as applicants are likely to have lost familiarity with school-leaving science content at the point of applying to medical school. In this instance, preparing for Section 2 presents useful washback as applicants focus on learning, or relearning, science content that will be foundational to pre-clinical course work undertaken in medical education. Indeed, for some admissions tutors using BMAT in graduate-entry courses, the test's role in promoting positive washback is a key reason for using the test.

For high-stakes exams such as A Levels, which follow a specific curriculum with formal teaching input, support for teachers is central to fostering positive impact. For BMAT this is not the case: specific teaching and specialist preparation is not required. The concentration on core biology, chemistry, mathematics and physics in BMAT Section 2 (endorsed by admissions tutors as important to success as a medical student) means that any revision done will support and complement candidates' preparation for school-leaving exams, rather than divert their attention from their studies. Furthermore, the fact that BMAT questions do not rely on factual recall alone, but require knowledge to be applied and recombined in novel ways to reach solutions makes preparation for BMAT useful for encouraging thinking skills conducive to university-level study.

The timing of BMAT is further also intended to minimise negative washback. In the UK, BMAT usually takes place on the first Wednesday in November each year, and has traditionally been timetabled in order to fit with the universities' schedules for shortlisting and interviewing applicants to medicine. As the majority of BMAT candidates are in their final year of school study, it has been considered important that preparation for the test would not affect their usual school performance nor eat into valuable study time – a concern mitigated by a test date early in the academic year.

As described previously, it is unlikely that BMAT would influence the larger system of secondary education, and washback in this context primarily concerns self-directed test preparation activities that students undertake. Nonetheless, applicants to medical school spend a substantial amount of time in self-preparation for an admissions test, so the considerations for optimising test washback are important. The following part of the chapter outlines some of the key findings on the consequential validity of BMAT.

7.5 How are candidates preparing for the test?

Key research study – An investigation into candidates' preparation for the BioMedical Admissions Test (Gallacher, McElwee and Cheung 2017)

Main findings

- The majority of students feel well prepared for BMAT.
- Attempting practice tests under timed conditions is associated with achieving better test scores.
- There are some gender differences in feelings of preparedness, test preparation strategies and test outcomes.
- Commercial courses and extra help from schools are not associated with better test outcomes.

Introduction

As described earlier in the chapter, understanding the ways that students prepare for BMAT is important in gaining a picture of the wider test impact and washback effects of BMAT. The research summarised below investigated candidates' preparation for BMAT and how preparation strategies may influence test performance. These studies investigated the role of help received through commercial preparation courses, from schools and self-preparation activities, such as self-directed study with the free preparation materials provided by Cambridge Assessment Admissions Testing.

The research was designed to explore the strategies and materials used by students to prepare for BMAT, as these are the main washback effects of tests. Furthermore, it was hypothesised that preparation would be influenced by background variables, such as socio-economic status and school type, and that the amount of preparation help available to candidates may influence their test scores. Better-resourced schools, especially in the independent sector, are often better placed to devote time to helping candidates with special tuition and exam techniques. Students from independent schools are already over-represented in professions such as medicine (Milburn 2012). It was therefore deemed important to investigate whether (a) there was any evidence of systematic preparation in the independent sector, and (b) whether this translated into better test scores for this cohort, which would threaten the differential validity of the test and its equity for all candidates. However, estimating the impact of preparation from schools and from commercial coaching organisations is tricky, and some large-scale US studies using data from Scholastic Aptitude Tests (SATs) and the American College Test (ACT) have found that coaching gains have been largely over-estimated (Briggs 2001, 2004).

Claims made by commercial organisations offering test preparation that boosts scores need careful critical analysis. Firstly, estimates of score gains from commercial coaching must be made in relation to a control group of similar students who did not prepare for the test with a commercial programme – without this control group, any test preparation 'effect' is misleading. A second, perhaps more challenging, problem is that the groups of students who opt to pay for commercial coaching or not are not assigned at random. Those who choose to pay for coaching are actively self-selected and, as a group, may differ on other important variables also related to admissions test performance such as conscientiousness, motivation, or family encouragement characteristics.

In order to address issues on consequential validity related to test preparation, Cambridge Assessment produces BMAT preparation materials and makes these freely available. These materials include specimen and past papers, worked examples, answer keys and, recently, the *BMAT Section 2: Assumed Subject Knowledge guide*, which is a revision tool focused on the science knowledge needed for Section 2. Making these freely available is intended to provide all students with equal access.

Cambridge Assessment Admissions Testing maintains that its policy of making BMAT preparation materials available for free on its website means that commercial preparation courses are unnecessary. The website states that:

> Anyone offering a paid service to help you pass your admissions test(s) will have no more knowledge than someone who has read this website and studied past papers. So while a learner's performance at any test will improve with some familiarisation or practice, we would not advise candidates to pay for such help.[2]

Box 7.5 Preparation resources provided on the BMAT website[3]

BMAT Preparation Guide
Practice papers for Sections 1, 2 and 3
Worked examples for Sections 1, 2, and 3
BMAT Section 2: Assumed Subject Knowledge guide
Sample essays with examiner comments for Section 3
Test specification
Short videos introducing the test and on student experience with the test

The study presented here was conducted to inform Cambridge Assessment practices and policies, and to provide an evidence base for the preparation

2 www.admissionstestingservice.org/for-test-takers/preparation-materials
3 All resources on the BMAT website are openly accessible and free of charge.

guidance given to candidates. In addition, the research aimed to estimate the prevalence of preparation course use in the BMAT candidature. After presenting the research study, we describe how these research findings have informed the development of free resources that are made available to test candidates.

Study aims

The analysis presented here draws from two surveys that investigated candidates' preparation behaviours and their feelings of preparedness. Survey responses were also linked to BMAT scores where possible, to explore the relationships between self-reports of preparation and performance on the test. The research aims of this analysis were:

- to gain an understanding of the preparation behaviours of BMAT candidates, including use of help beyond the support freely available on the Cambridge Assessment website
- to test for relationships between preparation behaviours and BMAT performance, including the use of help beyond the support freely available on the Cambridge Assessment website
- to gain an understanding of the feelings of preparedness, and how useful each source of help is in preparing for BMAT.

Study methods

The main survey consisted of items about demographic background, feelings of preparedness, use of preparation materials and details of external help received from either schools or commercial organisations. Online delivery was used to administer the questions and the survey was made available on the BMAT website after candidates had already taken the test; approximately half of respondents responded before knowing their BMAT scores, while the rest responded after test results were released. Participation was voluntary and results presented here are anonymous, but candidate details were collected to enable matching to BMAT results data from the November 2015 session. In addition to data from the 2015 survey, responses from a similar survey administered in 2007 and 2008 are reported (Emery 2010b). Although the surveys included similar questions, the sampling procedures were different between the studies: Emery (2010b) only included candidates who had successfully gained entry into medical study whilst the 2015 survey sampled candidates soon after sitting the test, some of whom may not have gone on to study medicine. Therefore, the results of the two studies should not be directly compared. The discussion here focuses primarily on findings from the 2015 survey; however results from the earlier survey are reported to triangulate findings across the studies.

Missing data was excluded from analysis on an analysis-by-analysis basis, instead of including only that with full sets of responses. Therefore the sample size 'n' varies considerably across analyses. This affects more complicated multivariate analyses more heavily than simple analyses, but allows maximal use of the data. The cohort is analysed as a whole, and also divided by gender and school type to investigate patterns of differential responses and scores.

Results

Feeling prepared for BMAT

Candidates were asked to report how prepared they felt before taking the test. These perceptions of preparedness were investigated across groups by gender and school category. The majority of respondents felt 'very well prepared' or 'quite well prepared' (66%), and a low proportion of respondents felt 'very under prepared' (6%). Figure 7.3 shows the distribution of responses from the 2015 and 2007 samples side by side, showing that they are broadly similar across the two administrations, with a slight increase in the proportion of respondents who felt very or quite prepared.

Figure 7.3 Feelings of preparedness for the 2015 sample and 2007 sample

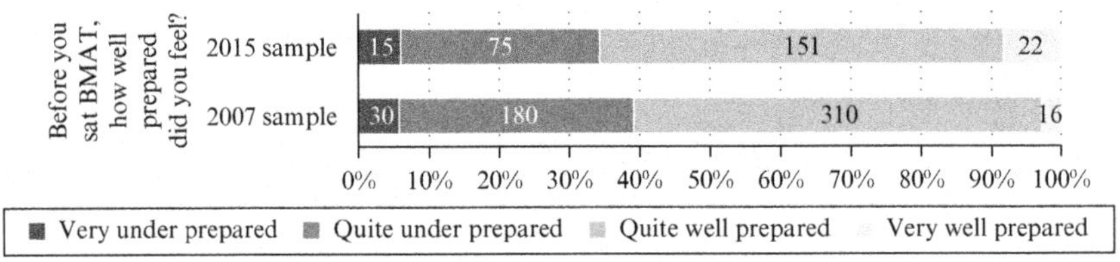

There were significant differences in feelings of preparedness across respondent backgrounds. Female respondents reported feeling less prepared than male respondents (Mann-Whitney $U = 6165$, $p = 0.038$), as can be seen in Figure 7.4: 72% of males felt very or quite well prepared compared to only 62% of females. Most of this difference is accounted for by the fact that males were more than twice as likely to report feeling very well prepared than females (12.8% versus 5.4%) Emery (2010b) found similar gender differences in feelings of preparedness in the 2007 sample.

Figure 7.4 Feelings of preparedness for the 2015 sample, by gender

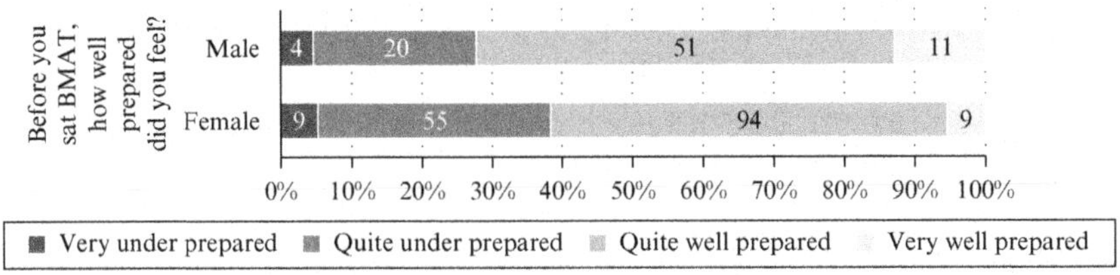

Whether this gender difference in self-reported preparedness is related to actual preparedness is unclear. Female respondents spent more time preparing for BMAT, on average, than males (see Figure 7.3), which might suggest that they were more prepared. The differences in reported preparedness might be related to gender differences in test anxiety or self-belief in their abilities. Female students score more highly on measures of test anxiety than males (Hembree 1988). Moreover, it is known that gender differences in self-belief persist, especially with respect to maths and science subjects at school. For instance, female students were found to be less confident of performing well on a maths test, despite negligible differences in actual test scores (Ross, Scott and Bruce 2012). This was found to be related to lower self-efficacy and a higher fear of failure in female students than in males.

It was found that there were significant differences in feelings of preparedness between respondents from different school types ($\chi^2 = 11.22$, $p = 0.011$). Despite the widely held assumption that students from independent schools receive more support in preparing for BMAT than state-schooled students, this was not borne out by the responses in the 2015 survey (Figure 7.5). UK state school respondents reported feeling better prepared than overseas students or respondents from independent schools. In contrast, the previous survey (Emery 2010b) found no association between school type and feelings of preparedness. In the intervening period, Cambridge Assessment Admissions Testing has improved the provision of preparation materials for test takers on their website, to include a *BMAT Section 2: Assumed Subject Knowledge guide*, explained answers for Sections 1 and 2 practice papers, and examples of Section 3 answers, with examiner comments. As these resources are freely available, state-schooled test takers may feel more reassured that they have been able to adequately prepare for BMAT, and this may be reflected in their responses in the 2015 survey.

Figure 7.5 Feelings of preparedness for the 2015 sample by school type

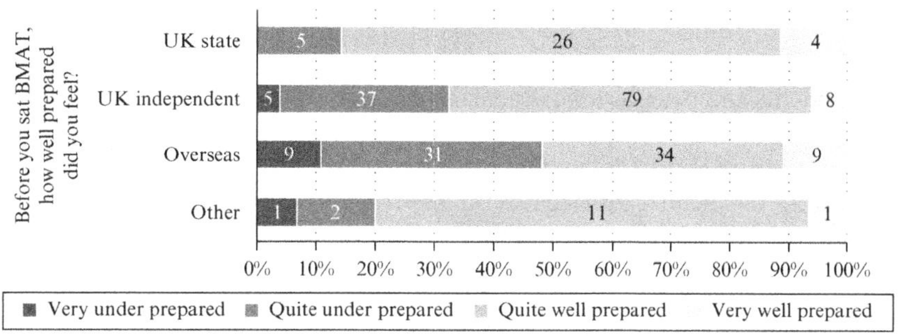

Across the entire 2015 survey sample, more hours of preparation was related to feeling more prepared generally. Moreover, those who felt more prepared were significantly more likely to perform better at BMAT Section 1 ($r_s = 0.164, p = 0.005$), Section 2 ($r_s = 0.164, p = 0.005$), and Section 3's quality of content ($r_s = 0.121, p = 0.031$) than respondents who felt under prepared. These effects of feelings of preparedness on test performance are small, but significant.

Participants were also likely to report feeling better prepared for BMAT if they had looked at the specimen tests on the BMAT website, had tried the specimen tests under timed conditions, or had used the BMAT preparation book. These ratings indicate that there are some very simple steps that candidates can take to feel better prepared for BMAT, which may positively impact their confidence on the test day.

Self-study for BMAT

Self-study was defined as using past papers, the *BMAT Section 2: Assumed Subject Knowledge guide*, and textbooks, but excluded time reported engaged in preparation support sessions delivered by schools or attending preparation courses. The median amount of self-study time reported for BMAT preparation was approximately 30 hours in the 2015 survey. This represents a considerable increase from the 2007 survey, when the median reported preparation time was eight hours (Emery 2010b). This could be a consequence of the additional preparation materials made available to test takers on the BMAT website. Out of 295 survey respondents, six respondents reported spending over 200 hours for BMAT overall (the maximum reported being 10,000 hours), so any value greater than 3 standard deviations from the median was treated as an outlier and excluded (greater than 216). Figure 7.6 displays the distribution of responses.

The time spent preparing for each BMAT section varied considerably (Table 7.2) with respondents spending much more time (on average) on Sections 1 and 2, than on Section 3. The difference between the time spent preparing for the different BMAT sections was more striking than in the previous survey (Emery 2010b): 2015 respondents spent (on average) 6-fold and 5-fold more time preparing for Sections 1 and 2, respectively, than the 2007 respondents and twice as long preparing for Section 3.

As mentioned above, female respondents reported spending more time preparing for BMAT (on average) than their male counterparts (Table 7.3). However, the gender differences in reported preparation time were not significant for Sections 1 and 2. This is in contrast to the previous study (Emery 2010b), which found that females reported a significantly greater number of hours preparing for BMAT Section 2 than males. From the 2015 sample, only the difference between genders in Section 3 preparation hours was significant (Mann-Whitney $U = 5664.5, p = 0.026$).

Figure 7.6 Hours spent preparing for the BMAT

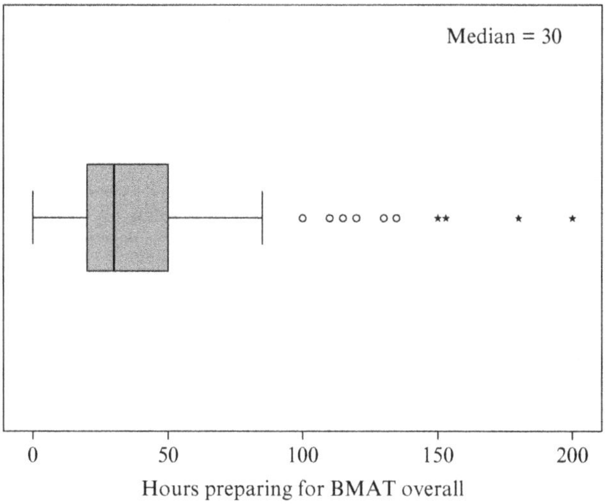

Table 7.2 Median numbers of hours' preparation for the 2015 sample and 2007 sample

Hours preparing for:	Median	
	2015 sample	2007 sample
BMAT overall	30	8
BMAT Section 1	12	2
BMAT Section 2	15	3
BMAT Section 3	4	2

Table 7.3 Median numbers of hours' preparation for the 2015 sample, by gender

Hours preparing for:	Median	
	Male	Female
BMAT overall	29	32
BMAT Section 1	10.5	11
BMAT Section 2	14	15
BMAT Section 3	3	5

Some interesting differences in the median number of hours spent preparing for BMAT were observed between different school types (Table 7.4). Respondents from the Other category (the majority of whom are 'mature' applicants over 21) reported spending the most time preparing for BMAT, followed by respondents from UK independent schools. However, the difference was only significant with respect to the number of hours spent preparing for Section 3 (Kruskall-Wallis test $\chi^2 = 10.87, p = 0.012$).

Table 7.4 Median numbers of hours' preparation for the 2015 sample, by school category

Hours preparing for	Median			
	UK state	UK independent	Overseas	Other
BMAT overall	29	35	31	42
BMAT Section 1	11	15	10	15
BMAT Section 2	14	15	15	20
BMAT Section 3	4	5	2	10

Almost all respondents (95%) reported that they used the BMAT website for preparation (Figure 7.7) and about 90% looked at the full specimen tests for Sections 1 and 2; whereas only 80% of respondents had used the Section 3 specimen paper (Figure 7.8).

Figure 7.7 Sources of help while preparing for BMAT 2015

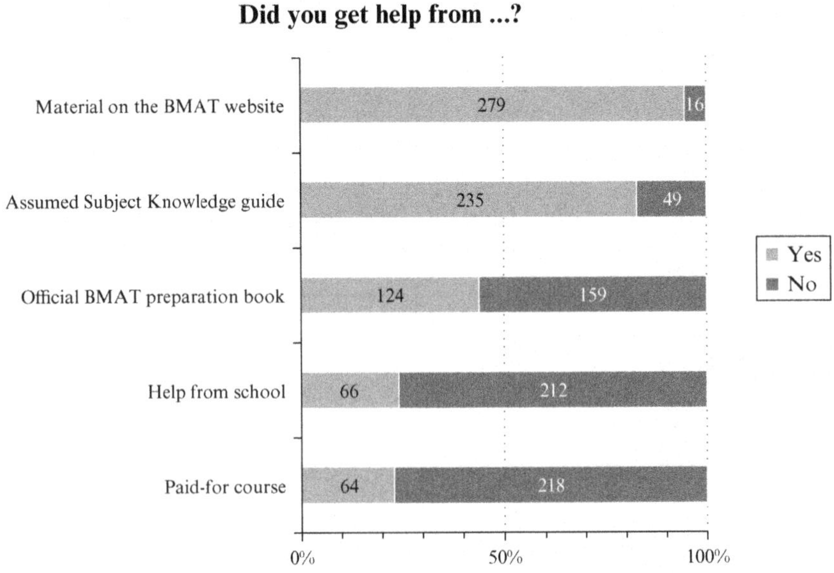

Figure 7.8 Use of Cambridge Assessment Admissions Testing material while preparing for BMAT by the 2015 sample

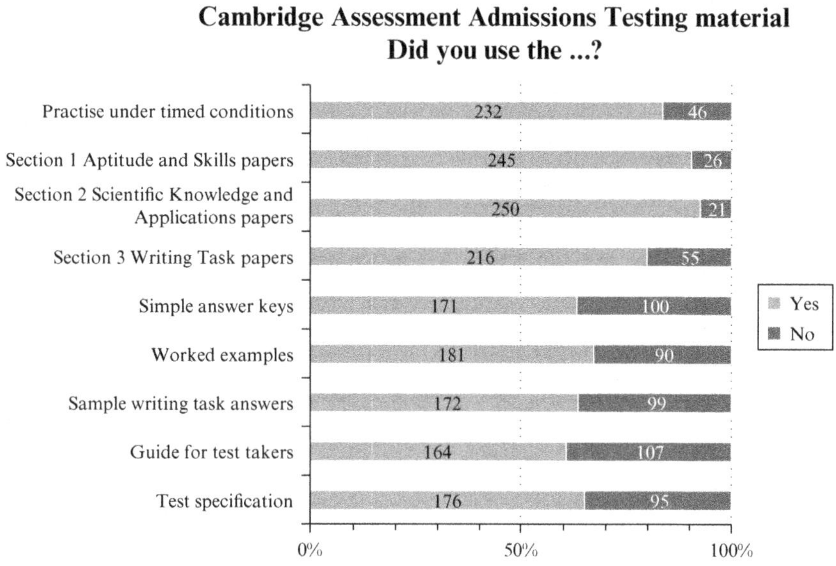

In the 2015 sample, the majority of candidates (83%) who looked at practice test papers reported practising under timed conditions (Figure 7.8). This suggests a change in test preparation behaviours, as Emery (2010b) found that only one third of students who reported using the specimen papers had practised them under timed conditions. Females reported lower rates of practising under timed conditions than did males. The reasons for this are unclear but could contribute to female respondents feeling less prepared for the test than males (see Figure 7.4).

External help preparing for BMAT

While the free materials provided by Cambridge Assessment Admissions Testing were widely used, only a minority of students in 2015 reported receiving help from their school or from commercial courses: overall, 24% of respondents reported getting help from their school and 23% reported attending a course (Figure 7.7). However, there was considerable difference between candidates from different school backgrounds in the likelihood of receiving external help. Overseas respondents were the least likely to access external help in preparing for BMAT, followed by those from the 'other' category. In common with the findings from the previous survey (Emery 2010b), candidates from UK independent schools were much more likely to receive help from their school, or attend a course, than respondents from other

Figure 7.9 Sources of help while preparing for BMAT, by school type

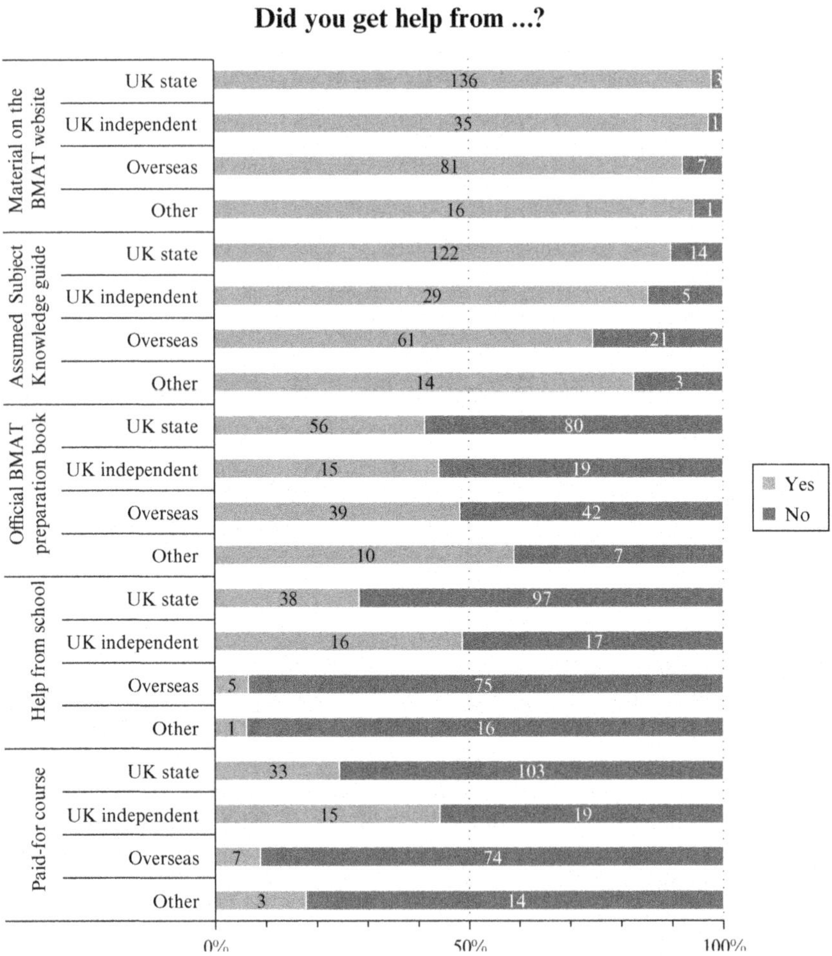

backgrounds. Almost half (48%) of UK independent school respondents had received help from their school, compared to 28% for UK state schools; and 6% each for overseas and 'other' (Figure 7.9). This may not be surprising, in light of other evidence that independent schools invest more time and effort in preparing their students for applying to medical school (Wright 2015). Similarly 44% of UK independent school respondents had attended a commercial course, compared to 24%, 9% and 18% for UK state schools, overseas and 'other' respectively (Figure 7.9). Again, this is perhaps unsurprising: parents who pay for their children's education are more likely to be able to afford to pay for a commercial course. The fact that independently schooled respondents were much more likely to access external help in preparing for BMAT could be perceived as affording them an additional advantage in applying to medical school. This could be a cause for concern for medical schools and candidates from outside of the UK independent school sector, but it should be noted that the results from the 2015 survey do not demonstrate any association between accessing these forms of external help and improved BMAT scores (see the next section).

The 2007 survey also found that there was considerable variation between different school backgrounds in the amount of school help accessed: for those students who *did* report receiving school help, the modal (most frequently reported) number of hours of help accessed was five to nine hours for independent school students, three to four hours for grammar/selective school students, and one hour for comprehensive school students (Emery 2010b). In this survey, the majority of respondents reported receiving no preparation help from their school. For those that did report receiving school help, this amounted to an average of three hours (which was the same for state and independent school students) and was most frequently in the form of advice on BMAT test contents rather than organised tuition/revision classes.

Relationships between types of preparation and BMAT scores

Relationships between preparation behaviours and BMAT performance were tested using correlations and hierarchical regression analysis. In each analysis, the impact of gender and school type was investigated, as well as the self-reports of test preparation behaviours from the survey.

When interpreting these findings it must be considered that there is no baseline measure of candidates' ability, and so it is unknown whether candidates choosing different methods of BMAT preparation were of equal ability at the outset. Choice of preparation method may be related to other characteristics that determine test performance that cannot be controlled for without additional data. *Causal* relationships between preparation methods and test performance should therefore not be inferred.

Bi-variate analysis shows that attempting practice tests under timed conditions was associated with higher tests scores on all sections of BMAT. In contrast, attempting practice tests without time constraints was associated with poorer test performance. Similarly, looking at practice papers without attempting to answer them was also associated with poorer performance on Sections 1 and 2. This finding was confirmed through multi-variate analysis; practising under timed conditions remained a significant predictor of test performance on all three sections of BMAT when controlling for other factors.

None of the following preparation behaviours was found to predict test performance in multi-variate models controlling for other factors: using materials from the BMAT website, accessing help from school or attending a commercial course. Moreover, no association was found between the hours spent preparing for BMAT and test scores.

Differential validity was also investigated. After controlling for test preparation behaviours, gender (male) was significantly associated with better performance on Section 2, though not on Sections 1 or 3. Issues relating to gender differences in test performance have been described in Chapter 2. In contrast, no association was observed between the following factors and better test performance: school type, help received at school or attending commercial preparation courses. This is encouraging in terms of social justice and access to the medical profession for state-schooled students from lower income backgrounds, who may attend schools that are less experienced in preparing their students to apply to medical school (Wright 2015) and who cannot afford to pay for a preparatory course.

Discussion

This study into BMAT preparation investigated consequential validity questions about how candidates are preparing for BMAT, feeling of preparedness and associations between preparation strategies and test performance. Throughout the analysis we investigated whether there were differential effects by gender or school type.

Candidates now spend 30 hours (on average) preparing for BMAT, a substantial increase from the reported average of eight hours in the 2007 survey (Emery 2010b). The reasons for this increase are not known but one possible explanation may be that there are now considerably more resources freely available on the BMAT website than there were at the time of the previous survey. As candidates are investing a substantial amount of time on test preparation, the issue of washback is particularly important to ensure that time spent on test preparation has educational value beyond performance on the test.

Attempting tests under timed conditions is associated with better test performance, and based on this finding the test preparation guidelines on the BMAT website encourage students to use this technique. Simply looking at papers without attempting them, or attempting papers without time constraints were both associated with poorer performance, suggesting that these are ineffective or even counterproductive preparation behaviours. If candidates become used to spending more time than realistic per question, they will be less able to answer the questions in the time available during the live administration, causing undue stress and underperformance compared to practice papers. We found that females are less likely to practise under timed conditions, and tend to have slightly lower scores on Section 2; however, we cannot infer causation between these findings.

While a quarter of students receive external help from either schools or commercial courses in test preparation, there was no evidence that this resulted in higher test scores when controlling for other variables. From this we conclude that while students from different socio-economic backgrounds engage in different test preparation strategies, there is not evidence that this systematically gives any group an advantage on test performance.

This study aimed to provide a picture of how candidates prepare for BMAT and demonstrated that there are some simple, and low-cost, ways to prepare for the test that impact upon candidates' sense of test-readiness. Any gains from commercial coaching, while difficult to estimate in a correlational design, were not apparent from this data.

7.6 How is the test perceived by stakeholders?

Key research study – Student perceptions of the medical admissions process (Emery and McElwee 2014)

Main findings

- Perceptions of admissions tests are not a deterrent to applying to medical study.
- Admissions tests are seen as 'daunting' for similar reasons as interviews.
- There are gender differences in how admissions test are perceived.

Introduction and context

A key group of BMAT stakeholders are the test candidates themselves – it is important to investigate whether candidates view BMAT as fair and whether their perceptions of the test pose a barrier to applying to university. A piece of research was carried out (Emery and McElwee 2014) to investigate candidates' perceptions of admissions tests within the wider context of the medical applications process.

Selection to study medicine in the UK is an area of particular challenge with respect to widening participation (that is, the desire to increase the proportion of students in higher education who come from traditionally under-represented – i.e. more socially disadvantaged – groups). A much higher proportion of students of medicine and dentistry in the UK come from the higher socio-economic groups (Steven, Dowell, Jackson and Guthrie 2016). In the late 1990s, students from social class I (whose parents have professional occupations) were 30 times more likely to gain a place at medical school than those from class V (whose parents have partly skilled or unskilled occupations) (Seyan, Greenhalgh and Dorling 2004). More recently, it was found that applicants from social class I still predominate and those from lower social classes are significantly under-represented in the applicant pool. Moreover, those from National Statistics Socio-economic Classification

(NS-SEC) class 1 are more likely to be successful in their application than those from the lowest social class (NS-SEC class V) (Steven et al 2016).

Widening participation (WP) in medicine has particularly difficult challenges to overcome. Entry requirements are competitive, with admissions tutors generally looking for three A grades at A Level as a minimum. This is an issue as A Level attainment is closely related to social class and it is acknowledged that candidates from WP backgrounds may have school grades that underestimate their potential for higher education study (Hoare and Johnston 2011). Applicants to medicine are also generally required to demonstrate that they have acquired work experience (usually unpaid) in a medical or community setting. This may also disadvantage students from WP backgrounds for various reasons: because they cannot afford to do voluntary work; public transport links are not suitable if they are from rural areas; or they have lesser access to personal or family connections through which they can organise suitable placements. Finally, the length of the degree course in medicine may be a deterrent in respect of the higher tuition fees and associated costs of accommodation.

With all of these competing issues, it is important that an admissions test such as BMAT does not pose an additional barrier to entry for students from WP backgrounds (or from state schools, who are also under-represented in medical study). Emery and McElwee's (2014) study aimed to take a 'student voice' perspective and explore how potential medicine applicants perceive admissions tests such as BMAT, as part of the applications process for medical study in the UK.

Research questions

1. Do students' views on admissions tests and other selection criteria for medical study differ according to their social and educational backgrounds?
2. Are students from WP backgrounds (or from state schools) more likely to view admissions tests as a deterrent to applying to study medicine?

Data collection and analyses

This study used a convergent mixed methods survey design to investigate students' perceptions of selection methods (academic achievement, admissions tests, traditional interviews and MMIs) and potential differences according to gender and socio-economic status. A survey including demographic items, Likert-rating scales and open-ended questions was distributed to students interested in applying to medical school. The survey was distributed at medical school 'open days' for perspective applicants, and on the BMAT website. Participation was voluntary.

WP indicators were collected; including whether the respondent was eligible for free school meals or education maintenance bursaries, or whether they were the first in their family to attend university. Students from state schools who also had met one of the WP indicators were considered as potentially having WP status for medical school admissions and were classified as WP in our analysis.

Questions on attitudes towards the selection criteria were mostly in Likert-scale format (ratings on a 5-point scale from 1 'not at all' to 5 'very'). These questions asked students about their perceptions of the fairness, usefulness and relevance of each of the criteria, how daunting they considered each to be, and their level of confidence that they could perform well on these. Open-ended questions were included for students to expand on their responses to Likert-scale questions.

Likert responses were analysed to calculate mean ratings for each selection method and these were used to investigate differences between groups. Responses to open-ended questions were analysed through a general inductive approach. In a second stage, quantitative and qualitative results were integrated and interpreted leading to a second round of qualitative analysis.

Throughout the survey, the questions referred to 'admissions tests' (or specific admissions test skills) rather than specifically asking about BMAT. A number of skills tested by the United Kingdom Clinical Aptitude Test (UKCAT, www.ukcat.ac.uk), another widely used admissions test for medicine in the UK, were also included to gain a more rounded picture of students' views overall. The selection criteria investigated were:

- GCSE grades
- A Level predicted grades
- personal statements
- teacher references
- relevant work experience
- admissions tests in general[†]
- admissions tests – verbal and numeric reasoning skills[†]
- admissions tests – abstract reasoning skills
- admissions tests – subject-specific reasoning skills[†]
- admissions tests – writing skills[†]
- admissions tests – behavioural skills
- traditional interviews
- MMIs.

A brief definition of each selection criterion was provided to ensure that all respondents understood what each element involved. The questionnaire was piloted and then distributed at open days at BMAT institutions, at an outreach summer school, and electronically via the BMAT website. In total,

[†] These are sections included in BMAT.

data from 749 respondents (63% female, 37% male) who indicated that they were considering applying to study medicine in the UK was included for analysis. Almost 55% indicated that they were in the second year of their A Levels (or equivalent), with the rest of the responses from candidates in the first year of A Levels, or with their secondary school education completed. Approximately 80% of respondents were based in the UK.

Results

Of the UK respondents, 79% were categorised as attending a state school and 21% as attending an independent (fee-paying) school. Of the two thirds of the sample who provided sufficient background data to enable classification, 39% were identified as potentially meeting WP criteria. The results below are organised according to specific questions from the questionnaire.

How daunting/scary do you think you would find the following admissions criteria?

Mean participant ratings for this question ranged from 2.07 (for relevant work experience) up to 3.89 (for admissions tests in general). All criteria, apart from relevant work experience, received median ratings of 3 or 4, suggesting that students find the applications process overall quite daunting. It is interesting to note that, although admissions tests in general received quite a high rating, the ratings for the individual admissions test skills were lower. Of the specific admissions test skills, abstract reasoning skills received the highest mean 'dauntingness' rating (3.51), with verbal and numeric reasoning skills and subject-specific reasoning skills, as tested in BMAT, receiving lower ratings (3.37 and 3.06 respectively). Students did report finding writing skills, also in BMAT, somewhat more daunting (mean rating of 3.40). Males reported finding every aspect of the selection process less daunting than did females. By contrast, there was no difference in ratings by students from state and independent schools, nor according to whether they were classified as from a WP background or not.

Qualitative analysis revealed that students find admissions tests, traditional interviews and MMIs daunting for similar reasons. These selection criteria are 'one-off' chances and are seen as challenging. Students worry about not performing to their 'true ability' due to test anxiety, illness or an unusually poor performance. Furthermore, interviews and admissions tests are seen as final 'hurdles' that must be cleared to gain entry to medical study. These issues are illustrated by the following quotes from applicants:

> Traditional interviews are very daunting and the fear of not portraying yourself well is always on your mind, and that your life could be changed by those 10 minutes.
> (Male student from a state school, first in family to attend university and eligible for free school meals)

> I feel that it's not fair, as you have achieved the grades, sorted your personal statement and work experience but fall at the last hurdle.
> (Male student from a sixth form college)

> These admissions tests are based on a one-chance day, and underperformance on one day could leave someone unable to get into their desired university, despite them having an excellent academic background and all the relevant work experience.
> (Female student from a comprehensive sixth form college)

How likely is it that the following admissions criteria would deter you from applying to study medicine at a particular institution?

Participants' ratings of the extent to which the various admissions criteria were a deterrent to application formed an interesting counterpoint to their ratings of how daunting they felt these to be. The modal rating for all criteria in this question was '1' (not at all). The picture that emerged from the data is that students may find the admissions process daunting but they are committed to the idea of applying to study medicine regardless. The qualitative comments supported this idea – when asked to comment on why certain aspects of the process might deter them, a significant proportion of those who commented remarked that nothing would deter them from applying.

Females rated the verbal and numeric reasoning, and the subject-specific aspects of admissions tests as slightly more of a deterrent than did males. However, the mean ratings were low for both genders. According to their ratings, students from state schools or from WP backgrounds are no more likely to be deterred by admissions tests than those from independent schools or non-WP backgrounds.

How fair is it to compare students from different educational and social backgrounds on each of the following admissions criteria?

Overall, respondents perceived all admissions criteria to be somewhere between 'somewhat fair' (score of 3) and 'fair' (score of 4). On average, none of the criteria was perceived to be 'unfair' (2) or 'not at all fair' (1). The lowest mean fairness ratings were given to abstract reasoning skills (3.22), relevant work experience (3.24), and writing skills (3.25). Verbal and numerical reasoning skills, and subject-specific reasoning skills (as tested in BMAT Sections 1 and 2), received slightly higher fairness ratings of 3.35 and 3.51 respectively. Perhaps somewhat surprisingly, participants gave the highest mean fairness ratings to traditional interviews (3.92). This is in contrast to the published evidence that suggests that traditional interviews are not as effective or as fair as some other selection methods (Patterson et al 2016). However, participants who were classified as WP rated traditional interviews as slightly less fair than did candidates who were classified as non-WP.

Qualitative analysis revealed that students acutely perceive the social and educational inequities at play in the admissions process and that these produce perceptions of unfairness. This was often described as unequal access to resources, including financial resources (e.g. to be able to pay for a commercial course), educational resources (what type of school they attend) and cultural capital (the social networks and knowledge that students access from their friends and families). The following quote illustrates these issues:

> Whilst this is virtually impossible to resolve, there is a massive social bias towards wealthier, better educated candidates. This is particularly significant in assessing candidates on their relevant work experience, which is easiest to acquire if an applicant has contacts in the medical profession. I also believe that . . . individualism is quelled by advice given to candidates over personal statements and interview responses.
> (Male student from a state sixth form school)

How confident are you that you could perform well on the admissions criteria?

Overall, respondents expressed a relatively high level of confidence that they could perform well on every criterion. Mean participant ratings for the 'perform well' question ranged from 3.34 (for abstract reasoning skills) to 3.96 (for personal statements). The mean rating for traditional interviews was slightly higher than those for MMIs and admissions tests in general. Of the specific admissions test sections, behavioural skills and subject-specific skills received the highest mean ratings, followed by verbal and numeric reasoning skills and writing skills and, lastly, abstract reasoning skills. Females were less confident in their capacity to perform well than males – although both genders still gave relatively high confidence ratings. State school and WP respondents were slightly (but statistically significantly) less confident that they could perform well on admissions tests overall than were independent school and non-WP respondents; however, when their ratings for individual admissions test sections/skills were examined there was no significant difference between the groups.

In your opinion, to what extent is help and preparation from other sources (e.g. school, tutors, parents, preparation courses) likely to have a large impact on performance on the following admissions criteria?

Personal statements were rated as the aspect of the admissions process most likely to be influenced by external help (mean rating of 4.12), followed by interviews (3.80), MMIs (3.59) and securing work experience (3.58). All these criteria received higher ratings than admissions tests. Of the specific admissions test sections, subject-specific skills received the highest mean rating (3.45), followed by writing skills (3.37), verbal and numeric reasoning skills (3.23), abstract reasoning skills (3.13) and, lastly, behavioural skills (3.04).

A forced-choice question was also posed to respondents: 'If you had a choice, in addition to academic performance (e.g. GCSE and A Level grades), on which criteria would you prefer your medicine application to be considered?' An interesting school-type trend emerged in the responses, although it did not prove to be statistically significant. A greater proportion of state school students stated a preference to have their application considered on the basis of both interview performance and admissions test performance (53% of state school students, compared with 43% of independent school students), while students from private schools were more likely to choose interview performance only (43%).

Discussion

This study examined the views of potential medicine applicants towards the various admissions criteria that might be considered as part of their application process. Questions did not canvass views on specific admissions tests but rather focused on the skills assessed within these tests.

Views towards admissions tests, traditional interviews and MMIs were mixed, with students generally finding these selection criteria 'daunting' but fair. In assessing the impact of admissions tests on the process of selection for medicine it is particularly important to contrast responses to the question of *how daunting* certain aspects of the selection process seem to the question of *how much of a deterrent* to application those same aspects present. While admissions tests in general were rated as the most daunting of the criteria listed, their rating as a deterrent to application was low. In fact, the modal rating for this question was a '1' (i.e. 'not at all' a deterrent) for all criteria. The majority of respondents stated that they were 'quite sure' or 'very sure' that they wanted to study medicine. Thus a picture emerges of candidates who are committed to the idea of studying medicine and, while they may find aspects of the selection process daunting, they are not deterred from applying in pursuit of their ambition. Students from WP backgrounds and from state schools did not report finding the prospect of an admissions test to be more of a deterrent than did the non-WP and independent school respondents.

Overall, the results of this study suggest that there are very few differences in how students from different social and educational backgrounds view the admissions process to medicine and admissions tests, in particular. More pronounced were some of the gender differences: females rated most criteria as more daunting than did males. Females also made a greater number of qualitative comments about the competitiveness of the application process. For all the criteria listed, males rated higher confidence than females that they could perform well. This is of particular interest given the small but stable gender differences in BMAT performance, discussed in Chapter 2, that do not appear to stem from any discernible test bias.

What do these results contribute to our understanding of the consequential validity of admissions tests? For medical school applicants, who are determined to get into medical school regardless of the obstacles placed in their path, the importance of an admissions test that impacts on the success or failure of their application is self-evident. Candidates reported finding admissions tests relatively daunting, which is likely to be related to how difficult they perceive the test to be, but also reported feeling relatively confident of performing well. All of these findings are consistent with elements of positive washback, and therefore consequential validity, as described by Green (2013): that the test should be perceived to be both important and difficult (but attainable). It is important to acknowledge the limitations of this research: the timing of the questionnaire in the admissions cycle meant that a number of respondents had already taken an admissions test other than BMAT, which may have impacted their views of BMAT. Further, the fact that the questionnaire was distributed at university open days and on the BMAT website means that early prospective applicants who were truly deterred from applying to medicine would not have been included; reaching this particular group is difficult. Nonetheless, this study provides important insights into students' views of applying to medicine and the place of admissions tests within that process.

7.7 Chapter summary

Consequential validity is an element of test validation that is critical to the fitness for purpose of any assessment. To explore the consequential validity of BMAT we have reviewed the practices of test design, stakeholder engagement and empirical research using a socio-cognitive validity framework (O'Sullivan and Weir 2011) and addressed issues of washback, test score use, test preparation practices, perceptions of the test and differential validity. As consequential validity can only be established after a test has been developed and used, the principles of *impact by design* aim to anticipate outcomes and mitigate possible negative effects at the test development phase.

By conducting research on the consequences (both perceived and real) of test use, test developers can seek to understand the impact of decisions that result from a testing policy. In medical education research, consequential validity focuses on the decisions made by tutors about how to interpret test scores (Downing 2003). However, we have shown that the decisions made by test takers, medical students and prospective test takers can also be considered as part of consequential validity. In particular, it was noted that consequential validity could impact future admissions cycles and decisions of potential applicants about whether to apply for biomedical study. Our findings indicate that applicants to medical school view forms of selection as relatively daunting, but these methods do not pose a barrier to applying (Emery and McElwee 2014).

We have presented research into the preparation behaviours and test perceptions of different groups of applicants by gender and school status, and this is an important step in fully investigating the differential validity of BMAT. However, there is another group of applicants – mature students – that has not been as rigorously investigated. Due to the different backgrounds of this group of students, and efforts from medical schools to enrol mature students, further research is needed in this area.

Through monitoring test use and maintaining effective collaboration with stakeholders, consequential validity can feed into test or curriculum revisions. If test providers and stakeholders understand how students prepare for a test, they can also adopt measures designed to support positive test impact, such as those that encourage test preparation behaviours designed to have a beneficial educational impact. This chapter has described how Cambridge Assessment Admissions Testing seeks to ensure the positive impact of BMAT in these ways, by providing enhanced support materials (such as the Section 2 revision guide), through focused research with past and potential candidates, and by encouraging dialogue with (and between) stakeholder institutions.

Chapter 7 main points

- Washback impacts on education systems differently for admissions tests when compared to language tests.
- Practising tests under timed conditions is associated with higher test scores on all sections of BMAT, whereas school type and attending a course are not.
- Perceptions of admissions tests are not a deterrent to applying to medical study. Students are committed to the idea of applying regardless.
- Further work on consequential validity should investigate how the social consequences of test use interact with other aspects of validity.
- The social consequences of assessment should be considered as part of test design.

8 Conclusions and recommendations

Kevin Y F Cheung

Research and Thought Leadership Group, Cambridge Assessment Admissions Testing

Introduction

The socio-cognitive framework of test validity originally outlined by Weir (2005) has served as a springboard to investigate the examination of writing (Shaw and Weir 2007), reading (Khalifa and Weir 2009), speaking (Taylor 2011) and listening (Geranpayeh and Taylor (Eds) 2013). These previous volumes have contributed to Cambridge English Language Assessment's approaches to test development and revision by comprehensively evaluating Cambridge English examinations. Similarly, the present volume represents a stock-taking of Cambridge Assessment Admissions Testing's approach to assessment, focusing on the potential for biomedical study as conceptualised in the BioMedical Admissions Test (BMAT). The issues identified here serve as a focal point for revising admissions tests in the future, and development of tests for other contexts.

Although the socio-cognitive framework was originally developed to evaluate language tests, Weir pointed out that the model would be useful in other fields of educational assessment: 'Though specifically framed with English for Speakers of Other Languages (ESOL) in mind, the blueprint has implications for all forms of educational assessment' (2005:2). In the present volume, we apply the framework to the admissions testing context. This extends use of the socio-cognitive framework outside of the language testing domain, but we are admittedly not the first to do so. According to O'Sullivan and Weir (2011), the socio-cognitive framework has been applied to examinations assessing art, physics and ophthalmology, due to its usefulness for guiding discussions of validity. However, to my knowledge, this volume represents the most comprehensive application of Weir's socio-cognitive framework to an assessment setting outside of the language testing domain.

As one might expect, some issues relating to the validity of tests are different in the admissions testing context when compared with language testing. Notably, cognitive validity is particularly complex in admissions testing, due to the range of constructs that are plausible to assess in this context. Another way that the field of admissions testing diverges from language testing is the focus on prediction when investigating criterion-related validity. Also, the concepts of consequential validity and washback for admissions testing stakeholders are different from the topics commonly explored in language learning. These differences have not been barriers to applying the socio-cognitive framework; instead, they have highlighted that the aspects of validity identified by Weir (2005) can manifest in various ways, and that these aspects are important to consider across all assessments. Perhaps more surprisingly for readers, there are numerous areas where the issues in language testing and admissions testing are similar.

The chapters of this volume have highlighted one important parallel between language testing and admissions testing – the advantage of adopting holistic perspectives when evaluating tests and their use. The range of topics covered by authors for this volume has vanquished the myth of the validated admissions test, by showing that the test itself is one part of a much larger context that responsible test providers must consider. Only focusing on the test in isolation could result in claims about the assessment that are not defensible once the situation surrounding the test administration is taken into account. By assuming that tasks assess relevant cognitive processes or ignoring the testing context, test developers can risk unintended consequences arising from introduction of an assessment, particularly one that is used for high-stakes purposes. In this regard, an approach to evaluating the entire testing policy has been adopted throughout this volume, as advocated by Newton and Shaw (2014). Unlike Newton and Shaw, however, we propose that an existing framework of validity, Weir's (2005) socio-cognitive model, is a sufficient starting point for this approach, as it already extends evaluation of validity beyond the technical aspects of a test.

Many of Weir's (2005) ideas regarding validity and language testing can be applied appropriately to admissions tests; however, there is one place where the Cambridge Assessment Admissions Testing position diverges from the perspective adopted by Weir. He argues that 'practicality is simply not a necessary condition for validity' (2005:49). Whilst I agree that the test provider must focus on the construct to ensure that practicality does not intrude and distort what we are aiming to assess, validity lies in the appropriateness of inferences made using the assessment, and practical issues can impact on these. For example, if universities do not receive results of an admissions test within a timeframe that supports their shortlisting decisions, the validity of the test is compromised. Therefore, the practical aspects of marking and returning results must be considered as part of validity, and we have included them in Chapters 4 and 5 on context validity and scoring validity. Similarly, the cost of producing and marking an admissions test must not make registration prohibitively expensive for candidates, as this would impact on interpreting results where the self-selected candidate pool has been unduly shaped by factors not relevant to the test constructs, such as socio-economic status. These issues are apparent in the context of selection to study medicine, where widening access to higher education is emphasised. Many of these topics are touched upon in Chapter 7's exploration of consequential validity.

Notwithstanding the divergent views on practicality, the arguments made by Weir (2005) about language testing are remarkably similar to those presented throughout this volume on an admissions testing context. This applies to the current approach adopted when developing admissions tests and also to earlier work, particularly in relation to BMAT. The history behind various aspects of BMAT's validity has been presented in this volume and this represents a snapshot of a moment in the lifetime of the test. There are currently 17 universities in the UK and internationally who use BMAT for admission to more than 25 courses of medical, biomedical or dentistry study. This number is steadily growing and it is likely that new developments in the administration, delivery and scoring of BMAT will emerge in the coming years, as it serves an increasingly global higher education arena. Further challenges are potentially on the horizon that will need to be addressed with an evidence-based approach that considers all the aspects of validity identified in the socio-cognitive framework.

The rest of this final chapter turns to each aspect of the socio-cognitive framework to summarise the validity of BMAT viewed through the lens of Weir's (2005) model. Importantly, these summaries also identify areas for future research that can support investigation of validity going forward. Validity exists on a continuum and should not be regarded as a binary concept (Messick 1989); therefore, it is important to acknowledge that continuing efforts are needed to ensure BMAT's fitness for purpose.

Test taker characteristics

Cambridge Assessment Admissions Testing routinely monitors the test taker population and their performance on the three sections of BMAT. This approach acknowledges that the test taker is at the heart of the assessment and that test development should recognise the physiological, psychological and experiential issues that can impact performance. An understanding of the test taker population is important for considering all aspects of validity identified in the socio-cognitive framework. From a quality assurance perspective, information about test takers' gender and school background is used to check for bias in test items. In the context of BMAT, the predictive equity of test scores for different groups is an issue to consider and continue investigating, particularly as the population taking BMAT changes. The authors of Chapter 2 highlight the need to understand shifting educational contexts to guide this work going forward. As changes to education policy can influence the ways that certain groups are categorised or focused upon, the practical issues involved in classifying students should be carefully considered for future work. To support this, engagement with the users of an admissions test is crucial. Many of Chapter 2's more nuanced observations about proxies for socio-economic status came from Brenda Cross, whose experiences as a seasoned medical school admissions tutor revealed the care that medical schools take when selecting applicants, and the complex array of considerations that they face. Admissions tests are always situated in a wider selection process that can include access arrangements and influence from government education policies. These issues are easily missed by a test developer without the input of users who are actually making selection decisions, and Cambridge Assessment's approach recognises the need to engage with admissions tutors as part of understanding the test taker.

There are avenues for research on BMAT's test taker characteristics that would contribute to literature outside the admissions testing domain. Linking Cambridge Assessment data to other sources, such as UCAS data, could be useful for understanding group differences, not just in BMAT performance, but also in the choices made by school leavers and applicants to medical school. Some research on university choice indicates that there are complex relationships between gender, distance of the institution from home and A Level choice (Gill, Vidal Rodeiro and Zanini 2015). Monitoring of the test taker population is also crucial for evaluating the performances of an international candidature with a diverse educational background. Over the last five years, an increasing number of medical schools have recognised the attributes assessed by BMAT as important and decided to include the test as part of their selection procedures. Departments in the Netherlands, Spain, Malaysia, Thailand and Singapore now require BMAT to be taken as part of the selection process. Universities in other countries are also at various stages of trialling and evaluating how BMAT fits into their procedures and policies. Monitoring the test taker characteristics of future sessions will contribute to understanding the specific challenges of assessing candidates from different education systems. Furthermore, an understanding of how international group performance interacts with more traditional group differences, such as gender, will be crucial to ensuring that BMAT remains fit for purpose.

Cognitive validity

Understanding the cognitive processes elicited by BMAT tasks is crucial to investigating the validity of the test. As Weir and Taylor (2011:299) point out: 'It is hard to see how one can build a convincing validity argument for any assessment practice without assigning cognitive processing a central place within that argument.' Suitable interpretation of test scores relies on extrapolating from performance on test tasks to real-world behaviours. Therefore, BMAT should elicit the kinds of mental operations that are relevant for biomedical study. Chapter 3 uses cognitive validity as conceptualised in the socio-cognitive framework to present a key question for developers of admissions tests: what are the skills and cognitive processes that a test should aim to elicit and assess?

In the case of BMAT, this question is answered by presenting the rationale for assessing the skills targeted by the test, and the theoretical basis for conceptualising each skill as potential for biomedical study. The rationales for assessing generic thinking skills, scientific knowledge and application, and written argument were considered when designing BMAT as a successor to two earlier tests used for selection to medical study. The Oxford Medical Admissions Test (OMAT) and the Medical and Veterinary Admissions Test (MVAT) were used to select undergraduate students and deal with increasingly large pools of applicants. Both of these tests were designed to assess specific abilities theorised as important in biomedical study (James and Hawkins 2004, Massey 2004), which was identified as the real-world situation relevant for evaluating a biomedical admissions test. In Chapter 3, the original rationales were re-examined in the context of contemporary understandings of biomedical study. Although a wide range of topics are included in biomedical study, various sources agree that core skills are relevant for biomedical study. Trainee clinicians are engaged in rigorous learning and need to develop problem solving skills (Quality Assurance Agency 2015), scientific reasoning (General Medical Council 2009) and writing abilities (Goodman and Edwards 2014, McCurry and Chiavaroli 2013). This confirmed that the skills assessed by BMAT remain relevant to the contexts that the test is used for.

Relevant theoretical models were used to examine the thinking skills assessed by Section 1, the scientific reasoning skills assessed by Section 2, and the written communication targeted in Section 3. Theories of critical thinking and problem solving were used to present the cognitive processes assessed by Section 1 as abilities that can be developed, and to distinguish the test construct from models of intelligence (Black 2012, Fisher 1992). This exercise raised some interesting issues. In particular, we identified a need to explicitly define terms commonly used to describe the constructs assessed by admissions tests, and to situate BMAT in relation to these terms. Based on a review of literature from educational psychology and assessment (e.g. Kaplan and Saccuzzo 2012, Newton and Shaw 2012, Stemler 2012), key terms used in admissions testing were defined and applied to BMAT. As a result, the title of BMAT's Section 1 is currently being reviewed, to evaluate whether 'aptitude' is a suitable description of the abilities that are being assessed. Think-aloud studies conducted by Cambridge Assessment researchers on item types from Section 1 were also presented. This illustrated one of the ways that cognitive processes elicited by a test can be investigated, and also demonstrated how findings from research can inform the processes used in test design.

Theories of scientific problem solving (e.g. Dunbar and Fugelsang 2005) were used to consider the cognitive processes involved in answering Section 2 items, and to conceptualise them as searches in a problem space (Simon and Newell 1971). Linking Section 2 to theoretical perspectives on scientific reasoning identified complex interactions between subject-specific knowledge and more domain-general reasoning abilities (Klahr and Dunbar 1988, Zimmerman 2000), which are components acknowledged as important to consider during Cambridge Assessment's item authoring processes. However, it is recognised that further investigation of the balance between knowledge and novel problem solving could be beneficial for assessing scientific reasoning. This presents a possible avenue for further research that might be supported by technological advancements, which have been used to investigate scientific problem solving (Tsai, Hou, Lai, Liu and Yang 2011).

Consideration of the theories underpinning Section 3 was heavily informed by Shaw and Weir's (2007) work on examining writing. Section 3's Writing Task was investigated in terms of the cognitive processes that it aims to elicit. In particular, the discussion focused on knowledge transforming processes that are commonly assessed at higher levels of language proficiency (Scardamalia and Bereiter 1987). However, the retrospective review of example responses to BMAT Section 3 could be complemented with further research on the cognitive writing processes activated when responding to tasks. Key logging, eye tracking and verbal protocol analysis could potentially be used to investigate how candidates plan, organise and monitor whilst writing. The skills assessed by Section 3 are also regarded as examples of test takers' productive reasoning abilities, drawing on critical thinking and assessment research recommending that constructed responses are used to complement other formats commonly used in standardised testing (Butler 2012, Liu et al 2014).

The conceptualisation of BMAT sections as assessments of separate skills has also been investigated as part of cognitive validity. A key study confirming that it was valid to interpret Sections 1 and 2 as measures of two distinct skills was conducted by Emery and Khalid (2013a); this was presented to illustrate another method commonly used to investigate cognitive validity. Chapter 3 highlighted how important it is to consider the theory underlying an admissions test. It was argued that assessment providers have a responsibility to present theoretical reasons for assessing the cognitive processes targeted by examinations, and that theories should be investigated with research.

Context validity

BMAT's context validity was examined in Chapter 4, which stressed the relationship between context validity and cognitive validity. Designing tasks for an admissions test such as BMAT requires careful consideration of various features, because the response format, test timing and task content can all influence the skills assessed by a test. These issues were considered in some detail when developing guidelines used to support context validity, so they are explored in some detail. Multiple-choice questions (MCQs) and tasks requiring constructed responses have specific advantages and disadvantages, so BMAT uses a combination of these task types across its sections.

The number of tasks to include in a test section is another feature of context validity that was considered for BMAT Sections 1 and 2, alongside evaluations of the time needed to complete typical test items. These considerations were informed by early research studies that investigated speededness in BMAT (Shannon 2005), that ultimately led to changes in the number of items included in BMAT sections. More recent studies monitoring time pressure in BMAT have been conducted by analysing omission rates, and an example of this was presented as a key study (Emery 2013a).

A number of threats to validity can be introduced or overlooked when constructing test tasks, and various steps are used to ensure that BMAT assesses the correct skills as intended. Cambridge Assessment's approach to authoring tasks uses detailed test specifications, review by subject matter experts (SMEs) and standardised processes to safeguard against threats to context validity.

A particularly important feature checked for all tasks is the knowledge required to successfully complete the task. Some tests mistakenly claim to include tasks that do not require any knowledge, when they actually mean that test tasks assume a certain level of non-specialist knowledge. For BMAT, tasks destined for Section 1 or Section 3 are checked against a threshold of everyday knowledge. Section 2, on the other hand, assesses the ability to apply subject-specific science and maths knowledge to novel questions. This makes it important to identify the aspects and level of subject knowledge that a test taker is expected to have when they take BMAT. A recent review of the curriculum underpinning BMAT Section 2 was conducted and described in the chapter, to illustrate how assessment experts can explicitly define a pool of assumed knowledge for a test. Once defined, the subject knowledge curriculum was used to support suitable test taker preparation. Furthermore, it allowed SMEs to check the science needed to answer an item correctly against the topics included in the curriculum. However, the checks relating to subject knowledge are not the only ones required to ensure context validity.

BMAT items are commissioned and stored in item banks in preparation for constructing test papers. Various SMEs are recruited to author, edit and vet items before they are placed in a BMAT item bank. A description of the multi-stage question paper production process was presented to outline how different SMEs review specific issues, first in items, and then in papers. The checks conducted during item commissioning, item editing, paper construction and paper vetting were described, alongside rationales for their inclusion.

Another important part of context validity refers to the administration conditions associated with a test. For BMAT, it is critical that the test is administered securely and in a standardised way, so that test takers experience similar conditions when completing tasks. Cambridge Assessment's approach to administration uses strict test regulations and centre approval processes to monitor these issues. Furthermore, the advantages and disadvantages of various administration methods are continuously reviewed. For example, the possibility of using a computer-based (CB) testing model is regularly evaluated with consideration of the security and access issues associated with a change from paper-based (PB) testing. Although the discussion currently presented in Chapter 4 concludes that BMAT should continue to be administered in PB format, it is entirely possible that this will change at some point in the future. In terms of BMAT's context validity, this is one area that will undoubtedly require further research. In particular, the equivalence of completing CB and PB tasks will likely form the focus of future work on context validity.

Scoring validity

Chapter 5 focused on the processes used to minimise error and ensure that BMAT scores are meaningful. A range of statistical methods are used to safeguard BMAT from threats to scoring validity, and these are presented to provide the reader with an overview of operational validation processes that monitor BMAT sessions.

For the MCQ sections of BMAT, analysis is used to check that items are appropriately difficult and that they discriminate between test takers with low and high abilities. This ensures that the test is targeted to a suitable level for Sections 1 and 2. Rasch analysis is used to score these sections and report them. The approach to scoring taken by Cambridge Assessment produces a scale ranging from 1.0 to 9.0, where equal intervals in BMAT scale scores represent equal differences in candidate ability.

In addition to analysis that is used to monitor and produce scores, a number of analyses are conducted regularly on BMAT Sections 1 and 2. These show that BMAT sections have acceptable internal consistency and also indicate that items are free from bias in relation to gender and school type. The limitations of commonly used statistical coefficients are also relevant to discussions of internal consistency, so they are presented with some of the reasons that estimates of reliability are necessary, but not sufficient, indicators of test quality. Although the internal consistency coefficients of the sections could be improved, this might not be appropriate for BMAT due to the relatively multidimensional nature of the sections and the cognitive validity arguments for designing the sections in this way. Interestingly, there are parallels between recent developments in admissions testing and shifts in language testing observed by Weir (2005) over a decade ago. An overview of these issues is used to contextualise the approach to scoring validity adopted by Cambridge Assessment Admissions Testing, and to distinguish it from a more psychometrically led approach that is prevalent in the US.

For the scoring validity of BMAT Section 3, the marking criteria and marker training procedures are crucial. These safeguard scoring validity by systematically monitoring and evaluating the subjective marks awarded by examiners. These are detailed in Chapter 5 alongside some of the statistical procedures used to review marker reliability. These marker standardisation and training procedures for BMAT Section 3 are informed by research from language testing contexts (Shaw and Weir 2007). However, there are opportunities for further investigation of this area, because the impact of training on Section 3 examiners has not been investigated directly.

It should be noted that the procedures used to evaluate BMAT's scoring validity are designed specifically for the context of the test's administration. Future changes to BMAT's administration may require greater focus on scoring validity. For example, BMAT's use in an increasing number of territories may require alternative scoring procedures to be considered. To date, groups of candidates have not been considered across BMAT sessions that occur at different points in a year, because these tend to take place in different locations and are accepted by different university departments. However, increasing globalisation and student mobility may necessitate scoring procedures that enable precise comparability of scores across sessions, most likely with statistical equating. These procedures sometimes require additional data to be collected, so developments will need careful consideration of logistical and security issues. Furthermore, Cambridge Assessment researchers may need to develop innovative methods of scoring to deal with use of BMAT in new contexts, and this represents a significant focus for development of the test.

Criterion validity

Investigating the relationships between test scores and other variables is a key consideration for assessments used in selection contexts, such as admissions tests. In particular, predictive validity is prioritised over many other aspects of validity when selecting applicants for job roles and university places. In medical selection, some researchers refer to correlations between on-course performance and test scores as 'the validity coefficient' (Cleland et al 2012:11), and predictive validity is emphasised over other forms when discussing admissions tests (e.g. McManus, Dewberry, Nicholson, Dowell et al 2013). In line with these established conventions, Cambridge Assessment has placed a historical emphasis on this aspect of validity. In particular, our researchers have focused on BMAT's predictive validity and equity in published research (Emery and Bell 2009, Emery et al 2011). However, Cambridge Assessment Admissions Testing's contemporary approach to validity adopts the socio-cognitive framework (O'Sullivan and Weir 2011) and acknowledges that other aspects of validity are also relevant to admissions tests. This contrasts with the approach adopted by some other researchers, who treat predictive validity as the only form of validity that matters in selection contexts (e.g. Hopkins et al 1990).

In considerations of criterion-related validity, we heed Weir's (2005:13) warnings that 'no single validity can be considered superior to another. Deficit in any one raises questions as to the well-foundedness of any interpretation of test scores.' The tendency to primarily consider one type of validity over others has also been a concern for experts in the wider educational assessment community, who have reflected on some historical practices that prioritised particular forms of validity. For example, Newton and Shaw (2014) describe how conceptualisations of validity as the hypothetical agreement between test scores and a theoretical true proficiency led to an early focus on criterion validity. This developed almost accidentally, as researchers overlooked the limitation that operationalised criterion measures were flawed representations of true proficiency.

Therefore, Cambridge Assessment researchers consider a wide range of methodological and theoretical issues when planning predictive validity studies. A critical approach is required because various issues reduce the strength of relationships in selection contexts. Whilst corrections for attenuated coefficients are available (e.g. Sackett and Yang 2000), applying them uncritically in pursuit of a stronger 'validity coefficient' may not be appropriate in complex selection contexts. Indeed, corrected coefficients can hinder, rather than support, meaningful interpretation if applied without an understanding of common methodological challenges and how they might have impacted on the specific selection context of the study. In addition, concurrent validity in the context of BMAT was discussed to highlight that various admissions tests used for healthcare selection are assessing quite different constructs, rendering comparability studies unsuitable. Furthermore, there is little agreement on how potential for medical study should be conceptualised for an admissions test, so there is not an external framework suitable for benchmarking BMAT in concurrent validity studies. Development of a framework for selection to healthcare courses is a suitable area for medical educators to explore.

The authors of Chapter 6 present conceptual overviews of the theoretical issues and methodological challenges relevant to investigating criterion-related validity in selection contexts. Illustrative examples are used to introduce the issues to those who are unfamiliar with them, recognising that they tend to be exacerbated by common selection practices, and the impact of these procedures is easy to overlook.

Cambridge Assessment's approach to conducting and reporting predictive studies is also presented, in order to contextualise the research summarised in the chapter. This approach advocates reporting uncorrected coefficients alongside known information about the selection procedures used, which can be achieved by conducting situated studies in collaboration with admissions tutors. However, this is not presented as the only appropriate way of investigating criterion-related validity. Recently, Cambridge Assessment has been collaborating with the General Medical Council (GMC) to provide data for a UK Medical Education Database (UKMED). This initiative is described to illustrate how big data approaches can also contribute to understanding the relationships between test scores and other outcomes.

These developments present future research opportunities to investigate the criterion-related validity of admissions tests, particularly because inclusion of various other selection criteria could enable researchers to accurately describe the procedures that are used in practice. However, it must be recognised that large datasets do not eliminate the need to collaborate closely with admissions tutors and understand issues specific to their contexts. Therefore, the challenge for researchers conducting further work in this area is to embrace the opportunities provided by these developments, whilst remaining cautious in case of spurious findings that are not explained by theory. This can be achieved by guiding statistical analysis with *a priori* consideration of theory, and by complementing large-scale studies with smaller ones.

Consequential validity

In Chapter 7, the social impact of using BMAT was unpacked using the concept of consequential validity from the socio-cognitive framework. By applying a broad conceptualisation of consequential validity to the admissions testing context, McElwee, Fyfe and Grant extend arguments made in the field of language testing to the sphere of admissions testing, and also into medical education. In this regard, the social and ethical issues related to a test's use should be considered part of overall validity rather than as a separate element. Whether assessment experts refer to these issues as validity or not, it is generally agreed that they are important for the test developer to consider (Newton and Shaw 2014). In our view, omitting consequential validity from models of validity would allow test developers to argue that this aspect of assessment rests solely with test users, and this stance would be detrimental to educational assessment; therefore, consideration of social and ethical consequences should be integrated into models of validity. Integration with other aspects of validity is particularly important because the analysis of consequential validity presented in Chapter 7 showed that test use can impact on issues recognised as central to validity.

In previous applications of the socio-cognitive framework, much has been stated about the symbiotic relationship between cognitive, context and scoring validity (e.g. Khalifa and Weir 2009) because these aspects constitute the core of construct validity. Revisions of the socio-cognitive framework have reflected this by explicitly referring to the two-way relationship between context and cognitive validity (O'Sullivan and Weir 2011). Similarly, this volume has emphasised how these elements interact for an admissions test; however, the admissions testing context presents an opportunity to identify other interactions that further extend the socio-cognitive framework, particularly in relation to consequential validity.

Methods used to select university applicants inevitably impact on widening access initiatives in higher education, which are important issues for policy-makers and society. In terms of access to the medical profession, the emphasis on widening participation is even stronger than in other disciplines. In a close examination of BMAT's consequential validity, the authors of Chapter 7 point out that consequential validity is considered not only as *a posteriori* to a test event as conceptualised in Weir's original framework, but also *a priori* due to the impact on following selection rounds and future cohorts of applicants. In this regard, it should be recognised that the test's impact on wider society can change the test taker population for further administrations of an admissions test. How the test is perceived can potentially change the applicant pool, which might have a knock-on effect for a professional workforce. Therefore, it is particularly important to investigate consequential validity and recognise this mechanism in the admissions testing context by revising the socio-cognitive framework (see Figure 8.1).

Cambridge Assessment has not ignored the consequential validity of admissions tests, and the key studies presented in the volume are evidence of that, but it is fair to say that this area has only been focused on relatively recently. This has partly been prompted by adoption of the socio-cognitive framework, but also because BMAT users have sought to understand how prospective medical students prepare their applications for medical school. This trend is reflected more widely in recent medical education research looking at selection, which has investigated how assessments are perceived by applicants and members of the medical profession (Cleland, French and Johnston 2011, Kelly, Gallagher, Dunne and Murphy 2014, Stevens, Kelly, Hennessy, Last, Dunne and O'Flynn 2014). Despite general worries that selection procedures might deter potential applicants from certain groups, these issues have not been viewed as aspects of validity. In medical education, consequential validity is only used to refer to issues that stem from test score interpretation (Downing 2003). We argue that conceptualising consequential validity in a broader sense would support the development of theoretical frameworks about the consequences of test use in medical education, where there have been calls for more theory when evaluating initiatives to widen access (Nicholson and Cleland 2015). This theory-based approach has

Figure 8.1 A revised socio-cognitive framework

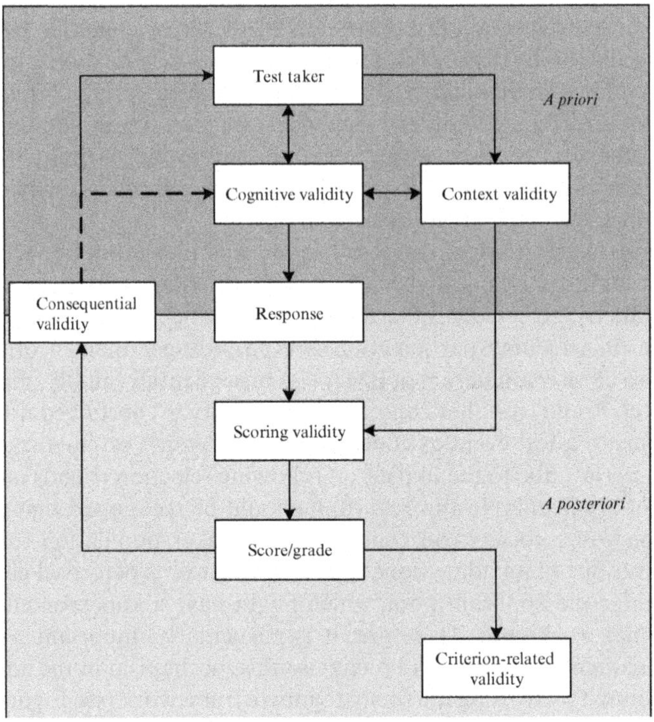

been adopted by some medical education researchers looking at admissions; Niessen, Meijer and Tendeiro (2017) framed qualitative findings on the consequences of using selection methods as part of organisational justice theory. Survey research on test taker perceptions of selection methods was presented as a key study in Chapter 7 (Emery and McElwee 2014) and it may be useful to consider the results in light of wider social theories.

Selection to study medicine and dentistry is a key place where attention to theory can have an important impact. In addition to considering the technical and predictive components of selection methods, policy-makers should recognise that assessments at this stage potentially shape the attitudes and beliefs of future healthcare professionals (Röding and Nordenram 2005). In the Netherlands, research has compared the motivation and self-beliefs of medical students entering through competitive selection with those selected by lottery. Wouters et al (2016) found that the strength of motivation was higher in competitively selected students. Although these differences were not shown to be pervasive in the long term, they do warrant further investigation in other selection contexts. There is also evidence that the relationship between selection procedures and motivation varies across studies, indicating that contextual factors could be important when investigating motivation in medical students (Wouters, Croiset, Schripsema, Cohen-Schotanus, Spaai, Hulsman and Kusurkar 2017).

Research from educational psychology may also present insights into these issues. Experimental work with children indicates that motivation and resilience are influenced by beliefs about the fixedness of their academic abilities (Dweck 2012, Yeager and Dweck 2012). Whilst it would be a mistake to apply these ideas uncritically to adolescents applying for university study, we should consider the self-beliefs promoted by selection procedures, and whether their impact might differ on the subgroups present in applicant pools. Consequential validity poses specific questions about how the constructs we assess can influence those being assessed. Answering these theoretical questions can potentially inform the ways that universities communicate about selection to prospective applicants.

Researchers should investigate how assessment constructs are perceived, not just by university stakeholders, but also by test takers. Cambridge Assessment's approach to admissions testing recognises that scores on all such tests, even those grounded in the psychometric approach to intelligence, are 'a function of innate talent, learned knowledge and skills, and environmental factors that influence knowledge and skill acquisition' (Kuncel and Hezlett 2010:339). Therefore, Cambridge Assessment's admissions tests, which are constructed with a focus on skills that can be developed, should not be conceptualised purely as measures of innate attributes. This has been communicated to admissions tutors and other assessment experts; however, we do not fully understand how test takers perceive tests such as BMAT and, importantly, how they understand their performances on them. Despite BMAT's explicit focus on skills that can be developed, do admissions tests encourage biomedical trainees to believe they were born smart enough to become a doctor or dentist, and that other people were not? If so, what is the impact of this, if any, on their learning and their future clinical practice? Perhaps even more crucially, what impact is there on test takers who come to believe they were not born with the genetic endowment to become a doctor? Furthermore, these considerations must inform the current search for evidence-based 'non-cognitive' criteria (Hecker and Norman 2017). Bearing in mind that tutors will need to communicate decisions to those who are ultimately unsuccessful at entering the healthcare professions, what does it mean to not have the integrity for entering medical study? Understanding these issues can potentially develop theories about student motivation and also inform higher education policy.

The reflections on consequential validity presented in this volume, and particularly in Chapter 7, are initial steps towards addressing this aspect of validity in admissions tests. There are many directions and areas of investigation that stem from the questions posed by consequential validity. One example is represented by the dashed line (to indicate a tentative relationship for investigation) linking consequential validity to cognitive validity in Figure 8.1. In the admissions context, if the selection policy of a university treats an assessment in a way that is incompatible with the targeted construct, then the meaning of the score can potentially be changed. Consider a university's policy on accepting results from examinations that have been sat more than once. If the assessment targets an ability that is beneficial for a particular field of study, the rationale for using the selection method is normally that the ability is associated with study success, either incrementally or to a pre-requisite level. In this situation, previously achieved scores are indicators of ability from earlier in the developmental process; they are not relevant to decision making at the point of application, and the selector should accept results from the most recent sitting of the exam.

One example that illustrates how this issue manifests in practice is when universities decide whether to accept A Level grades achieved in resits. If the grade at first attempt is the only one considered, this changes the nature of the construct that the score represents. The A Level cannot be conceptualised as mastery of a knowledge-based curriculum in this situation, because the policy dictates that the first attempt stands. Mastery of a knowledge-based curriculum can theoretically be improved upon and developed, but the policy has instead changed the meaning of the A Level grade that is accepted. Of course, A Level grades at first attempt are influenced by many different factors and universities may have good reasons for treating them in this way. McManus et al (2005) observe that A Levels could be indirect indicators of motivation or commitment, and conceptualising them in this way may be predicated on the applicant studying multiple subjects at the same time. However, universities should consider the theoretical reasons for using an assessment outcome in a particular way.

These issues also apply to assessments that claim to assess innate abilities. For these measures, as the trait being assessed is theoretically fixed, test scores should not vary across multiple attempts. In fact, multiple test attempts can be conceptualised as parallel evaluations of the same innate trait, and the most valid score to consider would be some kind of average across the attempts. Decisions about accepting resits are often made due to practical concerns about the number of applications that a university can consider in a cycle. Biomedical courses sometimes provide empirical reasons for not recognising A Levels that have been re-examined, using data to show poorer outcomes for students admitted with resits. However, policy-makers should also attempt to understand the mechanisms that drive these outcomes. The idea that consequential validity can influence cognitive validity highlights the need to reflect on the ways that commonly used selection criteria are conceptualised. The interactions between consequential validity, other aspects of validity and wider social theory represent areas to be explored with future research.

Conclusion

In Chapter 1, Saville proposed that the socio-cognitive framework developed in language testing could guide comprehensive evaluation of BMAT's validity. This volume has used Weir's (2005) socio-cognitive framework to present key aspects of test validity, and demonstrated how they can be used to consider validity of an assessment used in selection for medical study. Application of the socio-cognitive framework to BMAT demonstrates its flexibility as a model for test evaluation, and provides an example of how it can be used to focus attention on aspects of validity, in an assessment other than a language test. Some aspects of validity identified in the socio-cognitive framework are commonly overlooked in the admissions testing context, despite being considered regularly by researchers working in language testing. However, none of the issues covered can be considered trivial and each chapter successfully argues that the aspect of validity focused upon is important. By considering each aspect in turn, we have shown how they relate to the ways BMAT was developed, how it is currently administered, and how its validity is continuously monitored.

Throughout the volume, we have reiterated that the separate chapters of the book do not represent isolated issues relating to the use of BMAT. Rather, the chapters, and the socio-cognitive framework itself, provide a structure for systematic investigation of validity as a unitary concept. Nevertheless, organising the issues in this way can give the mistaken impression that they are discrete topics. Therefore, it is important to reiterate that the aspects of validity described throughout this volume are interconnected. This volume demonstrates that Cambridge Assessment's approach to admissions testing fits particularly well with a socio-cognitive framework that conceptualises validity as unitary. Various aspects of BMAT's validity are considered necessary but not sufficient to ensure that inferences based on test scores are valid. In this approach, validity is conceptualised on a continuum, but test quality is not linked simply to isolated coefficients representing psychometric quality. Evidence that each aspect of validity has been considered for BMAT contributes cumulatively to the confidence associated with use of test scores. This dissuades test developers from focusing blindly on one or two aspects of validity at the cost of others, which has been a historical issue in educational assessment, as demonstrated by a quote from the 1966 edition of the *Standards*: 'Too frequently in educational measurement attention is restricted to criterion-related validity' (1966:6).

This collection of chapters is not intended to be an exhaustive compilation of research on BMAT, but rather to give an insight into some of the ways that the test has been evaluated. Hopefully, readers from various disciplines will have found the description and discussion of Cambridge Assessment's approaches useful. This volume has demonstrated how a multidisciplinary approach spanning language testing and admissions testing can be beneficial. It would be good if sharing this work with medical educators, language testing researchers and admissions test developers could encourage collaboration across subgroups of educational assessment experts, to share expertise and best practice in a way that benefits various forms of assessment.

References

Admissions Testing Service (2016a) *BMAT Section 1 Question Guide*, available online: www.admissionstestingservice.org/images/324081-bmat-section-1-question-guide.pdf

Admissions Testing Service (2016b) *Biomedical Admissions Test (BMAT) Test Specification*, available online: www.admissionstestingservice.org/images/47829-bmat-test-specification.pdf

American Educational Research Association, American Psychological Association and National Council on Measurement in Education (1966) *Standards for Educational and Psychological Testing*, Washington, DC: American Educational Research Association.

American Educational Research Association, American Psychological Association and National Council on Measurement in Education (1985) *Standards for Educational and Psychological Testing*, Washington, DC: American Educational Research Association.

American Educational Research Association, American Psychological Association and National Council on Measurement in Education (2014) *Standards for Educational and Psychological Testing*, Washington, DC: American Educational Research Association.

Anastasi, A and Urbina, S (1997) *Psychological Testing*, New York: Macmillan.

Andrich, D A (2004) Controversy and the Rasch model: A characteristic of incompatible paradigms? *Medical Care* 42 (1), 1–15.

Andrich, D A (2009a) *Interpreting RUMM2030 Part I: Dichotomous Data*, Perth: RUMM Laboratory.

Andrich, D A (2009b) *Interpreting RUMM2030 Part VI: Quantifying Response Dependence in RUMM*, Perth: RUMM Laboratory.

Angoff, W H (1974) The development of statistical indices for detecting cheaters, *Journal of the American Statistical Association* 69 (345), 44–49.

Arthur, N and Everaert, P (2012) Gender and performance in accounting examinations: Exploring the impact of examination format, *Accounting Education: An International Journal* 21 (5), 471–487.

Association of American Medical Colleges (2014) *Core Competencies for Entering Medical Students*, available online: www.staging.aamc.org/initiatives/admissionsinitiative/competencies/

Association of American Medical Colleges (2016) *Using MCAT® Data in 2017 Medical Student Selection*, available online: www.aamc.org/download/462316/data/2017mcatguide.pdf

Atkinson, R C and Geiser, S (2009) Reflections on a century of college admissions tests, *Educational Researcher* 38 (9), 665–676.

Bachman, L (1990) *Fundamental Considerations in Language Testing*, Oxford: Oxford University Press.

Bachman, L and Palmer, A (1996) *Language Testing in Practice*, Oxford: Oxford University Press.

Baldiga, K (2014) Gender differences in willingness to guess, *Management Science* 60, 434–448.
Ball, L J (2014) Eye-tracking and reasoning: What your eyes tell about your inferences, in Neys, W D and Osman, M (Eds) *New Approaches in Reasoning Research*, Hove: Psychology Press, 51–69.
Ball L J and Stupple, E J N (2016) Dual-reasoning processes and the resolution of uncertainty: The case of belief bias, in Macchi, L, Bagassi, M and Viale, R (Eds) *Cognitive Unconscious and Human Rationality*, Cambridge: MIT Press, 143–166.
Barrett, G V, Phillips, J S and Alexander, R A (1981) Concurrent and predictive validity designs: A critical reanalysis, *Journal of Applied Psychology* 66, 1–6.
Bax, S (2013) The cognitive processing of candidates during reading tests: Evidence from eye-tracking, *Language Testing* 30 (4), 441–465.
Bell, C (2015) A modern perspective on statistical malpractice detection, *Research Notes* 59, 31–35.
Bell, J F (2007) Difficulties in evaluating the predictive validity of selection tests, *Research Matters* 3, 5–9.
Bell, J F, Bramley, T, Claessen, M J A and Raikes, N (2007) Quality control of examination marking, *Research Matters* 4,18–21.
Bell, J F, Judge, S, Parks, G, Cross, B, Laycock, J F, Yates, D and May, S (2005) The case against the BMAT: Not withering but withered? available online: www.bmj.com/rapid-response/2011/10/31/case-against-bmat-not-withering-withered
Ben-Shakhar, G and Sinai, Y (1991) Gender differences in multiple-choice tests: The role of differential guessing tendencies, *Journal of Educational Measurement* 28, 23–35.
Best, R, Walsh, J L, Harris, B H J and Wilson, D (2016) UK Medical Education Database: An issue of assumed consent [Letter to the editor], *Clinical Medicine* 16 (6), 605.
Black, B (2008) *Critical Thinking – a definition and taxonomy for Cambridge Assessment: Supporting validity arguments about Critical Thinking assessments administered by Cambridge Assessment*, Paper presented at 34th International Association of Educational Assessment Annual Conference, Cambridge, 9 September 2008, available online: www.cambridgeassessmentjobs.org/Images/126340-critical-thinking-a-definition-and-taxonomy.pdf
Black, B (2012) An overview of a programme of research to support the assessment of critical thinking, *Thinking Skills and Creativity* 7 (2), 122–133.
Blanden, J and Gregg, P (2004) Family income and educational attainment: A review of approaches and evidence for Britain, *Oxford Review of Economic Policy* 20 (2), 245–263.
Bol'shev, L N (2001) Statistical estimator, in Hazewinkel, M (Ed) *Encyclopedia of Mathematics*, New York: Springer, available online: www.encyclopediaofmath.org/index.php/Statistical_estimator
Bond, T G and Fox, C M (2001) *Applying the Rasch Model: Fundamental Measurement in the Human Sciences*, Mahwah: Lawrence Erlbaum.
Borsboom, D, Mellenbergh, G J and van Heerden, J (2004) The concept of validity, *Psychological Review* 111 (4), 1,061–1,071.
Bramley, T and Oates, T (2011) Rank ordering and paired comparisons – the way Cambridge Assessment is using them in operational and experimental work, *Research Matters* 11, 32–35.
Bramley, T, Vidal Rodeiro, C L and Vitello, S (2015) *Gender differences in GCSE*, Cambridge: Cambridge Assessment internal report.

Bridges, G (2010) Demonstrating cognitive validity of IELTS Academic Writing Task 1, *Research Notes* 42, 24–33.

Briggs, D C (2001) The effect of admissions test preparation: Evidence from NELS:88, *Chance* 14 (1), 10–18.

Briggs, D C (2004) Evaluating SAT coaching: Gains, effects and self-selection, in Zwick, R (Ed) *Rethinking the SAT: The Future of Standardized Testing in University Admissions*, London: Routledge, 217–234.

British Medical Association (2009) *Equality and Diversity in UK Medical Schools*, London: British Medical Association.

Buck, G, Kostin, I and Morgan, R (2002) *Examining the Relationship of Content to Gender-based Performance Differences in Advanced Placement Exams*, College Board Research Report 2002-12, ETS RR-02-25, Princeton: Educational Testing Service.

Butler, H A (2012) Halpern critical thinking assessment predicts real-world outcomes of critical thinking, *Applied Cognitive Psychology* 25 (5), 721–729.

Butterworth, J and Thwaites, G (2010) *Preparing for the BMAT: The Official Guide to the BioMedical Admissions Test*, Oxford: Heinemann.

Cambridge Assessment (2009) *The Cambridge Approach: Principles for Designing, Administering and Evaluating Assessment*, Cambridge: Cambridge Assessment, available online: www.cambridgeassessment.org.uk/Images/cambridge-approach-to-assessment.pdf

Cambridge English (2014) *Instructions for Secure Administration of Admissions Tests*, Cambridge: UCLES.

Cambridge English (2016) *Principles of Good Practice: Research and Innovation in Language Learning and Assessment*, Cambridge: UCLES, available online: www.cambridgeenglish.org/images/22695-principles-of-good-practice.pdf

Cambridge International Examinations (2016) *Cambridge International AS and A Level Thinking Skills*, available online: www.cie.org.uk/images/329504-2019-syllabus.pdf

Chapman, J (2005) *The Development of the Assessment of Thinking Skills*, Cambridge: UCLES.

Cheung, K Y F (2014) *Understanding the authorial writer: A mixed methods approach to the psychology of authorial identity in relation to plagiarism*, unpublished doctoral thesis, University of Derby.

Cizek, G J (1999) *Cheating on Tests: How to Do It, Detect It, and Prevent It*, London: Lawrence Erlbaum.

Cizek, G J (2012) Defining and distinguishing validity: Interpretations of score meaning and justifications of test use, *Psychological Methods* 17 (1), 31–43.

Cleary, T A (1968) Test bias: Prediction of grades of Negro and white students in integrated colleges, *Journal of Educational Measurement* 5, 115–124.

Cleland, J A, French, F H and Johnston, P W (2011) A mixed methods study identifying and exploring medical students' views of the UKCAT, *Medical Teacher* 33 (3), 244–249.

Cleland, J, Dowell, J S, McLachlan, J C, Nicholson, S and Patterson, F (2012) *Identifying best practice in the selection of medical students (literature review and interview survey)*, available online: www.gmc-uk.org/Identifying_best_practice_in_the_selection_of_medical_students.pdf_51119804.pdf

Coates, H (2008) Establishing the criterion validity of the Graduate Medical School Admissions Test (GAMSAT), *Medical Education* 42, 999–1,006.

College Board (2015) *Test Specifications for the Redesigned SAT*, New York: College Board.

Council of Europe (2001) *Common European Framework of Reference for Languages: Learning, Teaching, Assessment*, Cambridge: Cambridge University Press.

Cronbach, L J (1951) Coefficient alpha and the internal structure of tests, *Psychometrika* 16 (3), 297–334.

Cronbach, L J (1998) *Essentials of Psychological Testing*, New York: Harper and Row.

Cronbach, L J and Shavelson, R J (2004) My current thoughts on coefficient alpha and successor procedures, *Educational and Psychological Measurement* 64 (3), 391–418.

Department for Education (2014) *Do academies make use of their autonomy?*, available online: www.gov.uk/government/uploads/system/uploads/attachment_data/file/401455/RR366_-_research_report_academy_autonomy.pdf

Department of Labor, Employment and Training Administration (1999) *Testing and Assessment: An Employer's Guide to Good Practices*, Washington, DC: Department of Labor, Employment and Training Administration.

DeVellis, R F (2012) *Scale Development: Theory and Applications* (3rd edition), London: Sage Publications.

Devine, A and Gallacher, T (2017) *The predictive validity of the BioMedical Admissions Test (BMAT) for Graduate Entry Medicine at the University of Oxford*, Cambridge: Cambridge Assessment internal report.

Dowell, J S, Norbury, M, Steven, K and Guthrie, B (2015) Widening access to medicine may improve general practitioner recruitment in deprived and rural communities: Survey of GP origins and current place of work, *BMC Medical Education* 15 (1), available online: bmcmededuc.biomedcentral.com/track/pdf/10.1186/s12909-015-0445-8?site=bmcmededuc.biomedcentral.com

Downing, S M (2002) Construct-irrelevant variance and flawed test questions: Do multiple-choice item-writing principles make any difference? *Academic Medicine* 77, S103–S104.

Downing, S M (2003) Validity: On the meaningful interpretation of assessment data, *Medical Education* 37, 830–837.

Du Plessis, S and Du Plessis, S (2009) A new and direct test of the 'gender bias' in multiple-choice questions, *Stellenbosch Economic Working Papers* 23/09, available online: ideas.repec.org/p/sza/wpaper/wpapers96.html

Dunbar, K and Fugelsang, J (2005) Scientific thinking and reasoning, in Holyoak, K J and Morrison, R G (Eds) *The Cambridge Handbook of Thinking and Reasoning*, Cambridge: Cambridge University Press, 705–725.

Dweck, C S (2012) *Mindset: Changing the Way You Think to Fulfil Your Potential*, London: Little, Brown Book Group.

Ebel, R L and Frisbie, D A (1991). *Essentials of Educational Measurement* (5th edition), Englewood Cliffs: Prentice-Hall.

Eccles, J S (2011) Gendered educational and occupational choices: Applying the Eccles et al model of achievement-related choices, *International Journal of Behavioral Development* 35, 195–201.

Eccles, J S, Adler, T F, Futterman, R, Goff, S B, Kaczala, C M, Meece, J L and Midgley, C (1983) Expectations, values, and academic behaviors, in Spence, J T (Ed) *Achievement and Achievement Motives: Psychological and Sociological Approaches*, San Francisco: W H Freeman, 75–146.

Elliot, J and Johnson, N (2005) *Item level data: Guidelines for staff*, Cambridge: Cambridge Assessment internal report.
Elliott, M and Wilson, J (2013) Context validity, in Geranpayeh, A and Taylor, L (Eds) *Examining Listening: Research and Practice in Second Language Listening*, Studies in Language Testing volume 35, Cambridge: UCLES/ Cambridge University Press, 152–241.
Elston, M A (2009) *Women and medicine: The future. A report prepared on behalf of the Royal College of Physicians*, available online: www.learning.ox.ac.uk/ media/global/wwwadminoxacuk/localsites/oxfordlearninginstitute/documents/ overview/women_and_medicine.pdf
Emery, J L (2007a) *A report on the predictive validity of the BMAT (2004) for 1st year examination performance on the Veterinary Medicine course at the University of Cambridge*, Cambridge: Cambridge Assessment internal report.
Emery, J L (2007b) *A report on the predictive validity of the BMAT (2005) for 1st year examination performance on the Medicine and Veterinary Medicine course at the University of Cambridge*, Cambridge: Cambridge Assessment internal report.
Emery, J L (2007c) *Analysis of the relationship between BMAT scores, A level points and 1st year examination performance at the Royal Veterinary College (2005 entry)*, Cambridge: Cambridge Assessment internal report.
Emery, J L (2010a) *A Level candidates attaining 3 or more 'A' grades in England 2006-2009*, Cambridge: Cambridge Assessment internal report.
Emery, J L (2010b) *An investigation into candidates' preparation for the BioMedical Admissions Test (2007 session): A replication involving all institutions*, Cambridge: Admissions Testing Service internal report.
Emery, J L (2013a) *Are BMAT time constraints excessive?*, Cambridge: Cambridge English internal report.
Emery, J L (2013b) *BMAT test-taker characteristics and the performance of different groups 2003–2012*, Cambridge: Cambridge English internal report.
Emery, J L and Bell, J F (2009) The predictive validity of the BioMedical Admissions Test for pre-clinical examination performance, *Medical Education* 43 (6), 557–564.
Emery, J L and Bell, J F (2011) Comment on I C McManus, Eamonn Ferguson, Richard Wakeford, David Powis and David James (2011). Predictive validity of the BioMedical Admissions Test (BMAT): An Evaluation and Case Study. Medical Teacher 33 (1): (this issue), *Medical Teacher* 33, 58–59.
Emery, J L and Khalid, M N (2013a) *An investigation into BMAT item bias using DIF analysis*, Cambridge: Cambridge English internal report.
Emery, J L and Khalid, M N (2013b) *Construct investigation into BMAT using Structural Equation Modelling*, Cambridge: Cambridge English internal report.
Emery, J L and McElwee, S (2014) *Student perceptions of selection criteria for medical study: Are admissions tests a deterrent to application?*, Cambridge: Cambridge English internal report.
Emery, J L, Bell, J F and Vidal Rodeiro, C L (2011) The BioMedical Admissions Test for medical student selection: Issues of fairness and bias, *Medical Teacher* 33, 62–71.
Evans, J S B T and Ball, L J (2010) Do people reason on the Wason selection task? A new look at the data of Ball et al (2003), *The Quarterly Journal of Experimental Psychology* 63 (3), 434–441.

Evans, J S B T, Barston, J L and Pollard, P (1983) On the conflict between logic and belief in syllogistic reasoning, *Memory and Cognition* 11 (3), 295–306.
Facione, P A (1990) *Critical Thinking: A Statement of Expert Consensus for Purposes of Educational Assessment and Instruction*, California: The California Academic Press.
Facione, P A (2000) The disposition toward critical thinking: Its character, measurement, and relationship to critical thinking skill, *Informal Logic* 20 (1), 61–84.
Ferguson, E and Lievens, F (2017) Future directions in personality, occupational and medical selection: myths, misunderstandings, measurement, and suggestions, *Advances in Health Science Education* 22 (2), 387–399.
Field, A (2013) *Discovering Statistics Using IBM SPSS Statistics*, London: Sage.
Field, J (2011) Cognitive validity, in Taylor, L (Ed) *Examining Speaking: Research and Practice in Assessing Second Language Speaking,* Studies in Language Testing volume 30, Cambridge: UCLES/Cambridge University Press, 112–170.
Fisher, A (1990a) *Research into a higher studies test: A summary*, Cambridge: UCLES internal report.
Fisher, A (1990b) *Proposal to develop a higher studies test: A discussion document*, Cambridge: UCLES internal report.
Fisher, A (1992) *Development of the syndicate's higher education aptitude tests*, Cambridge: UCLES internal report.
Fisher, A (2005) *'Thinking skills' and admission to higher education*, Cambridge: UCLES internal report.
Fitzpatrick, A R (1983) The meaning of content validity, *Applied Psychological Measurement* 7 (1), 3–13.
Furneaux, C and Rignall, M (2007) The effect of standardisation-training on rater judgements for the IELTS Writing Module, in Taylor, L and Falvey, P (Eds) *IELTS Collected Papers*, Cambridge: UCLES/Cambridge University Press, Studies in Language Testing Volume 19, 422–445.
Galaczi, E and ffrench, A (2011) Context validity, in Taylor, L (Ed) *Examining Speaking: Research and Practice in Assessing Second Language Speaking,* Studies in Language Testing volume 30, Cambridge: UCLES/Cambridge University Press, 112–170.
Gale, M and Ball, L J (2009) Exploring the determinants of dual goal facilitation in a rule discovery task, *Thinking and Reasoning* 15 (3), 294–315.
Gallacher, T, McElwee, S and Cheung, K Y F (2017) BMAT 2015 test preparation survey report, Cambridge: Cambridge Assessment internal report.
Garner, R (2015) Number of pupils attending independent school in Britain on the rise, figures show, *The Independent*, 30 April 2015, available online: www.independent.co.uk/news/education/education-news/number-of-pupils-attending-independent-schools-in-britain-on-the-rise-figures-show-10215959.html
General Medical Council (2009) *Tomorrow's Doctors: Outcomes and Standards for Undergraduate Medical Education*, available online: www.gmc-uk.org/Tomorrow_s_Doctors_1214.pdf_48905759.pdf
General Medical Council (2011) *The State of Medical Education and Practice in the UK*, London: General Medical Council.
Geranpayeh, A (2013) Detecting plagiarism and cheating, in Kunnan, A J (Ed) *The Companion to Language Assessment*, London: Wiley Blackwell, 980–993.

Geranpayeh, A (2014) Detecting plagiarism and cheating: Approaches and development, in Kunnan, A J (Ed) *The Companion to Language Assessment Volume II*, Chichester: Wiley, 980–993.
Geranpayeh, A and Taylor, L (Eds) (2013) *Examining Listening: Research and Practice in Assessing Second Language Listening*, Studies in Language Testing volume 35, Cambridge: UCLES/Cambridge University Press.
Gilhooly, K J, Fioratou, E and Henretty, N (2010) Verbalization and problem solving: Insight and spatial factors, *British Journal of Psychology* 101 (1), 81–93.
Gill, T, Vidal Rodeiro, C L and Zanini, N (2015) *Students' choices in Higher Education*, paper presented at the BERA conference, Queen's University Belfast, available online: cambridgeassessment.org.uk/Images/295319-students-choices-in-higher-education.pdf
Goel, V, Navarrete, G, Noveck, I A and Prado, J (2017) Editorial: The reasoning brain: The interplay between cognitive neuroscience and theories of reasoning, *Frontiers in Human Neuroscience* 10, available online: journal.frontiersin.org/article/10.3389/fnhum.2016.00673/full
Goodman, N W and Edwards, M B (2014) *Medical Writing: A Prescription for Clarity*, Cambridge: Cambridge University Press.
Green, A (1992) *A Validation Study of Formal Reasoning Items*, Cambridge: UCLES internal report.
Green, A (2003) *Test impact and English for academic purposes: A comparative study in backwash between IELTS preparation and university professional courses*, Unpublished doctoral dissertation, University of Surrey.
Green, A (2006) Watching for washback: Observing the influence of the International English Language Testing System Academic Writing Test in the classroom, *Language Assessment Quarterly* 3 (4), 333–368.
Green, A (2007) Washback to learning outcomes: A comparative study of IELTS preparation and university pre-sessional language courses, *Assessment in Education: Principles, Policy and Practice* 1, 75–97.
Green, A (2013) Washback in language assessment, *International Journal of English Studies* 13 (2), 39–51.
Griffin, B and Hu, W (2015) The interaction of socio-economic status and gender in widening participation in medicine, *Medical Education* 49 (1), 103–113.
Halpern, D F (1999) Teaching for critical thinking: Helping college students develop the skills and dispositions of a critical thinker, *New Directions for Teaching and Learning* 80, 69–74.
Hambleton, R K and Traub, R E (1974) The effect of item order on test performance and stress, *The Journal of Experimental Education* 43 (1), 40–46.
Hambleton, R K, Swaminathan, H and Rogers, H (1991) *Fundamentals of Item Response Theory*, Newbury Park: Sage Publications.
Hamilton, J S (1993) *MENO Thinking Skills Service: Development and Rationale*, Cambridge: UCLES internal report.
Hawkey, R (2011) Consequential validity, in Geranpayeh, A and Taylor, L (Eds) *Examining Listening: Research and Practice in Assessing Second Language Listening*, Studies in Language Testing volume 35, Cambridge: UCLES/Cambridge University Press, 273–302.
Haynes, S N, Richard, D C S and Kubany, E S (1995) Content validity in psychological assessment: A functional approach to concepts and methods, *Psychological Assessment* 7 (3), 238–247.

Hecker, K and Norman, G (2017) Have admissions committees considered all the evidence? *Advances in Health Sciences Education* 22 (2), 573–576.
Hembree, R (1988) Correlates, causes, effects, and treatment of test anxiety, *Review of Educational Research* 58, 47–77.
Hirschfeld, M, Moore, R L and Brown, E (1995) Exploring the gender gap on the GRE subject test in economics, *Journal of Economic Education* 26 (1), 3–15.
Hoare, A and Johnston, R (2011) Widening participation through admissions policy – a British case study of school and university performance, *Higher Education Quarterly* 36, 21–41.
Hojat, M, Erdmann, J B, Veloski, J J, Nasca, T J, Callahan, C A, Julian, E R and Peck, J. (2000) A validity study of the writing sample section of the Medical College Admission Test, *Academic Medicine*, 75, 25S–27S.
Holland, P W and Thayer, D T (1988) Differential item performance and Mantel-Haenszel procedure, in Wainer, H and Braun, I (Eds) *Test Validity*, Hillsdale: Lawrence Erlbaum, 129–145.
Holland, P W and Wainer, H (Eds) (1993) *Differential Item Functioning*, Hillsdale: Lawrence Erlbaum.
Hopkins, K, Stanley, J, Hopkins, B R (1990) *Educational and Psychological Measurement and Evaluation*, Englewood Cliffs: Prentice-Hall.
Hu, L T and Bentler, P (1999) Cutoff criteria for fit indices in covariance structure analysis: Conventional criteria versus new alternatives, *Structural Equation Modelling* 6, 1–55.
Hughes, A (2003) *Testing for Language Teachers* (2nd edition), Cambridge: Cambridge University Press.
Hyde, J S, Lindberg, S M, Linn, M C, Ellis, A B, and Williams, C C (2008) Gender similarities characterize math performance, *Science* 321, 494–495.
Independent Schools Council (2015) *ISC Census 2015*, available online: www.isc.co.uk/media/2661/isc_census_2015_final.pdf
Independent Schools Council (2016) *ISC Census 2016*, available online: www.isc.co.uk/media/3179/isc_census_2016_final.pdf
James, W and Hawkins, C (2004) Assessing potential: The development of selection procedures for the Oxford medical course, *Oxford Review of Education* 30, 241–255.
Jencks, C and Crouse, J (1982) Aptitude vs. achievement: should we replace the SAT? *The Public Interest* 67, 21–35.
Joint Council for Qualifications (2016a) *Adjustments for candidates with disabilities and learning difficulties: Access arrangements and reasonable adjustments*, available online: www.jcq.org.uk/exams-office/access-arrangements-and-special-consideration
Joint Council for Qualifications (2016b) *General and vocational qualifications: General regulations for approved centres*, available online: www.jcq.org.uk/exams-office/general-regulations
Julian, E R (2005) Validity of the Medical College Admission Test for predicting medical school performance, *Academic Medicine* 80, 910–917.
Kane, M (2013) Validating the interpretations and uses of test scores, *Journal of Educational Measurement* 50, 1–73.
Kaplan, R M and Saccuzzo, D P (2012) *Psychological Testing: Principles, Applications, and Issues*, California: Wadsworth Publishing Company.
Katz, S and Vinker, S (2014) New non-cognitive procedures for medical applicant selection: A qualitative analysis in one school, *BMC Medical Education*, available online: www.ncbi.nlm.nih.gov/pubmed/25376161

Kellogg, J S, Hopko, D R and Ashcraft, M H (1999) The effects of time pressure on arithmetic performance, *Journal of Anxiety Disorders* 13 (6), 591–600.
Kelly, M E, Gallagher, N, Dunne, F and Murphy, A (2014) Views of doctors of varying disciplines on HPAT-Ireland as a selection tool for medicine, *Medical Teacher* 36 (9), 775–782.
Kelly, S and Dennick, R. (2009). Evidence of gender bias in True-False-Abstain medical examinations, *BMC Medical Education,* available online: www.ncbi.nlm.nih.gov/pmc/articles/PMC2702355/
Khalifa, H and Weir, C J (2009) *Examining Reading: Research and Practice in Assessing Second Language Reading*, Studies in Language Testing volume 29. Cambridge: UCLES/Cambridge University Press.
Klahr, D and Dunbar, K (1988) Dual space search during scientific reasoning, *Cognitive Science* 12 (1), 1–48.
Klein, S, Liu, O L, Sconing, J, Bolus, R, Bridgeman, B, Kugelmass, H and Steedle, J (2009) *Test Validity Study (TVS) Report*, Washington, DC: US Department of Education.
Koenig, T W, Parrish, S K, Terregino, C A, Williams, J P, Dunleavy, D M and Volsch, J M (2013) Core personal competencies important to enteringstudents' success in medical school: What are they and how could they be assessed early in the admission process? *Academic Medicine* 88 (5), 603–613.
Kreiter, C D and Axelson, R D (2013) A perspective on medical school admission research and practice over the last 25 years, *Teaching and Learning in Medicine* 25, S50–S56.
Ku, K Y L (2009) Assessing students' critical thinking performance: Urging for measurements using multi-response format, *Thinking Skills and Creativity* 4, 70–76.
Kuncel, N R and Hezlett, S A (2010) Fact and fiction in cognitive ability testing for admissions and hiring decisions, *Current Directions in Psychological Science* (19) 6, 339–345.
Kuncel, N R, Hezlett, S A and Ones, D S (2001) A comprehensive meta-analysis of the predictive validity of the Graduate Records Examinations: Implications for graduate student selection and performance, *Psychological Bulletin* 127, 162–181.
Kusurkar, R A, Ten Cate, T J, van Asperen, M and Croiset, G (2011) Motivation as an independent and a dependent variable in medical education: A review of the literature, *Medical Teacher* 33 (5), 242–262.
Lado, R (1961) *Language Testing: The Construction and Use of Foreign Language Tests. A Teacher's Book*, New York: McGraw Hill.
Landrum, R E and McCarthy, M A (2015) Measuring critical thinking skills, in Jhangiani, R S, Troisi, J D, Fleck, B, Legg, A M and Hussey, H D (Eds) *A Compendium of Scales for Use in the Scholarship of Teaching and Learning*, available online: teachpsych.org/ebooks/compscalessotp
Lawshe, C H (1975) A quantitative approach to content validity, *Personnel Psychology* 28, 563–575.
Leijten, M and Van Waes, L (2013) Keystroke logging in writing research: Using inputlog to analyze and visualize writing processes, *Written Communication* 30 (3), 358–392.
Linacre, J M (2014) *Facets computer program for many-facet Rasch measurement*, version 3.71.4, Beaverton: Winsteps.com.
Linacre, J M (2016) *Winsteps® Rasch Measurement Computer Program User's Guide*, Beaverton: Winsteps.com.

Linn, R L (2009) Considerations for college admissions testing, *Educational Researcher* 38 (9), 677–679.

Liu, O L, Frankel, L and Roohr, K C (2014) Assessing critical thinking in higher education: Current state and directions for next-generation assessment, *ETS Research Report Series* 1, 1–23.

Long, R (2017)GCSE, AS and A Level reform, House of Commons briefing paper Number SN06962, available from: researchbriefings.parliament.uk/ResearchBriefing/Summary/SN06962

Lord, F M and Novick, M R (1968) *Statistical Theories of Mental Test Scores*, Reading: Addison-Wesley.

Lu, Y and Sireci, S G (2007) Validity issues in test speededness, *Educational Measurement: Issues and Practice* 26, 29–37.

Luxia, Q (2007) Is testing an efficient agent for pedagogical change? Examining the intended washback of the writing task in a high-stakes English test in China, *Assessment in Education: Principles, Policy and Practice* 1, 51–74.

Mantel, N and Haenszel, W (1959) Statistical aspects of the analysis of data from retrospective studies of disease, *Journal of the National Cancer Institute* 22 (4), 719–748.

Massey, A J (2004) *Medical and veterinary admissions test validation study*, Cambridge: Cambridge Assessment internal report.

Mayer, R E, Larkin, J H and Kadane, J (1984) A cognitive analysis of mathematic problem-solving ability, in Sternberg, R J (Ed) *Advances in the Psychology of Human Intelligence*, Hillsdale: Lawrence Erlbaum, 231–273.

McCarthy, J M and Goffin, R D (2005) Selection test anxiety: Exploring tension and fear of failure across the sexes in simulated selection scenarios, *International Journal of Selection and Assessment* 13 (4), 282–295.

McCurry, D and Chiavaroli, N (2013) Reflections on the role of a writing test for medical school admissions, *Academic Medicine* 88 (5), 568–571.

McDonald, A S (2001) The prevalence and effects of test anxiety in school children, *Educational Psychology* 21 (1) 89–101.

McDonald, R P (1981) The dimensionality of tests and items, *British Journal of Mathematical and Statistical Psychology* 34 (1), 100–117.

McManus, I C, Dewberry, C, Nicholson, S and Dowell, J S (2013) The UKCAT-12 study: Educational attainment, aptitude test performance, demographic and socio-economic contextual factors as predictors of first year outcome in a collaborative study of twelve UK medical schools, *BMC Medicine* 11, available online: bmcmedicine.biomedcentral.com/articles/10.1186/1741-7015-11-244

McManus, I C, Dewberry, C, Nicholson, S, and Dowell, J S, Woolf, K and Potts, H W W (2013) Construct-level predictive validity of educational attainment and intellectual aptitude tests in medical student selection: Meta-regression of six UK longitudinal studies, *BMC Medicine* 11, available online: bmcmedicine.biomedcentral.com/articles/10.1186/1741-7015-11-243

McManus, I C, Powis, D A, Wakeford, R, Ferguson, E, James, D and Richards, P (2005) Intellectual aptitude tests and A Levels for selecting UK school leaver entrants for medical school, *BMJ* 331, 555–559.

Medical Schools Council (2014) *Selecting for Excellence Final Report*, London: Medical Schools Council.

Mellenbergh, G J (2011) *A Conceptual Introduction to Psychometrics. Development, Analysis, and Application of Psychological and Educational Tests*, The Hague: Eleven International Publishing.
Messick, S (1989) Validity, in Linn, R L (Ed) *Educational Measurement* (3rd edition), Washington DC: The American Council on Education and the National Council on Measurement in Education, 13–103.
Messick, S (1995) Validity of psychological assessment: Validation of inferences from person's responses and performance as scientific inquiry into scoring meaning, *American Psychologist* 9, 741–749.
Milburn A (2012) *Fair access to professional careers – A progress report by the Independent Reviewer on Social Mobility and Child Poverty*, London: Cabinet Office.
Morris, B J, Croker, S, Masnick, A M and Zimmerman, C (2012) The emergence of scientific reasoning, in Kloos, H, Morris, B J and Amaral, J L (Eds) *Current Topics in Children's Learning and Cognition*, Rijeka: InTech, 61–82.
Ndaji, F, Little, J and Coe, R (2016) *A comparison of academic achievement in independent and state schools: Report for the Independent Schools Council January 2016*, Durham: Centre for Evaluation and Monitoring, Durham University, available online: www.isc.co.uk/media/3140/16_02_26-cem-durham-university-academic-value-added-research.pdf
Newble, D (2016) Revisiting 'The effect of assessments and examinations on the learning of medical students', *Medical Education* 50 (5), 498–501.
Newble, D I and Jaeger, K (1983) The effect of assessments and examinations on the learning of medical students, *Medical Wducation* 17 (3), 165–171.
Newton, P and Shaw, S D (2014) *Validity in Educational and Psychological Assessment*, London: Sage.
Nicholson, S and Cleland, J (2015) Reframing research on widening participation in medical education: using theory to inform practice, in Cleland, J and Durning, S J (Eds) *Researching Medical Education*, Oxford: Wiley Blackwell, 231–243.
Niessen, A S M and Meijer, R R (2016) Selection of medical students on the basis of non-academic skills: is it worth the trouble? *Clinical Medicine* 16(4), 339–342.
Niessen, A S M, Meijer, R B and Tendeiro, J N (2017) Applying organizational justice theory to admission into higher education: Admission from a student perspective, *International Journal of Selection and Assessment* 25 (1), 72–84.
Norris, S P (1990) Effect of eliciting verbal reports of thinking on critical thinking test performance, *Journal of Educational Measurement* 27 (1), 41–58.
Novick, M R (1966) The axioms and principal results of classical test theory, *Journal of Mathematical Psychology* 3 (1), 1–18.
Nowell, A and Hedges, L V (1998) Trends in gender differences in academic achievement from 1960 to 1994: An analysis of differences in mean, variance, and extreme scores, *Sex Roles* 39 (1/2), 21–43.
O'Hare, L and McGuiness, C (2009) Measuring critical thinking, intelligence and academic performance in psychology undergraduates, *The Irish Journal of Psychology* 30, 123–131.
O'Hare, L and McGuiness, C (2015) The validity of critical thinking tests for predicting degree performance: A longitudinal study, *International Journal of Educational Research* 72, 162–172.
O'Sullivan, B and Weir, C J (2011) Test development and validation, in O'Sullivan, B (Ed) *Language Testing: Theories and Practices*, Basingstoke: Palgrave Macmillan, 13–32.

Palmer, E J and Devitt, P G (2007) Assessment of higher order cognitive skills in undergraduate education: modified essay or multiple choice questions? *BMC Medical Education* 7, bmcmededuc.biomedcentral.com/articles/10.1186/1472-6920-7-49
Papp, S and Rixon, S (forthcoming 2017) *Assessing Young Language Learners: The Cambridge English Approach*, Studies in Language Testing volume 47, Cambridge: UCLES/Cambridge University Press.
Patel, V L, Arocha, J F and Zhang, J (2005) Thinking and reasoning in medicine, in Holyoak, K J and Morrison, R G (Eds) *The Cambridge Handbook of Thinking and Reasoning*, Cambridge: Cambridge University Press, 727–750.
Patterson, F, Knight, A, Dowell, J S Nicholson, S., Cousans, and Cleland, J. (2016). How effective are selection methods in medical education? A systematic review, *Medical Education* 50, 36–60.
Paul, R and Elder, L (2007) *Critical Thinking Competency Standards (For Educators)*, Tomales: Foundation for Critical Thinking.
Pearson VUE (2017) *UK Clinical Aptitude Test (UKCAT) Consortium UKCAT Examination Executive Summary Testing Interval: 1 July 2016–4 October 2016*, available online: www.ukcat.ac.uk/media/1057/ukcat-2016-technical-report-exec-summary_v1.pdf
Pelacia, T and Viau, R (2017) Motivation in medical education, *Medical Teacher* 39 (2), 136–140.
Plass, J A and Hill, K T (1986) Children's achievement strategies and test performance: The role of time pressure, evaluation anxiety and sex, *Developmental Psychology* 22 (1), 31–36.
Powis, D A (2015) Selecting medical students: An unresolved challenge, *Medical Teacher* 37 (3), 252–260.
Quality Assurance Agency (2002) *Subject Benchmark Statement: Medicine*, available online: www.qaa.ac.uk/en/Publications/Documents/Subject-benchmark-statement-Medicine.pdf
Quality Assurance Agency (2015) *Subject Benchmark Statement: Biomedical Sciences*, available online: www.qaa.ac.uk/en/Publications/Documents/SBS-Biomedical-sciences-15.pdf
Ramsay, P A (2005) *Admissions tests (Cambridge TSA and BMAT) and disability*, Cambridge: University of Cambridge internal report.
Rasch, G (1960/1980) *Probabilistic Models for Some Intelligence and Attainment Tests*, Chicago: University of Chicago Press.
Rasch, G (1961) On general laws and meaning of measurement in psychology, in *Proceedings of the Fourth Berkeley Symposium on Mathematical Statistics and Probability* (4), Berkeley: University of California Press, 321–333.
Rasch, G (2011) *All statistical models are wrong!*, available online: www.rasch.org/rmt/rmt244d.html
Reibnegger, G, Caluba, H-C, Ithaler, D, Manhal, S, Neges, H M and Smolle, J (2010) Progress of medical students after open admission or admission based on knowledge tests, *Medical Education* 44, 205–214.
Röding, K and Nordenram, G (2005) Students' perceived experience of university admission based on tests and interviews, *European Journal of Dental Education* 9 (4), 171–179.
Rodriguez, M C (2003) Construct equivalence of multiple-choice and constructed-response items: A random effects synthesis of correlations, *Journal of Educational Measurement, 40*(2), 163–184.

Ross, J A, Scott, G and Bruce, C D (2012) The gender confidence gap in fractions knowledge: Gender differences in student belief–achievement relationships, *School Science and Mathematics* 112 (5), 278–288.

Sackett, P R and Yang, H (2000) Correction for range restriction: An expanded typology, *Journal of Applied Psychology* 85, 112–118.

Sam, A, Hameed, S, Harris, J, Meeran, K (2016) Validity of very short answer versus single best answer questions for undergraduate assessment, *BMC Medical Education* 16 (1), available online: bmcmededuc.biomedcentral.com/articles/10.1186/s12909-016-0793-z

Saville, N and Hawkey, R (2004) The IELTS impact study: Investigating washback on teaching materials, in Cheng, L, Watanabe, Y and Curtis, A (Eds) *Washback in Language Testing: Research Context and Methods*, London: Lawrence Erlbaum, 73–96.

Saville, N (2003) The process of test development and revision within UCLES EFL, in Weir, C J and Milanovic, M (Eds) *Continuity and Innovation: Revising the Cambridge Proficiency in English Examination 1913–2002*, Studies in Language Testing volume 15, Cambridge: UCLES/Cambridge University Press, 57–120.

Saville, N (2012) Applying a model for investigating the impact of language assessment within educational contexts: The Cambridge ESOL approach, *Research Notes* 50, 4–8.

Scardamalia, M and Bereiter, C (1987) Knowledge telling and knowledge transforming in written composition, in Rosenberg, S (Ed) *Advances in Applied Psycholinguistics, Volume 2: Reading , Writing and Language Learning*, Cambridge: Cambridge University Press, 142–175.

Schwartzstein, R, Rosenfeld, G, Hilborn, R, Oyewole, S and Mitchell, K. (2013) Redesigning the MCAT exam: balancing multiple perspectives, *Academic Medicine* 88 (5), 560–567.

Scorey, S. (2009a) *Investigating the predictive validity of the BMAT: An analysis using examination data from the Royal veterinary College BVetMed course for the 2005, 2006 and 2007 BMAT cohorts*, Cambridge: Cambridge Assessment internal report.

Scorey, S (2009b) *Investigating the predictive validity of the BMAT: An analysis using examination data from the University College London course for the 2003 to 2007 BMAT cohorts*, Cambridge: Cambridge Assessment internal report.

Seyan K, Greenhalgh T and Dorling D (2004) The standardised admission ratio for measuring widening participation in medical schools: analysis of UK medical school admissions by ethnicity, socioeconomic status, and sex, *British Medical Journal* 328, 1,545–1,546.

Shannon, M D (2005) *Investigation of possible indictors of excessive time pressure in BMAT*, Cambridge: Cambridge Assessment internal report.

Shannon, M D and Scorey, S (2010) *BMAT Section 3 marking trial March 2010 – Marker reliability analysis*, Cambridge:Cambridge Assessment internal report.

Shannon, M D (2010) (Ed) *Preparing for the BMAT: The Official Guide to the BioMedical Admissions Test*. Oxford: Heinemann.

Sharples, J M, Oxman, A D, Mahtani, K R, Chalmers, I, Oliver, S, Collins, K, Austvoll-Dahlgren, A and Hoffmann, T (2017) Critical thinking in healthcare and education, *BMJ* 357, available online: www.bmj.com/content/357/bmj.j2234.long

Shaw, S D (2002) The effect of standardisation on rater judgement and inter-rater reliability, *Research Notes* 8, 13–17.

Shaw, S D and Weir, C J (2007) *Examining Writing: Research and Practice in Assessing Second Language Writing*, Studies in Language Testing volume 26, Cambridge: UCLES/Cambridge University Press.
Shea, J and Fortna, G (2002). Psychometric methods, in Norman, G R, van der Vleuten, C P and Newble, D I (Eds) (2012) *International Handbook of Research in Medical Education (Vol. 7)*, New York: Springer Science and Business Media, 97–126.
Shultz, M M and Zedeck, S (2012) Admission to law school: New measures, *Educational Psychologist* 47 (1), 51–65.
Simon, H A and Newell, A (1971) Human problem solving: The state of the theory in 1970, *American Psychologist* 12 (2), 145–159.
Sireci, S G (1998) The construct of content validity, *Social Indicators Research* 45, 83–117.
Sjitsma, K (2009) On the use, misuse, and the very limited usefulness of Cronbach's alpha, *Psychometrika* 74 (1), 107–120.
Soares, J A (2012) The future of college admissions: Discussion, *Educational Psychologist* 47 (1), 66–70.
Stegers-Jager, K M, Steyerberg, E W, Lucieer, S M and Themmen, A P N (2015) *Medical Education* 49 (1), 124–133.
Stemler, S E (2012) What should university admissions tests predict? *Educational Psychologist* 47 (1), 5–17.
Steven, K, Dowell, J S, Jackson, C and Guthrie, B (2016) Fair access to medicine? Retrospective analysis of UK medical schools application data 2009–2012 using three measures of socioeconomic status, *BMC medical education* 16 (1), available online: bmcmededuc.biomedcentral.com/articles/10.1186/s12909-016-0536-1
Stevens L, Kelly M E, Hennessy M, Last J, Dunne F, O'Flynn S (2014) Medical students' views on selection tools for medical school – a mixed methods study, *Irish Medical Journal* 107 (8), 229–231.
Stoet, G and Geary, D C (2013) Sex differences in mathematics and reading achievement are inversely related: within- and across-nation assessment of 10 Years of PISA data, *PLOS ONE*, available online: journals.plos.org/plosone/article/file?id=10.1371/journal.pone.0057988&type=printable
Stupple, E J N, Maratos, F A, Elander, J, Hunt, T E, Cheung, K Y F and Aubeeluck, A V (2017) Development of the Critical Thinking Toolkit (CriTT): A measure of student attitudes and beliefs about critical thinking, *Thinking Skills and Creativity* 23, 91–100.
Tai, R H, Loehr, J F and Brigham, F J (2006) An exploration of the use of eye-gaze tracking to study problem-solving on standardized science assessments, *International Journal of Research and Method in Education* 29 (2), 185–208.
Taylor, L (Ed) (2011) *Examining Speaking: Research and Practice in Assessing Second Language Speaking,* Studies in Language Testing volume 30, Cambridge: UCLES/Cambridge University Press.
Thissen, D, Steinberg, L and Wainer, H (1993) Detection of differential item functioning using the parameters of item response models, In Holland, P and Wainer, H (Eds) *Differential Item Functioning.* Hillsdale: Lawrence Erlbaum, 67–113.
Thomson, A and Fisher A (1992) *MENO: A validation study of informal reasoning items*, Norwich: University of East Anglia internal report.
Tiffin, P A, McLachlan, J C, Webster, L and Nicholson, S (2014) Comparison of the sensitivity of the UKCAT and A Levels to sociodemographic

characteristics: A national study, *BMC Medical Education* 14, available online: bmcmededuc.biomedcentral.com/articles/10.1186/1472-6920-14-7
Tighe, J, McManus, I C, Dewhurst, N G, Chis, L and Mucklow, J (2010) The standard error of measurement is a more appropriate measure of quality for postgraduate medical assessments than is reliability: an analysis of MRCP (UK) examinations, *BMC Medical Education* 10, available online: bmcmededuc.biomedcentral.com/articles/10.1186/1472-6920-10-40
Trainor, S (2015) Student data privacy is cloudy today, clearer tomorrow, *The Phi Delta Kappan* 96 (5), 13–18.
Tsai, M-J, Hou, H-T, Lai, M-L, Liu, W-Y and Yang, F-Y (2012) Visual attention for solving multiple-choice science problem: An eye-tracking analysis, *Computers and Education* 58 (1), 375–385.
Universities and Colleges Admissions Service (2016) *Applicant numbers to 'early deadline' university courses increase by 1%, UCAS figures reveal today*, available online: www.ucas.com/corporate/news-and-key-documents/news/applicant-numbers-%E2%80%98early-deadline%E2%80%99-university-courses-increase
Weigle, S C (1994) Effects of training on raters of ESL compositions, *Language Testing* 11 (2), 197–223.
Weigle, S C (1999) Investigating rater/prompt interactions in writing assessment: Quantitative and qualitative approaches. *Assessing Writing* 6 (2), 145–178.
Weigle, S C (2002) *Assessing Writing*, Cambridge: Cambridge University Press.
Weir, C J (2005) *Language Testing and Validation: An Evidence-based Approach*, Basingstoke: Palgrave Macmillan.
Weir, C J and Taylor, L (2011) Conclusions and recommendations, in Taylor, L (Ed) *Examining Speaking: Research and Practice in Assessing Second Language Speaking*, Studies in Language Testing Volume 30, Cambridge: UCLES/Cambridge University Press, 293–313.
Wilhelm, O and Oberauer, K (2006) Why are reasoning ability and working memory capacity related to mental speed? An investigation of stimulus–response compatibility in choice reaction time tasks, *European Journal of Cognitive Psychology* 18 (1), 18–50.
Willmott, A (2005) *Thinking Skills and admissions: A report on the validity and reliability of the TSA and MVAT/BMAT assessments*, Cambridge: Cambridge English internal report.
Woolf, K, Potts, H W W, Stott, J, McManus, I C, Williams, A and Scior, K (2015) The best choice? *The Psychologist* 28, 730–735.
Wouters, A, Croiset, G, Galindo-Garre, F and Kusurkar, R A (2016) Motivation of medical students: Selection by motivation or motivation by selection, *BMC Medical Education* 16 (1), available online: www.ncbi.nlm.nih.gov/pubmed/26825381
Wouters, A, Croiset, G, Schripsema, N R, Cohen-Schotanus, J, Spaai, G W G, Hulsman R L and Kusurkar, R A (2017) A multi-site study on medical school selection, performance, motivation and engagement, *Advances in Health Sciences Education* 22 (2), 447–462.
Wright, S (2015) Medical school personal statements: a measure of motivation or proxy for cultural privilege? *Advances in Health Sciences Education* 20, 627–643.
Yeager, D S and Dweck, C S (2012) Mindsets that promote resilience: When students believe that personal characteristics can be developed, *Educational Psychologist, 47*(4), 302–314.

Yu, G, He, L and Isaacs, T (2017). *The Cognitive Processes of taking IELTS Academic Writing Task 1: An Eye-tracking Study*, IELTS Research Reports Online Series, British Council, IDP: IELTS Australia and Cambridge English Language Assessment, available online: www.ielts.org/-/media/research-reports/ielts_online_rr_2017-2.ashx
Zeidner, M (1998) *Test Anxiety: The State of the Art*, New York: Plenum.
Zimmerman, C (2000) The development of scientific reasoning skills, *Developmental Review* 20, 99–149.
Zimmerman, C (2007) The development of scientific thinking skills in elementary and middle school, *Developmental Review* 27, 172–223.
Zinbarg, R E, Revelle, W, Yovel, I and Li, W (2005) Cronbach's α, Revelle's β, and McDonald's ωH: Their relations with each other and two alternative conceptualizations of reliability, *Psychometrika* 70 (1), 123–133.
Zohar, A and Peled, B (2008) The effects of explicit teaching of metastrategic knowledge on low- and high-achieving students, *Learning and Instruction* 18 (4), 337–352.
Zumbo, B D and Rupp, A A (2004) Responsible modelling of measurement data for appropriate inferences: Important advances in reliability and validity theory, in Kaplan, D (Ed) *The SAGE Handbook of Quantitative Methodology for the Social Sciences*, Thousand Oaks: Sage Press, 73–92.
Zwick, R (Ed) (2004) *Rethinking the SAT: The Future of Standardized Testing in University Admissions,* London: Routledge.
Zwick, R and Ercikan, K (1989) Analysis of differential item functioning in the NAEP history assessment, *Journal of Educational Measurement* 26, 55–66.
Zwick, R, Thayer, D T and Lewis, C (1999) An empirical Bayes approach to Mantel-Haenszel DIF analysis, *Journal of Educational Measurement* 36 (1), 1–28.

Author Index

Subject Index

Lightning Source UK Ltd.
Milton Keynes UK
UKOW01f1905080917
308807UK00005B/125/P

9 781108 439312